SYNTEX LABORATORIES, INC.
3401 HILLVIEW AVENUE, P.O. BOX 10850
PALO ALTO, CALIFORNIA 94303

(415) 855-5545
TELEX 4997273 SYNTEX PLA

LOUIS HAGLER, M.D., DIRECTOR
JOAN DORFMAN, M.D., ASSOC. DIR.
RONALD H. LEWIS, M.D., ASSOC. DIR.
MEDICAL SERVICES DEPARTMENT

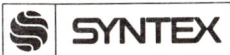

Dear Doctor:

Preparation for specialty boards is an intimidating experience. We at Syntex would like to make the process a little less traumatic by providing you with a copy of <u>Comprehensive Gynecology Review</u> that can help to organize and facilitate your preparation.

The <u>Review</u> has been written to complement Droegemueller's <u>Comprehensive Gynecology</u>, a standard and respected textbook. As you work through the broad collection of board-type questions and answers, you can identify areas in which your knowledge is adequate and others in which additional study might be required. Each answer is explained in a detailed comment which reinforces the learning process. Even if you are not planning to take the board exam this year, the <u>Review</u> can still serve as a valuable tool for self assessment.

We hope you find the <u>Review</u> useful. Good luck at examination time.

Sincerely,

Louis Hagler, M.D., Director
Medical Services Department

P.S.   We at Syntex look forward to continuing our close relationship with you throughout your career, by keeping you updated on support services, and providing product information on and samples of our OB/GYN products: TRI-NORINYL® (norethindrone and ethinyl estradiol), ANAPROX® DS (naproxen sodium), and FEMSTAT® Prefill (butoconazole nitrate).

Please see enclosed full prescribing information.

COMPREHENSIVE GYNECOLOGY REVIEW

COMPREHENSIVE GYNECOLOGY REVIEW

Gerald B. Holzman, M.D.
Professor and Vice-Chairman
Department of Obstetrics and Gynecology
Medical College of Georgia
Augusta, Georgia

Frank W. Ling, M.D.
Associate Professor
Division of Gynecology
Department of Obstetrics and Gynecology
University of Tennessee College of Medicine
Memphis, Tennessee

Douglas W. Laube, M.D.
Professor
Department of Obstetrics and Gynecology
University of Iowa Hospitals and Clinics
Iowa City, Iowa

Louis O. Vontver, M.D.
Professor
Department of Obstetrics and Gynecology
University of Washington School of Medicine
Seattle, Washington

With 123 illustrations

The C. V. Mosby Company
St. Louis • Washington, D.C. • Toronto 1988

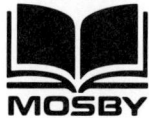

A TRADITION OF PUBLISHING EXCELLENCE

Editor: Stephanie Bircher
Assistant editor: Anne Gunter
Project manager: Mark Spann
Editing and production: Publication Services

Copyright ©1988 by The C.V. Mosby Company

All rights reserved. No part of this publication may be reproduced, stored in a retrieval system, or transmitted in any form or by any means, electronic, mechanical, photocopying, recording, or otherwise, without prior written permission from the publisher.

Printed in the United States of America

The C.V. Mosby Company
11830 Westline Industrial Drive, St. Louis, Missouri 63146

Library of Congress Cataloging-in-Publication Data

Comprehensive gynecology review.

  Intended to complement: Comprehensive gynecology / William Droegemueller ... [et al.]. c1987.

  1. Gynecology–Examinations, questions, etc.
I. Holzman, Gerald B., 1933–   . II. Comprehensive gynecology. [DNLM: 1. Genital Diseases, Female.
2. Gynecology—methods. WP 140 C737 Suppl.]
RG101.C726 1987 Suppl.   618.1   87-24808
ISBN 0-8016-2445-2

PS/PS/MV 9 8 7 6 5 4 3 2   01/A/070

PREFACE

Comprehensive Gynecology Review has been written to complement *Comprehensive Gynecology* and is intended for practicing physicians, residents, and students interested in gynecology. It can be used to identify areas of weakness, to reinforce new information obtained by reading the textbook, or to reassure oneself that the subject matter is understood. The format should be familiar: it is the standard testing format used by the National Board of Medical Examiners. *Comprehensive Gynecology Review* chapters follow the textbook chapters exactly. The questions within the chapters have been scrambled, and the answers appear in a separate section. Each answer includes a page reference in *Comprehensive Gynecology*, occasionally an additional reference, and a comment. Questions were chosen for a variety of reasons. Since the book is to help learn, the questions are not always of the same difficulty that a certifying examination would accept. The purpose of a certifying examination is to assure an agency that the examinee has attained a requisite amount of knowledge. The examination must discriminate between those who know and those who do not know. Questions that everyone should be able to answer are not included. Since this *Guide* is not written with a specific "level" of physician in mind, it was not possible to eliminate a question that everyone might know. Besides, one purpose of the *Guide* is to reinforce knowledge. Thus, there are easy questions. Likewise, in a certifying examination one must avoid the controversial; such questions are not avoided in this *Guide*. In practice, one has to treat the controversial. For this reason, some readers will disagree with some of our answers. This is a self-assessment instrument.

An attempt has been made to put the subject in a clinical perspective and to clarify. There are many illustrations that require interpretation. Unfortunately, there is a certain amount of cueing in each chapter that would not exist in a certifying examination. In organizing the book by chapters, this could not be avoided, as the most likely answer for a question in the chapter on endometriosis is likely to be endometriosis.

To simulate test conditions, an examinee should take 45 to 60 seconds to answer each question. Answer all the questions in a chapter before verifying the answers. To reinforce the material, read all the comments.

We wish to thank the authors of *Comprehensive Gynecology*, William Droegemueller, Arthur L. Herbst, Daniel Mishell, Jr., and Morton Stenchever, for suggesting the *Review* and then inviting us to write it. Our thanks to our families for their patience and support, and our gratitude to our editor, Stephanie Bircher, for her encouragement.

Gerald B. Holzman
Frank W. Ling
Douglas W. Laube
Louis O. Vontver

Contributors

David Muram, M.D.
Associate Professor of Obstetrics and Gynecology
University of Tennessee, School of Medicine
Memphis, Tennessee

Roger P. Smith, M.D.
Associate Professor of Obstetrics and Gynecology
Medical College of Georgia
Augusta, Georgia

Contents

PART ONE   BASIC SCIENCES

1. Embryology, 1
2. Genetics, 5
3. Anatomy, 13
4. Reproductive Endocrinology, 21

PART TWO   APPROACH TO THE PATIENT

5. History and Examination of the Patient, 29
6. Significant Symptoms and Signs in Different Age Groups, 33
7. Counseling the Patient, 37
8. Diagnostic Procedures, 42

PART THREE   GENERAL GYNECOLOGY

9. Congenital Abnormalities, 52
10. Pediatric Gynecology, 58
11. Contraception, Sterilization, and Pregnancy Termination, 64
12. Rape, Incest, and Abuse, 69
13. Breast Diseases, 75
14. Problems of Prenatal DES Exposure, 81
15. Abortion, 88
16. Ectopic Pregnancy, 97
17. Benign Gynecologic Lesions, 106
18. Endometriosis and Adenomyosis, 113
19. Disorders of Abdominal Wall and Pelvic Support, 121
20. Gynecologic Urology, 129
21. Infections of the Lower Genital Tract, 135
22. Upper Genital Tract Infections, 142
23. Preoperative Management, 148
24. Postoperative Complications, 154

PART FOUR — GYNECOLOGIC ONCOLOGY

25 Principles of Radiation Therapy and Chemotherapy in Gynecologic Cancer, 160
26 Intraepithelial Neoplasia of the Cervix, 166
27 Malignant Disease of the Cervix, 174
28 Neoplastic Diseases of the Uterus, 179
29 Neoplastic Diseases of the Ovary, 188
30 Premalignant and Malignant Diseases of the Vulva, 197
31 Premalignant and Malignant Diseases of the Vagina, 204
32 Malignant Disease of the Fallopian Tube, 210
33 Gestational Trophoblastic Disease, 214

PART FIVE — ENDOCRINOLOGY AND INFERTILITY

34 Dysmenorrhea and Premenstrual Syndrome, 221
35 Abnormal Uterine Bleeding, 226
36 Amenorrhea, 232
37 Hyperprolactinemia, Galactorrhea, and Pituitary Adenoma, 238
38 Hyperandrogenism, 245
39 Infertility, 252
40 Menopause, 257

PART ONE BASIC SCIENCES

CHAPTER 1 Embryology

DIRECTIONS: Select the one best answer or completion.

1. Human chorionic gonadotrophin reaches its peak at which week of pregnancy?
   A. 3–4
   B. 9–10
   C. 20–21
   D. 28–30
   E. 38–40
2. The sequence of development of fetal epithelium is
   A. mesoderm, ectoderm, endoderm.
   B. mesoderm, endoderm, ectoderm.
   C. ectoderm, mesoderm, endoderm.
   D. endoderm, mesoderm, ectoderm.
   E. ectoderm, endoderm, mesoderm.
3. The first functioning organ system in the embryo is the
   A. nervous
   B. digestive
   C. cardiovascular
   D. genitourinary
   E. skeletal
4. Blood formation in the embryo occurs first in the
   A. liver
   B. spleen
   C. bone marrow
   D. lymph nodes
   E. heart

DIRECTIONS: For each numbered item, select the one heading most closely associated with it. Each lettered heading may be used once, more than once, or not at all.

5–8. Match the stages of the first meiotic division with the appropriate description.
   (A) Chromosome pairs in contact
   (B) Condensation of chromatin as thread-like material
   (C) Development of chiasmata
   (D) Migration of chromosomes to equatorial plate

5. Leptotene
6. Zygotene
7. Pachytene
8. Diplotene

9–10. Match the postovulatory day with the appropriate event.
   (A) 3–4
   (B) 6–7
   (C) 9–10
   (D) 12–13
   (E) 15–16

9. Implantation
10. Venous sinuses formed

11–15. Match the male and female homologous structures.
   (A) Vagina
   (B) Labia majora
   (C) Ovarian follicles
   (D) Clitoris
   (E) Round ligament

11. Scrotum
12. Penis
13. Prostatic utricle
14. Seminiferous tubules
15. Gubernaculum testis

16–18. Match the congenital abnormality with the embryonic developmental failure.
   (A) Sinovaginal bulb fails to canalize
   (B) Paramesonephric duct does not develop
   (C) Paramesonephric duct does not fuse
   (D) Failure of rupture of anal membrane

16. Absence of uterus
17. Uterus didelphys
18. Transverse vaginal septum

DIRECTIONS: Each question contains four suggested answers of which one or more is correct. Choose the answer
   A if 1, 2, and 3 are correct
   B if 1 and 3 are correct
   C if 2 and 4 are correct
   D if 4 only is correct
   E if all are correct

19. Arrest of oocyte meiosis occurs at the
    1. metaphase of the first meiotic division.
    2. metaphase of the second meiotic division.
    3. telophase of the second meiotic division.
    4. prophase of the first meiotic division.
20. True statements concerning oocyte meiosis include:
    1. Meiotic-inducing substance originates in the rete cords.
    2. During telophase I, the two daughter cells receive an equal amount of cytoplasm.
    3. The oocyte and the first polar body are contained within the zona pellucida.
    4. The second meiotic division precedes ovulation.
21. True statements regarding fertilization include:
    1. Capacitation occurs in the sperm as they are transported up the female genital tract.
    2. Both the male and female pronuclei contain a haploid set of chromosomes.
    3. Fertilization usually occurs in the ampulla of the fallopian tube.
    4. A significant proportion of fertilized ova do not complete cleavage.
22. Effects of a teratogen depend on
    1. duration of exposure of teratogen.
    2. stage of embryonic development.
    3. dose of teratogen.
    4. individual's genetic make-up.
23. True statements concerning development of the excretory system include:
    1. The pronephros and its ducts serve as the first fetal kidney.
    2. The mesonephros produces urine for several weeks.
    3. Production of urine is an important excretory function of the fetal kidney.
    4. The metanephros begins as a pelvic organ.
24. True statements concerning the development of the genital duct system include:
    1. Mesonephric (wolffian) duct development precedes paramesonephric (müllerian) duct development.
    2. Leydig cells of the fetal testes produce testosterone while Sertoli cells produce MIF (müllerian inhibiting factor).
    3. The paramesonephric duct develops if no gonads are present.
    4. Structures developing from both mesonephric and paramesonephric ducts occur in the female.
25. True statements about sex differentiation include:
    1. If testes are to develop, H-Y antigen must be activated.
    2. The ovary differentiates at approximately the 11th week.
    3. A Y chromosome is required for the development of the testes.
    4. Ovarian development is normal if a single X chromosome is present.

ANSWERS

1. **B**, Page 9. Human chorionic gonadotrophin doubles every 1.2 to 2 days with its peak being reached at 7 to 9 weeks of pregnancy.
2. **E**, Page 10. During the third week after fertilization, a primitive streak forms in the caudal portion of the embryonic disk. The outward-facing epithelium is considered ectoderm, while the epithelium facing the yolk sac is endoderm. By the 16th day postconception, the intraembryonic mesoderm begins to form between the ectoderm and endoderm.
3. **C**, Page 10. Blood vessel formation (angiogenesis) is seen in the extraembryonic mesoderm by day 15 or 16. By the 21st day, the primitive heart is connected with blood vessels of the embryo to become the first functioning organ system.
4. **A**, Page 10. Blood vessel formation begins in the extraembryonic mesoderm of the yolk sac by day 15 or 16. Embryonic vessels are seen approximately 2 days later. In the embryo, blood formation does not begin until the second month of gestation, occurring first in the developing liver.
5–8. 5, **B**; 6, **D**; 7, **A**; 8, **C**; Page 4. In the earliest stage, the leptotene stage, chromatin material condenses into threadlike structures. During zygotene, migration to the equatorial plate occurs and homologous chromosomes pair up to form bivalents. At the end of this phase, tight pairing of the chromosomes along their entire length, *synapsis*, takes place. During the subsequent pachytene stage, each chromosome splits into two chromatids united at the centromere. The bivalent is thus transformed into tetrads. There are 23 tetrads in the human ovum. During diplotene, the chromosomes of the bivalents are held together at points called *chiasmata*, where crossing over of genetic material occurs between chromatids of homologous chromosomes.
9–10. 9, **B**; 10, **C**; Pages 6, 9. Subsequent to the first mitotic division, the cells continue to divide as the embryo passes along the fallopian tube and into the uterus. This takes 3 to 4 days after fertilization, and the embryo enters the uterus in any form, from 32 cells to the early blastula stage. Implantation typically occurs 3 days after the embryo enters the uterus. Invading syncytiotrophoblast comes in inti-

mate contact with endometrial capillaries to form venous sinuses at 7 1/2 to 9 days after conception.

11–15. 11, **B**; 12, **D**; 13, **A**; 14, **C**; 15, **E**; Table 1-2, page 15. There are homologous male and female derivatives for each embryonic structure. Paired structures include scrotum/labia majora, penis/clitoris, prostatic utricle/vagina, seminiferous tubules/ovarian follicles, and gubernaculum testis/round ligaments.

16–18. 16, **B**; 17, **C**; 18, **A**; Page 14. Abnormalities in specific developmental processes can result in discrete congenital abnormalities. If the paramesonephric duct does not develop, absence of the uterus occurs. Uterus didelphys is a result of lack of fusion of the paramesonephric duct. A transverse vaginal septum results from failure of the sinovaginal bulb to canalize.

19. **C** (2, 4), Page 4. At approximately 5 months gestation, oocytes enter the process of meiosis and progress to the prophase of the first meiotic division before entering the first arrest, which lasts for several years. Maturation continues to the second meiotic metaphase, when the second arrest occurs. This lasts, of course, until the oocyte is activated by fertilization.

20. **B** (1, 3), Pages 5, 6. The meiotic process occurs as a result of stimulation by a meiotic-inducing substance, which originates in the rete cords derived from the developing mesonephric tubules. Meiosis-preventing substance is probably produced by the granulosa cells of the differentiated ovarian follicle. In telophase I, one daughter cell receives the majority of the cytoplasm and the second daughter cell becomes the first polar body. Both the oocyte and the polar body are surrounded by the zona pellucida. From here, the oocyte advances to metaphase II of the second meiotic division, during which time ovulation occurs. The second meiotic division continues in the oviduct following sperm penetration.

21. **E** (All), Page 6. As the spermatozoa are transported through the cervical mucus, uterus, and fallopian tubes, they undergo capacitation and acrosome reaction, thus activating enzyme systems to make it possible for the sperm to penetrate the barrier of the zona pellucida. Once the sperm enters the cytoplasm of the egg, the sperm head swells and gives rise to the male pronucleus. The egg casts off the second polar body and the female pronucleus is formed. The pronuclei contain the haploid sets of chromosomes of maternal and paternal origin. Although the two do not fuse, the nuclear membranes surrounding them disappear, and the chromosomes reestablish the diploid complement of chromosomes. Cleavage gives rise to the two-cell embryo in the fallopian tube where fertilization occurred. Due to failure of chromosome arrangement on the spindle, gene defects, and environmental factors, a significant number of fertilized ova do not complete cleavage. Twinning may occur at any point until the blastula is formed.

22. **E** (All), Pages 10–11. All organ systems are usually formed from the fourth to the seventh week of gestation. A teratogenic event occurring during this time will result in malformation related to the organ systems developing at the time of insult. In addition, the effects of a teratogen depend on dose and duration of exposure to the teratogen, as well as the genetic makeup of the individual. Therefore, cardiovascular abnormalities are expected if a teratogen is to take effect early in the embryonic period. Teratogens may be chemical substances, their by-products, or physical conditions such as temperature elevation and irradiation. Agents applied after the 49th day usually will not be responsible for specific malformations. But they may kill or injure the embryo or cause developmental and growth retardation.

23. **C** (2, 4), Pages 11–12. Three sets of excretory ducts and tubules develop bilaterally in the fetus. First, the pronephros forms at about the fourth week after conception. The associated tubules probably have no excretory function. Late in the fourth week, the mesonephric tubules develop. The mesonephros functions as a fetal kidney, producing urine for 2 or 3 weeks. The permanent kidney, the metanephros, originally a pelvic organ, begins development in the fifth week and by differential growth it ultimately relocates in the lumbar region. The fetus produces urine throughout gestation, but the placenta handles the excretory functions of the fetus.

24. **E** (All), Pages 12, 14. The mesonephric duct development precedes the para-mesonephric duct development with the latter set developing on each side from evaginations of the coelomic epithelium. The mesonephric duct differentiates into the vas deferens, epididymis, and seminal vesicles. Leydig cells produce testosterone and the Sertoli cells of the testes produce MIF. In the presence of ovaries or if no gonads are present at all, the mesonephric ducts regress and the paramesonephric ducts develop. Structures developing from both mesonephric and paramesonephric duct systems do occur in adult females.

25. **A** (1, 2, 3), Pages 18, 20. Genes on the Y chromosome are either responsible for the development of the H-Y antigen or for activator genes that will induce production of the H-Y antigen. In some rare instances, the H-Y antigen may express itself in the absence of the Y chromosome. In such cases, the gene for H-Y antigen expression is expected

to be found on another chromosome, probably the X chromosome. In order for testes to be formed, however, the H-Y antigen must be activated. For normal male development, the testes must differentiate and function normally. The ovary, which develops at the 11th or 12th week, requires two functional X chromosomes. In cases where one X chromosome is missing, ovaries are almost invariably lacking oocytes. Conversely, germ cells in testes develop best when only one X chromosome is present.

CHAPTER 2

Genetics

DIRECTIONS: Select the one best answer or completion.

1. The pedigree in Figure 2-1 suggests the inheritance of a trait that is
   A. autosomal dominant.
   B. autosomal recessive.
   C. X-linked recessive.
   D. X-linked dominant.
   E. male-limited autosomal dominant.

2. Assume the trait is fully penetrant. The pedigree in Figure 2-2 is most consistent with a gene that is a(n)
   A. autosomal dominant.
   B. autosomal recessive.
   C. X-linked recessive.
   D. X-linked dominant.
   E. male-limited autosomal dominant.

3. A couple who had a barren marriage for 10 years now have had two spontaneous abortions at 6 and 8 weeks. A karyotype was done on both the husband and wife. He is 46 XY, and her karyotype is reproduced on page 6 (Figure 2-3). She is 30 and he is 32. Which of the following statements are correct and should be mentioned during counseling?
   A. No one with her karyotype has carried to term.
   B. No one with her karyotype has given birth to a chromosomally normal neonate.
   C. They might have a chromosomally abnormal neonate, but it would be identical to that of its mother.

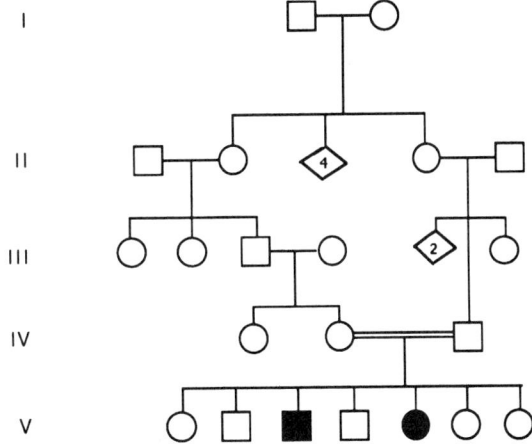

FIGURE 2-2.

   D. There is an increased risk of having a child with a trisomy.
   E. There is no chromosomal explanation for their poor reproductive history.

4. A couple who have had recurrent abortions had a karyotype done on the last abortus. The karyotype was 47 XX +16. Given this information, you would tell the couple that the chance of delivering a live-born infant with a trisomy is approximately
   A. 0.1%
   B. 1%
   C. 10%
   D. 25%

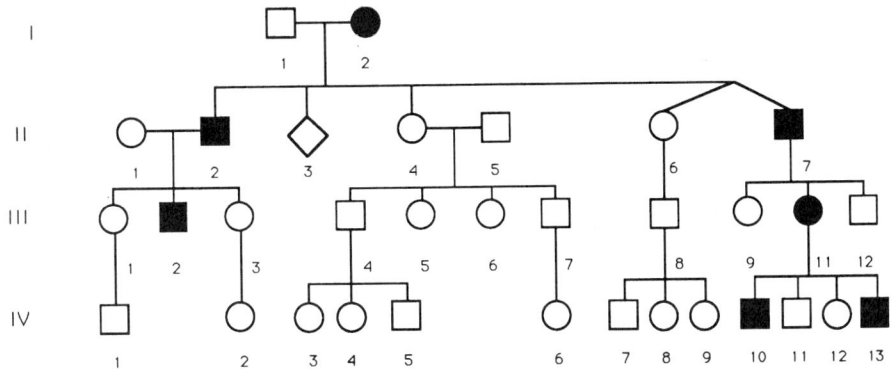

FIGURE 2-1.

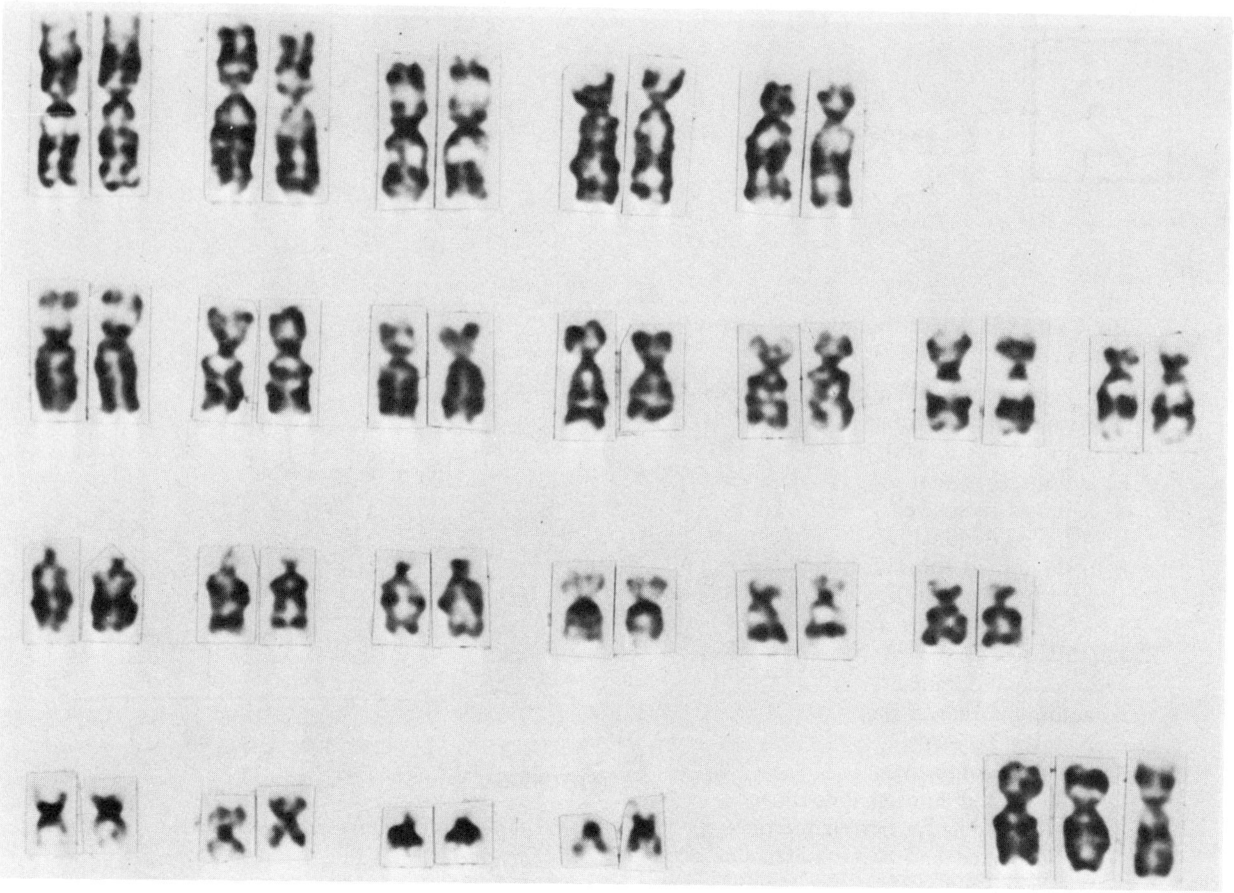

FIGURE 2-3.

5. Figure 2-4 represents a(n)
   A. Robertsonian fusion (translocation).
   B. isochromosome.
   C. reciprocal translocation.
   D. pericentric inversion.
   E. paracentric inversion.

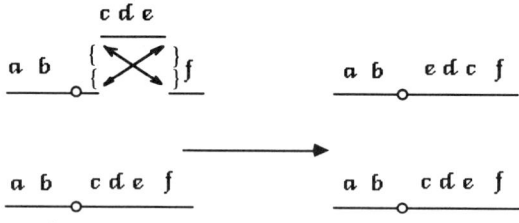

FIGURE 2-4

6. A prenatal patient has had her karyotype reported as containing a Robertsonian fusion (translocation). Theoretically, the likelihood of her having a conceptus with a trisomy is
   A. none
   B. 25%
   C. 50%
   D. 75%
   E. 100%

7. The spontaneous abortion figure quoted in most textbooks is 10% to 20%. If this figure includes all ova penetrated by sperm that do not result in live-born infants, the number
   A. is correct.
   B. should be 35–40%.
   C. should be 45–50%.
   D. should be 55–60%.
   E. should be 65–70%.

8. The sonographic study pictured in Figure 2-5 is associated with an abnormal fetal karyotype. All four views were taken from the same patient. You would anticipate that karyotype to be
   A. 45, X.
   B. 47, XX, +21.
   C. 47, XYY.
   D. 45, X/46, XY.
   E. 69, XXX.

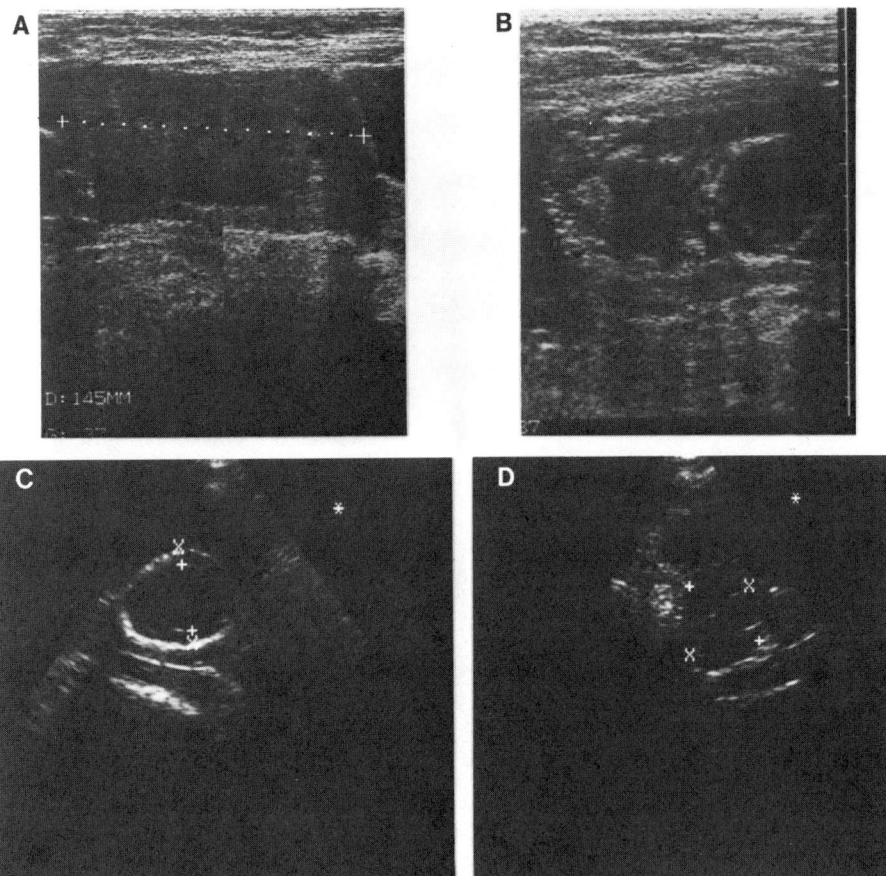

FIGURE 2-5.
Ultrasound through a pregnant uterus and adnexa. (A) A longitudinal section through the placenta. Distance = 145 mm. (B) A longitudinal section through the fetus. (C) Coronal section through the fetal skull. Calipers indicate a mantle of 25 mm. (D) The left adnexa. Calipers measure 45 by 55 mm.

9. Following delivery of the pregnancy depicted in question 8, one should order a(n)
   A. beta subunit Human Chorionic Gonadotrophin, serially.
   B. hematocrit.
   C. BUN.
   D. uric acid.
   E. HLA antigen.

DIRECTIONS: For each numbered item, select the one heading most closely associated with it. Each lettered heading may be used once, more than once, or not at all.

(A) Nondisjunctional event identified in abortus material
(B) Nondisjunctional event not identified in living or abortus material
(C) Patau syndrome
(D) Edwards' syndrome
(E) Down's syndrome

10. Trisomy 15
11. Trisomy 17

Partial Deletions of Chromosome

(A) 4
(B) 5
(C) 18
(D) Short arm X
(E) Long arm X

12. Shortness of stature
13. Wolf syndrome
14. Cri-du-chat syndrome

Match the specific chromosomal abnormality with its frequency of occurrence in chromosomally abnormal *abortal material*.

(A) 50%
(B) 20%
(C) 14–19%
(D) 3–6%
(E) 3–4%

15. Turner's syndrome
16. Triploidy
17. Trisomy

(A) <1%
(B) 3%
(C) 20%
(D) 32%
(E) 55%

Live-born infants with a chromosomal abnormality
18. Unbalanced translocation
19. 45 X

DIRECTIONS: For each numbered item, indicate whether it is associated with
A. only (A)
B. only (B)
C. both (A) and (B)
D. neither (A) nor (B)

(A) Meiosis
(B) Mitosis
(C) Both
(D) Neither

20. Nondisjunction
21. 47 XYY
22. 46,XY/45,X

DIRECTIONS: Each question contains four suggested answers of which one or more is correct. Choose the answer
A if 1, 2, and 3 are correct
B if 1 and 3 are correct
C if 2 and 4 are correct
D if 4 only is correct
E if all are correct

23. A 35-year-old primigravida had an amniocentesis 3 weeks ago. The karyotype is reproduced in Figure 2-6. A description of the phenotype should state that the
    1. sex is male.
    2. adult is severely mentally handicapped.
    3. adult is usually tall.
    4. neonate will have significant gynecomastia.

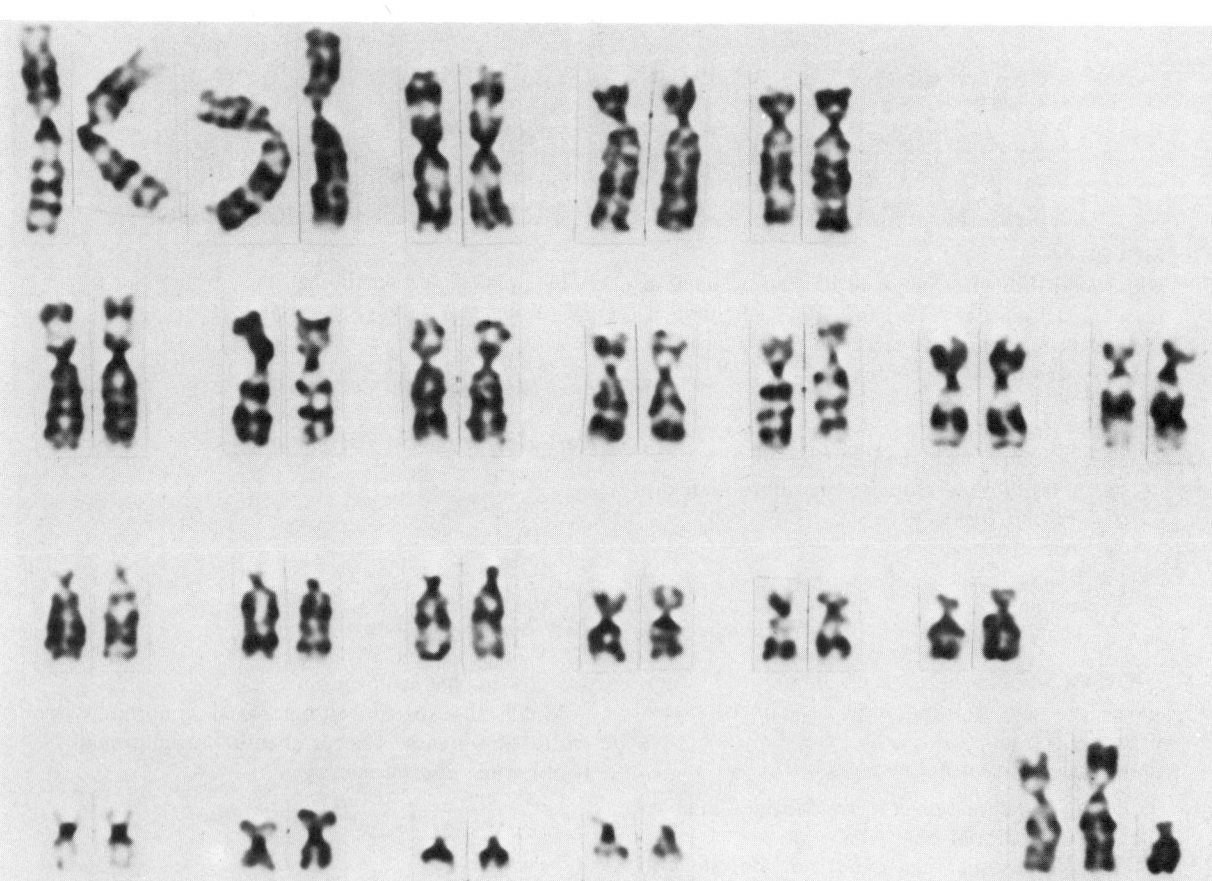

FIGURE 2-6

24. A couple, both of whom have achondroplasia, seek genetic counseling. Facts that you should mention include:
    1. 75% of the offspring will be abnormal.
    2. 50% of the offspring will have a more severe form.
    3. 25% of the offspring will be homozygous for the gene.
    4. 50% of the males will have the more severe form of the disease.
25. A family is suspected of carrying an X-linked recessive abnormality. One female member exhibits the trait. If this *were* an X-linked recessive, the possible explanations are
    1. complete penetrance of the trait.
    2. a function of the Lyon hypothesis.
    3. nondisjunction and deletion.
    4. a female who is homozygous.
26. An 18-year-old paraplegic seeks genetic counseling during the 22nd week of her pregnancy. She is the only member of her family who has this condition, which is due to a meningomyelocele repaired at birth. There is no history of a neural tube defect (NTD) on the husband's side of the family. You should advise this patient
    1. to take folate.
    2. there is a 2% risk of recurrence.
    3. to have a serum alpha-fetoprotein drawn.
    4. to have an amniocentesis for determination of amniotic fluid alpha-fetoprotein.
27. A woman who has had three spontaneous abortions is found to have the karyotype shown in Figure 2-7. Options available to this couple include:
    1. amniocentesis and selective abortion.
    2. ovum donation and embryo transplant.
    3. utilizing a surrogate mother.
    4. donor insemination.
28. Messenger RNA is different from DNA in that messenger RNA
    1. is a double helix.
    2. contains uracil.
    3. is not found in the nucleus.
    4. attaches to ribosomes.

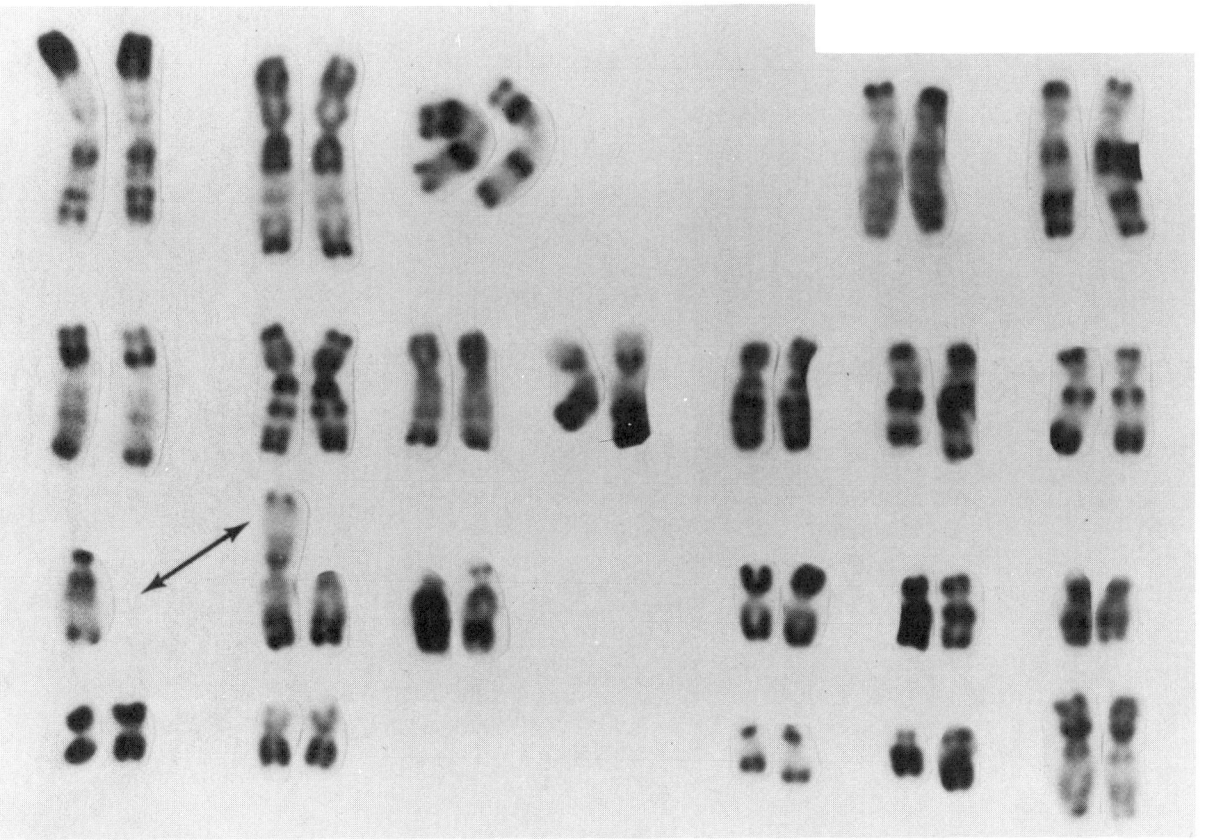

FIGURE 2-7.

29. A chromosome break may result in
    1. complete healing.
    2. a point mutation.
    3. partial deletion.
    4. a balanced translocation.
30. True statements about Tay-Sachs disease include:
    1. It is an autosomal recessive condition.
    2. It is most common in Jews of Eastern European origin.
    3. The carrier state can be detected by determining the individual's level of serum hexosaminidase A.
    4. Death usually occurs in the second decade.
31. True statements about the karyotype depicted in Figure 2-8 include:
    1. It is associated with severe mental retardation.
    2. It is usually but not always lethal.
    3. It is the most common karyotype associated with a stillborn.
    4. It is noted in about one third of trisomic abortus material.
32. True statements about couples with recurrent abortions include:
    1. Recurrent abortions occur in one out of every 200 couples attempting pregnancy.
    2. The percentage of women with chromosomal abnormalities in this group is 2.4%.
    3. The percentage of men with chromosomal abnormalities in this group is 2.4%.
    4. The most frequent parental chromosomal abnormality seen in this group is a sex chromosome trisomy.
33. A hydatidiform mole is usually
    1. 46 XX.
    2. made up of genetic material foreign to the mother.
    3. associated with loss of the maternal pronucleus.
    4. associated with advanced maternal age.

ANSWERS

1. **A,** Pages 25, 39. Usually, if 50% of the protein produced by the gene pair is enough to give the usual phenotype, the condition is dominant. In this case, no generation is spared, the condition is equally represented between males and females, and all affected individuals have at least one affected parent.

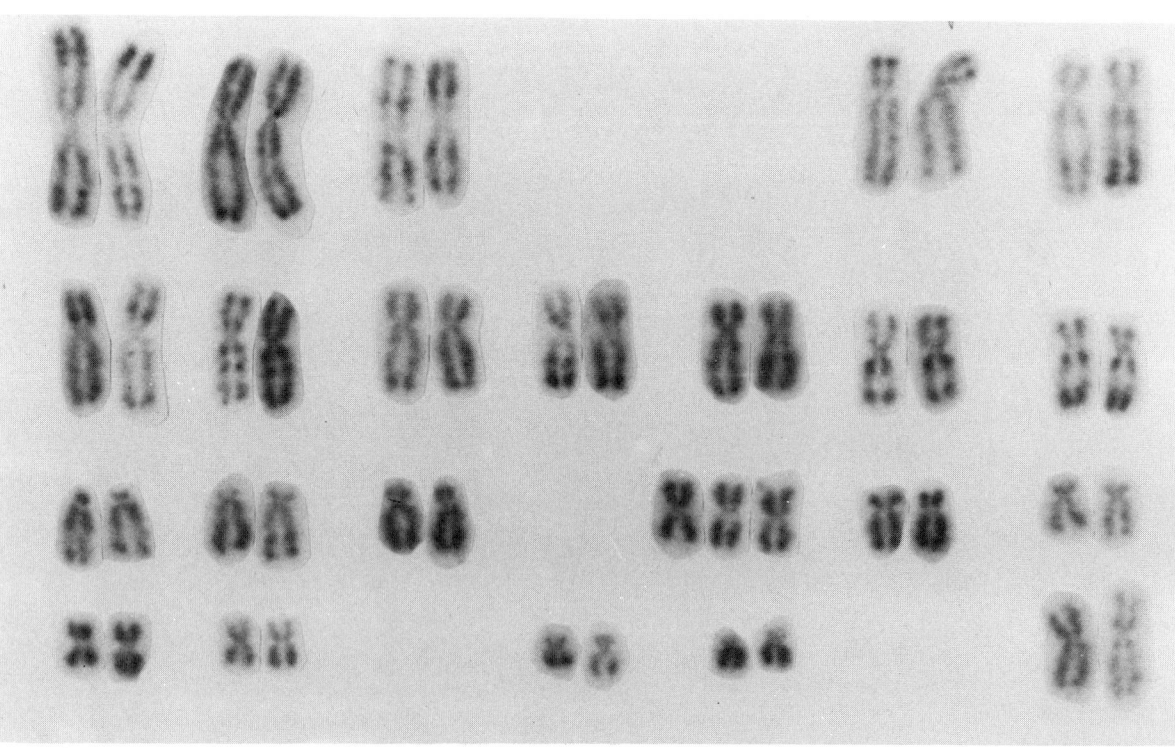

FIGURE 2-8.

Male-to-male transmission rules out X-linked dominant inheritance.

2. **B**, Pages 26, 39. Since there is full penetrance, an autosomal dominant is unlikely. Both sexes are affected, making X-linked inheritance extremely unlikely. The parents are consanguineous and must be presumed carriers. Two of seven children are affected. With an autosomal recessive trait, one would expect 25% of the children to be affected on the basis of segregation.

3. **D**, Page 31. The karyotype is 47, XXX. Fifty percent of these women are fertile. While most of the offspring produced are normal, there is a slight increase of an offspring produced with nondisjunctional events involving both the sex chromosomes and the autosomes.

4. **B**, Page 35. In women who have produced a conception which is trisomic, the risk of a subsequent trisomic event is 2–5%. The risk of delivering a live-born infant with a trisomy is 1%, however. The most common trisomy is 16, but none survive.

5. **E**, Pages 23, 24, 33, 34. In Robertsonian translocation (central fusion), two acrocentric chromosomes, such as 14 and 21, are involved. An isochromosome is the result of a transverse split rather than a longitudinal split of a metacentric chromosome during meiosis. The daughter chromosome has either two long or two short arms. With a reciprocal translocation, chromatin material is exchanged, but the chromosomal number does not change. When a chromosome breaks and turns on its axis, as is the case in this question, there is an inversion. In this example, the centromere was not involved, so the inversion is called *paracentric*. When the centromere is included, it is a *pericentric* inversion.

6. **B**, Pages 33, 34. One would expect that 25% would be normal, 25% carriers, 25% unbalanced and affected, and 25% monosomic. If this involved the 21 chromosome, one would be dealing with Down's syndrome. Since monosomy is lethal, the theoretical liveborn risk is 33% normal, 33% carriers, and 33% Down's syndrome. Even this does not turn out to be the case—the observed *live-born* risk of Down's is 10% if the mother has the translocation, and 2–3% if the father is the carrier.

7. **E**, Pages 34, 40. It has been estimated that about 15% of ova penetrated by sperm failed to divide. Another 15% failed to implant, and 25% to 30% are aborted spontaneously at previllous stages. Of the roughly 40% of fertilized ova that survive the first missed menstrual period, as many as 25% are aborted spontaneously, so that only about 30% to 35% of all ova penetrated by sperm actually result in live-born infants.

8. **E**, Pages 35–36, 38. Full explanation of the answer to this question follows the next question.

9. **A**, Pages 35–36, 38. In panel A of the sonogram in Figure 2-5, question 8, the placenta is large and contains several echolucent areas. In panel B, note the oligohydramnios. Panel C suggests hydrocephaly or holoprosencephaly. The ovary in panel D is enlarged and cystic, which is compatible with thecal lutein cysts. Given this, one should predict that the karyotype is triploidy. The latter is associated with a partial hydatidiform mole and should be followed like a hydatidiform mole.

10–11. 10, **A**; 11, **B**; Pages 30, 31, 40. Trisomy 13 (Patau syndrome) is incompatible with extended life. Trisomy 18 is Edwards' syndrome, also incompatible with extended life, while trisomy 21 is the more common and familiar Down's syndrome. Nondisjunctional events resulting in a trisomy have been described in every autosome except 1 and 17.

12–14. 12, **D**; 13, **A**; 14, **B**; Page 34. With loss of the short arm of the X chromosome, the individual has many of the findings associated with Turner's syndrome, including shortness of stature. Wolf's syndrome is due to the loss of a portion of the short arm of chromosome 4, and cri-du-chat syndrome to the loss of the short arm of chromosome 5.

15–17. 15, **B**; 16, **C**; 17, **A**; Pages 34, 35, 40. Half of the abortuses with chromosomal abnormalities have an autosomal trisomy; 20% have the karyotype 45, X; 14–19% triploidy; 3–6% tetraploidy; and chromosome rearrangements in 3–4%.

18–19. 18, **B**; 19, **A**; Pages 37, 40. (Ratcliffe S: Postnatal chromosome abnormalities. In Boyce HJ, ed: Chromosome variations in human evolution, London, Taylor & Francis, 1975.) Of live-born infants with chromosomal abnormalities, about 0.8 to 1% have 45, X, 36.8% have other sex chromosome abnormalities, 21% have autosomal trisomies of chromosomes 13, 18, and 21, and balanced chromosome translocations occur in 32.4%. There are 3.2% with unbalanced translocation abnormalities.

20–22. 20, **C**; 21, **A**; 22, **B**; Pages 24, 28, 31, 32. Nondisjunction is the faulty separation of chromosome pairs at anaphase in either meiosis or mitosis. Nondisjunction during spermatogenesis (meiosis) involving the Y chromosome can lead to the karyotype 47, XYY. Nondisjunctional events during mitosis in the early embryo will frequently produce individuals with cell populations containing different chromosome numbers.

23. **B** (1, 3), Pages 30, 31. The karyotype is that of 47, XXY, Klinefelter's syndrome. They are characterized by tall stature and azoospermia. Although they may be mentally retarded, this

is usually not severe. Gynecomastia is present in about one third of all cases, but it is unlikely to manifest itself in the neonate beyond that normally seen in a newborn male.

24. **B** (1, 3), Page 26. Each parent carries this autosomal dominant gene. It is highly unlikely that either is homozygous for the gene, since in that condition survival past infancy rarely, if ever, occurs. The gene is not on the X or Y chromosome. The sex ratio for heterozygotes is one male to one female. The gametes will be as pictured in Figure 2-9. Twenty-five percent will be normal (aa), 75% will be abnormal (AA or aA), 50% will have achondroplasia (aA), and 25% will be homozygous for this dominant gene and will have the lethal form (AA).

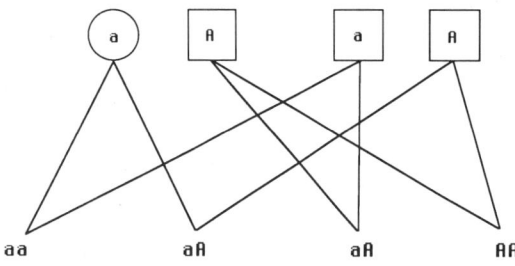

FIGURE 2-9

25. **C** (2, 4), Pages 24, 27. Penetrance is the percentage of individuals in a population with the mutation who actually demonstrate the phenotypic change. Nondisjunction and deletion would lead to monosomy 45, X—which is not the case in this example. In this case, the female either has the recessive gene on both chromosomes or the "normal" X is the one deactivated during "Lyonization." Usually the abnormal X is inactivated.

26. **C** (2, 4), Pages 28, 40. Although it has been suggested that neural tube defects might be prevented by administering folate supplements, these must be given preconceptually and during early gestation. The neural tube is formed by 4 weeks (postconception). This is a multifactorial disorder. The risk of recurrence in the United States is 11 times the population risk, which is approximately 2%. The sensitivity of amniotic fluid alpha-fetoprotein is better than maternal serum. Maternal serum alpha-fetoprotein is meant to be a screening test for a low risk population. Thus, amniocentesis is preferred in patients at risk, especially this late in pregnancy. Another possibility at 20 weeks is an ultrasound evaluation, but this was not an option.

27. **A** (1, 2, 3), Pages 37–38. The karyotype is of a Robertsonian fusion (translocation), 45, XX, t(13q14q). (From Stenchever MA: Contemp OB/GYN 17:38, April 1981.) This is maternal so that donor insemination will not help. Identifying an abnormal fetus and selective abortion or bypassing the abnormal mother are the only logical options listed.

28. **C** (2, 4), Pages 24, 25, and Figure 2-1 (from Drogemueller). RNA, unlike DNA, is a single strand whose sequence is encoded in the nucleus (messenger RNA). In the RNA molecule, uracil is substituted for thymine. Messenger RNA attaches to the ribosome and then attracts amino acids via smaller RNA molecules known as transfer RNA.

29. **E** (All), Page 32. A chromosome break may simply heal, with or without a point mutation at the point of breakage. If a segment of the chromosome is lost during this healing process, partial deletion of chromatin material may take place. If two chromosomes break, they may exchange chromosome arms and give rise to a translocation.

30. **A** (1, 2, 3), Page 27. Tay-Sachs disease is an autosomal recessive condition that is found most often in Jews of Eastern European origin. The carrier state can be detected by measuring serum hexosaminidase A. Death usually occurs by age 3 or 4.

31. **D** (4), Page 34. Figure 2-8 depicted a 47, XX16$^+$ karyotype. (From Stenchever MA: Contemp OB/GYN 17:38, April 1981.) A trisomy of chromosome 16 has been noted in about one third of trisomic abortus material. Since this has never been seen in living individuals, it must be considered universally lethal.

32. **B** (1, 3), Pages 37, 38. Roughly one in every 200 couples suffers from multiple abortions. Simpson discovered that the prevalence of chromosome abnormalities in women with chronic spontaneous abortion problems was about twice that of males (4.8% vs. 2.4%). The majority demonstrate either balanced reciprocal translocations or Robertsonian fusion.

33. **E**, (All), Pages 38, 40. It has been shown, using Q and R banding techniques, that most hydatidiform moles are 46, XX. It appears likely that in the formation of a hydatidiform mole, the female pronucleus is lost and the male pronucleus duplicates, so that *all* genetic material is foreign to the mother. With partial moles, a fetus is present and the karyotype is triploidy. Epidemiologic risk factors include extremes of age in the reproductive years.

CHAPTER 3

Anatomy

DIRECTIONS: Select the one best answer or completion.

1. On examination you find that a 40-year-old patient's uterus is anteflexed, firm, and approximately 9 cm long, 6 cm wide, and 4 cm thick, with an estimated weight of approximately 110 g. From this information alone you would be able to say that the patient was
   A. nulligravid.
   B. multigravid.
   C. 8 weeks pregnant.
   D. afflicted with adenomyosis.
   E. none of the above.

2. A 63-year-old asymptomatic woman is found to have a 3×2×3 cm left adnexal mass that feels cystic. The most likely etiology is
   A. enlarged follicle cyst.
   B. paraovarian cyst.
   C. corpus luteum cyst.
   D. hydrosalpinx.
   E. ovarian neoplasm.

3. At term, the pregnant uterus will increase in weight over the normal nonpregnant uterine weight approximately
   A. 2–3 times.
   B. 4–5 times.
   C. 10–20 times.
   D. 30–50 times.
   E. 100 times.

4. A 24-year-old patient is seen for a routine exam and a 2 cm asymptomatic cystic structure is found submucosally at the junction of the lower and middle third of the vagina at approximately 10 o'clock. The most likely etiology is
   A. vaginal inclusion cyst.
   B. clear cell adenocarcinoma.
   C. Gartner's duct cyst.
   D. Skene's duct cyst.
   E. Bartholin's duct cyst.

5. After a radical hysterectomy a patient complains of numbness over the medial aspect of her thigh. No muscle weakness is noted. This is most likely due to
   A. transection of the obturator nerve.
   B. nonpermanent injury to the obturator nerve.
   C. transection of the femoral nerve.
   D. nonpermanent injury to the femoral nerve.
   E. nonpermanent injury to the pudendal nerve.

6. The correct sequence of the arterial blood supply to the uterus begins with the aorta and continues through the
   A. internal iliac, common iliac, uterine.
   B. common iliac, hypogastric, uterine.
   C. external iliac, internal iliac, uterine.
   D. obturator, hypogastric, uterine.
   E. common iliac, pudendal, uterine.

7. A patient is most apt to have a tracholectomy performed if she
   A. is of Greek heritage.
   B. has had a prior subtotal hysterectomy.
   C. has a benign ovarian tumor.
   D. has an unusual retroperitoneal pelvic mass.
   E. has repeated episodes of dysfunctional uterine bleeding, unresponsive to D&C.

8. A woman who has endometrial cancer can have metastases to the inguinal nodes, transported via which lymphatic chain?
   A. Para aortic
   B. Obturator
   C. Round ligament
   D. Lumbar
   E. Iliac

9. A woman who has a vasovagal response during dilation of the cervix for a suction D&C done in the office is responding to stimulation of which of the following nerves?
   A. Pudendal
   B. Obturator
   C. Sciatic
   D. Femoral
   E. Frankenhauser's ganglion

10. The fallopian tube is anatomically divided into four segments. The longest segment is the
    A. interstitial.
    B. isthmic.
    C. ampullary.
    D. infundibular.
11. The major blood supply to the ovary arises from the
    A. common iliac artery.
    B. internal iliac artery (hypogastric).
    C. obturator artery.
    D. external iliac artery.
    E. aorta.
12. A woman complains of sudden onset of pain beneath the umbilicus, which then moves to the right lower quadrant. She denies nausea, vomiting, or fever. Her last menstrual period was 7 weeks ago, and she has been sexually active without contraception. Assuming she has a right tubal pregnancy, how do you account for the initial subumbilical pain?
    A. The tube was located anatomically in the midline.
    B. Tubal pain is transmitted via L2, 3, 4.
    C. Tubal pain is transmitted via S2, 3, 4.
    D. Tubal pain is transmitted via T11–12.
    E. Tubal pain is transmitted via C2, 3, 4.

DIRECTIONS: For each numbered item, select the one heading most closely associated with it. Each lettered heading may be used once, more than once, or not at all.

13–15. Match the female genital structure with the homologous male structure.
    (A) Prostate
    (B) Penis
    (C) Scrotum
    (D) Penile urethra
    (E) Cowper's gland
    13. Labia majora
    14. Skene's glands
    15. Labia minora
16–18. Match the following with the labeled portions of Figure 3–1.
    16. Zona basalis
    17. Myometrium
    18. Endometrium
19–21. Match the following structures with the labeled portions of Figure 3–2.
    19. Ovarian ligament
    20. Cervical portio
    21. Fimbria ovarica

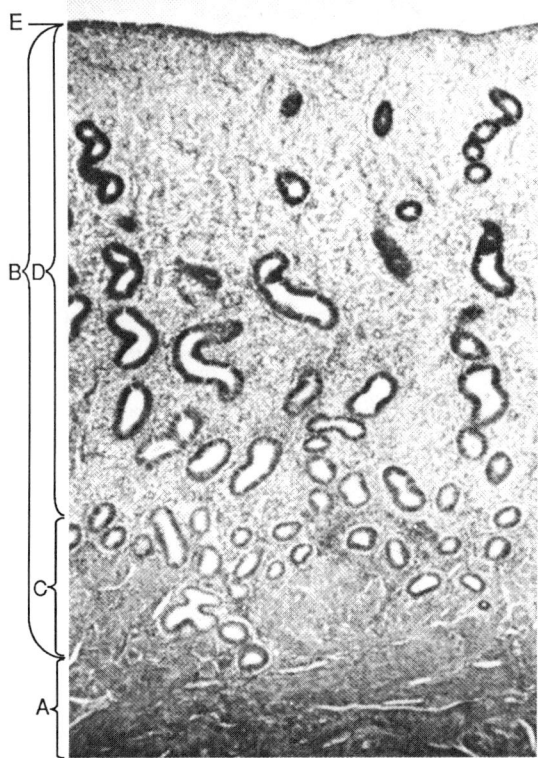

FIGURE 3-1.
A histologic view of the endometrium during the proliferative phase, demonstrating the strata in the endometrium.

(From Demopoulos Rl: Normal endometrium. In Blaustein A, ed. Pathology of the female genital tract, 2nd ed. New York, Springer-Verlag, 1982, p. 216.)

22–24. Match the anastomotic connection with the following pelvic vessels.
    (A) Superior gluteal artery
    (B) Uterine artery
    (C) Middle hemorrhoidal artery
    (D) Inferior vesical artery
    (E) Obturator artery
    22. Inferior mesenteric artery
    23. Deep iliac circumflex artery
    24. Medial femoral circumflex artery
25–27. Match the nodes with the labeled areas in Figure 3–3.
    25. Interiliac
    26. Common iliac
    27. Aortic

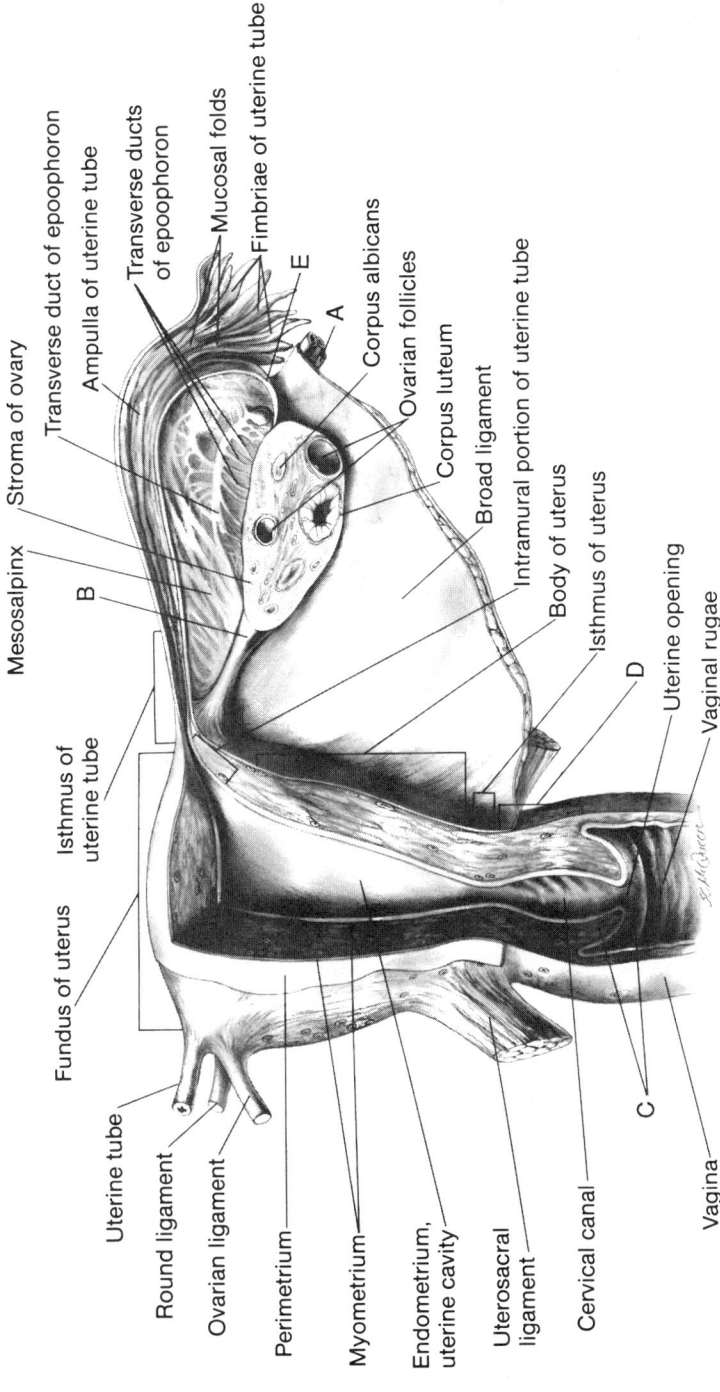

FIGURE 3-2.
A schematic drawing of a posterior view of the cervix, uterus, fallopian tube, and ovary. (Redrawn from Clemente CD: Anatomy: A regional atlas of the human body, 3rd edition. Baltimore-Munich, Urban & Schwarzenberg, 1987.)

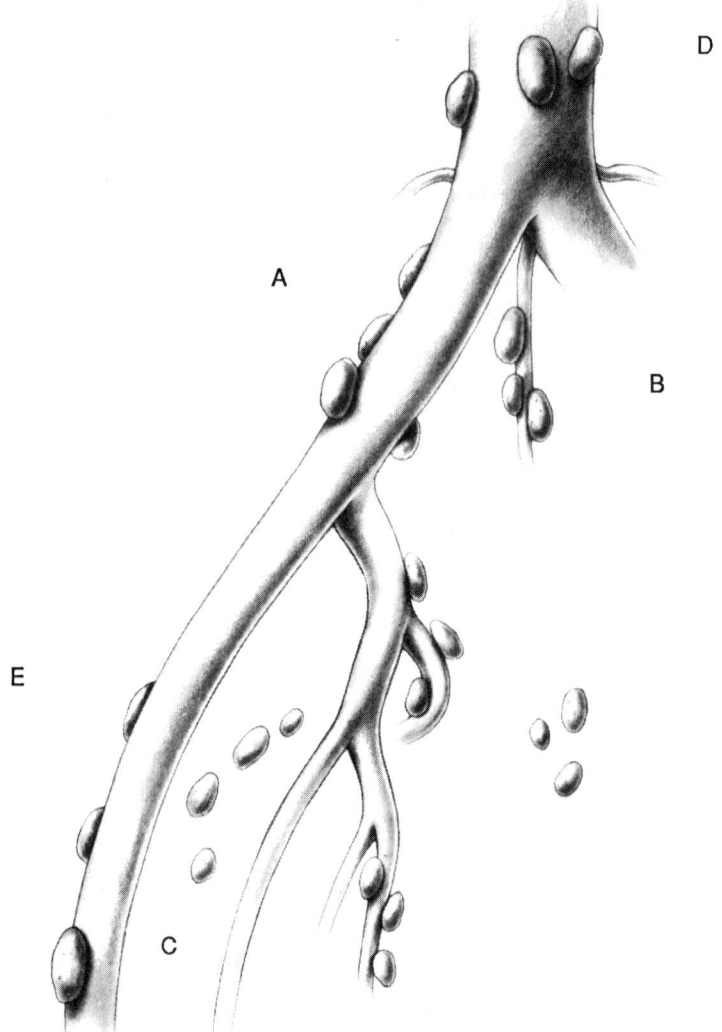

FIGURE 3-3.
Schematic view of the pelvic lymph nodes.
(From Plentl AA, Friedman EA: Lymphatic system of the female genitalia. Philadelphia, W.B. Saunders Co., 1971, p. 13.)

DIRECTIONS: Each question contains four suggested answers of which one or more is correct. Choose the answer
  A if 1, 2, and 3 are correct.
  B if 1 and 3 are correct.
  C if 2 and 4 are correct.
  D if 4 only is correct.
  E if all are correct.

28. True statements about the normal cervix include:
   1. The cervical stroma is 60% connective tissue and 40% smooth muscle.
   2. The endocervical columnar epithelium has secretory, ciliated, and intercalated cells.
   3. The endocervical lining is made up of many glands imbedded in the cervical stroma.
   4. Sperm may be stored in the lining folds of the endocervix for at least 48 hours.

29. When a woman coughs or strains, the pelvic diaphragm prevents the abdominal contents from being extruded through the pelvic cavity. This pelvic diaphragm is made up of which muscles?
   1. Coccygeus
   2. Deep transverse perineal
   3. Levator ani
   4. Psoas and iliacus

30. True statements about the vagina include:
    1. The upper portions of the vagina are supported by the cardinal ligaments.
    2. The anterior wall of the vagina is longer than the posterior wall.
    3. The endopelvic fascia supports the vaginal walls.
    4. Innervation arises from L2–4.
31. Patients with carcinoma of the cervix are likely to have metastases to the lymph nodes draining the cervix. These nodes include
    1. internal iliac.
    2. visceral nodes of the parametria.
    3. external iliac.
    4. obturator.
32. After ligating the uterine arteries and removing the uterus from the abdominal cavity, the vaginal cuff was noted to bleed. Possible sources of this bleeding are
    1. pudendal artery.
    2. middle hemorrhoidal artery.
    3. inferior vesical artery.
    4. inferior mesenteric artery.
33. Which of the following structures are parts of the normal ovary *and* have neoplastic potential?
    1. Stroma
    2. Epithelium
    3. Ova
    4. Granulosa cells
34. Following a rapid delivery, a large cervical tear is found to be bleeding. The vessels supplying blood to this site are
    1. descending branch of the uterine artery.
    2. pudendal artery.
    3. middle hemorrhoidal artery.
    4. obturator artery.
35. Sympathetic nerve fibers to the pelvis
    1. are part of the autonomic nervous system.
    2. originate from the cranial and sacral nerve roots.
    3. generally cause vasoconstriction and muscle contraction.
    4. enter the pelvis with large nerves such as the sciatic or femoral nerve.
36. A woman has a uterus measuring 6 cm in length, 3 cm in width, and 1.5 cm in thickness, with a weight of 30 g. This is consistent with
    1. menopause.
    2. adenomyosis.
    3. amenorrhea.
    4. pregnancy.

ANSWERS

1. **E**, Page 51. Although the size, shape, and consistency suggest a multigravid uterus, any of the listed possibilities could be true because of the great individual variation in anatomic size and configuration. It would not be possible to state that any one of the given reasons, or some other entity such as leiomyoma or a tumor was the reason for the upper limits of normal size and weight of this uterus.
2. **E**, Page 56. The size of the cystic structure would be normal in a menstruating female, but in a postmenopausal woman it is clearly abnormal, as no follicle or corpus luteum cysts should be present. Although the mass could be either a paraovarian cyst or a hydrosalpinx, these entities are very rare in postmenopausal women. Therefore, an ovarian neoplasm is the most likely finding. A malignant neoplasm is a definite concern. This finding in a postmenopausal patient warrants laparotomy.
3. **C**, Page 51. The normal nonpregnant uterus weighs 40–100 g. At term pregnancy, the uterus weighs 800–1000 g, which is a 10–20 fold increase. This increase is due to both hypertrophy and hyperplasia of muscle fibers, as well as an increase in decidua and blood volume contained within the uterus. Postpartum, the uterus decreases in both size and weight, so that by 6–10 weeks postpartum it is back to a normal prepregnancy weight, though usually slightly larger than a nulligravid uterus.
4. **C**, Page 48. The anterior lateral position, size, lack of symptoms, and age of the patient make the most likely diagnosis Gartner's duct cyst. Skene's ducts and glands are more anterior and distal in the vagina. Bartholin's gland is distal and posterior and inclusion cysts generally are found in areas of prior trauma, such as childbirth tears or episiotomy. The patient's age and description of a cyst make clear cell adenocarcinoma unlikely. Gartner's duct cyst is a dilation of a remnant of the embryonic mesonephros.
5. **B**, Page 66. The obturator nerve is motor to the adductor muscles of the thigh and sensory to the medial thigh. If it had been transected, motor weakness of the adductors would be present. Pressure injury, which involves the sensory fibers only or causes mild muscle weakness, will usually disappear in a few days or weeks. The femoral nerve is motor to the extensors of the leg and to the skin of the anterior thigh. The pudendal nerve is sensory to the perineum.
6. **B**, Pages 52, 58. The blood flows from the aorta to the common iliac to the hypogastric. The hypogastric (or internal iliac) has several branches that should be known by pelvic surgeons. They are superior gluteal, inferior gluteal, lateral sacral, uterine, internal pudendal, middle vesical, inferior vesical, ilial lum-

bar, middle hemorrhoidal, and vaginal. The obturator and superior vesical arteries may also arise from the hypogastric artery. The hypogastric artery ends as the obliterated umbilical artery. Arterial blood that supplies the uterus does not flow directly through the external iliac, obturator, or pudendal artery.

7. **B,** Page 48. The Greek word for neck is *trachēlos*. The word *cervix* originates from the Latin word for neck. Therefore, the surgical removal of the cervix is called *trachelectomy*, which is most apt to be performed in a woman whose cervix was left behind during a prior subtotal hysterectomy. Subtotal hysterectomies are done infrequently now and only if severe patient problems mandate rapid completion of surgery or if massive adhesions or other conditions prevent total removal of the uterus. These situations are very rare. Removal of a normal residual cervix is unnecessary.

8. **C,** Page 52. The inguinal nodes are not commonly involved with endometrial cancer, but the potential is present via the round ligament lymphatics. More commonly, the mode of spread is laterally through the lymphatics surrounding the iliac vessels and extending into the para aortic chain. Direct extension can also occur if the tumor penetrates the myometrium.

9. **E,** Page 51. The nerve supply to the cervix is via a plexus of nerves in the uterosacral ligaments, known as the paracervical or Frankenhauser's ganglion. These then innervate the endocervix. The efferent pathway from Frankenhauser's ganglion is to the hypogastric plexus and enters the spinal cord at T11–12. The vasovagal response of bradycardia with nausea, sweating, and sometimes syncope is occasionally seen with cervical or intrauterine manipulation, as parasympathetic fibers run together with the sympathetics.

10. **C,** Page 53. The whole fallopian tube is approximately 10–14 cm long. The ampullary portion is 4–6 cm long and is the segment where fertilization usually occurs. It has prominent folds, or plicae, which if disrupted by infection, inflammation, or trauma can result in blind pouches that can trap a fertilized ovum, leading to a tubal pregnancy. The other segments are shorter and have the following lengths: interstitial 1–2 cm, isthmic, 2–4 cm, infundibular, 1–2 cm.

11. **E,** Page 55. The major blood supply of the ovary arises from the aorta. In embryonic development, the gonads migrate caudally from their origin, bringing their blood supply, lymphatics, and nerves along with them. The right ovarian vein enters the inferior vena cava and the left ovarian vein enters the left renal vein. The lymphatics course cephalad in the infundibulo pelvic chain and join the para aortic nodes at the level of the renal pedicle. Approximately 20% of early ovarian cancer will have microscopic spread to the para aortic nodes.

12. **D,** Page 55. Pain fibers in the tube are stimulated by tubal distention with referred pain in the dermatomes supplied by the T11–12 cord segment as the tube developed as a midabdominal structure. Therefore, initial midabdominal pain can be appreciated when tubal distention is occurring. When inflammation or rupture occurs, there is irritation of the overlying peritoneum and localization of the pain to the right lower quadrant. The same sequence may occur with appendicitis.

13–15. 13, **C;** 14, **A;** 15, **D;** Pages 43–44. The homologous anatomic structures in the male are the scrotum, prostate, and the penile urethra for the labia majora, Skene's glands, and labia minora, respectively. Embryologic development of genital structures is influenced by the presence of testosterone. The sooner that excess androgen is present in embryonic development, the more likely it is that the configuration of the female genitalia will resemble the genitalia of a male. Knowledge of the homologous structures serves to remind us of this truism.

16–18. 16, **C;** 17, **A;** 18, **B;** Page 52. The zona basalis myometrium and endometrium are as shown in Figure 3–1. The endometrium does not have a basement membrane separating it from the myometrium. Rather, the basal endometrium inserts itself in the interstices between the muscle fibers of the myometrium. This results in the gritty sensation and sound when curettage is performed. The visceral peritoneum envelops the uterus, so that the uterus is, in fact, a retroperitoneal structure. The endometrium varies during the menstrual cycle from 1 to 6 mm in thickness, with most of the change occurring in the zona functionalis.

19–21. 19, **B;** 20, **C;** 21, **E;** Figure 3–5 (from Droegemueller). Pages 19–20.

19, **B,** Figure 3–5 (from Droegemueller). Page 55. The ovary is suspended by three ligaments: the infundibulopelvic ligament, which attaches the ovary to the pelvic side wall and contains the ovarian arteries, nerves and lymphatics; the utero ovarian ligament, which attaches the ovary to the uterus; and the mesovarium, which is part of the broad ligament and contains anastomotic branches from the uterine artery.

20, **C,** Figure 3–5 (from Droegemueller). The cervical portio is that part of the cervix that extends freely into the vaginal canal and is covered by squamous epithelium. It may have varying amounts of columnar epithelium extending onto its surface.

21, **E,** Figure 3–5 (from Droegemueller). The fimbria ovarica is the long tubal fimbria that attaches the infundibulum of the fallopian tube to the ovary.

22–24. 22, **C**; 23, **A**; 24, **E**; Table 3–1 (from Droegemueller). Pages 57, 58, 60. The high number of anastomoses in the pelvis allows many blood vessels to be sacrificed without ischemic compromise of the pelvic organs, particularly in younger women. For example, the inferior mesenteric artery can be ligated near the aorta without causing anoxic damage to the bowel, as anastomoses through the middle hemorrhoidal artery from the hypogastric and to the inferior hemorrhoidal artery from the pudendal maintains the blood supply. Venous return has an even greater number of anastomotic channels.

25–27. 25, **C**; 26, **A**; 27, **D**; Figure 3–15 (from Droegemueller) and Pages 60–64. The lymphatics of the pelvis are important because metastatic spread of pelvic malignancies occur along their path. Therefore, they must be sampled in cases of pelvic malignancy to determine optimum treatment. The interiliac nodes are found in the anatomic triangle made up of the external iliac artery, hypogastric artery, and pelvic sidewall. Deep femoral nodes are located in the femoral sheath and feed into the iliac and interiliac chains. Common iliac nodes are located adjacent to the common iliac artery. Aortic nodes are adjacent to the aorta and require meticulous technique for safe sampling. Parauterine nodes are found immediately lateral to the uterus and are removed during radical hysterectomy.

28. **D** (4), Page 50. The cervical stroma is 15% smooth muscle and 85% connective tissue. The epithelium has only two cell types, secretory and ciliated. Intercalated cells are found in the fallopian tube. The epithelium is arranged in folds and crypts which are not true glands, although the crypts are frequently referred to as such. Sperm storage in the mucus-filled crypts is a well-known phenomenon. Near midcycle, the sperm may persist in these crypts for several days.

29. **B** (1, 3), Pages 66, 67. The pelvic diaphragm is made up of the coccygeus and levator ani muscles. The levator ani is divided into three parts: the pubococcygeus, the puborectalis, and iliococcygeus. The deep transverse perineal muscle with its fascia make up the urogenital diaphragm, and the psoas and iliacus both lie cephalad and lateral to the true pelvis. The pelvic diaphragm resembles a derby hat placed upside down in the bony pelvic cavity.

30. **B** (1, 3), Pages 46–48. The vagina is supported by the cardinal ligaments and endopelvic fascia. Loss of this support can result in a cystocele and/or rectocele and/or prolapse. The anterior wall of the vagina is approximately 6–9 cm long, while the posterior wall of the vagina is approximately 8–12 cm long. The nerve supply to the vagina stems from S2–4.

31. **E** (All), Page 51. All of the listed nodes are part of the lymphatic drainage of the cervix. The visceral nodes of the parametria should be removed during radical hysterectomy. If lymphadenectomy is performed, the obturator, external and internal iliac nodes are also removed as curative surgery for carcinoma of the cervix. Other possible drainage channels include nodes in the common iliacs, superior and inferior gluteals, sacral, rectal, lumbar, and aortic chains, as well as nodes on the posterior surface of the bladder.

32. **A** (1, 2, 3), Page 47. Though the vaginal artery generally descends from the uterine artery, bleeding may still occur after the uterine artery has been ligated because of the highly developed collateral circulation. Collateral branches include the pudendal, middle hemorrhoidal, and inferior vesical arteries. The best method of achieving hemostasis is to suture the vaginal cuff.

33. **E** (All), Page 55. Fibrous tissue stroma forms the matrix of the ovary. The stroma surrounding the follicles makes up the theca interna and externa. The epithelium covering the ovary develops from the multipotential primitive coelomic epithelium, which during embryonic development also forms the lining of the tubes, uterus, and endocervix. Ova migrate to the ovary from the yolk sac during embryonic development. Occasionally, ova remain in a midline position in the embryo without entering the gonad. In this midline position, they can form teratomas or other germ cell tumors at a later date. Within the ovary, granulosa cells surround the ovum in a single layer. If this does not occur, the ovum does not survive.

All of these structures can develop neoplasms. The neoplasms formed often mimic structures that are formed normally by the multipotential originating cell. For example, the epithelial lining may form serous tumors that mimic tubal epithelium or the ovum can develop into an incomplete fetus with three germ layers. When the latter tumor is benign, it is called a benign cystic teratoma (dermoid).

34. **A** (1, 2, 3), Page 51. The descending branches of the uterine artery form the cervical artery. The pudendal artery feeds the vaginal artery, which anastomoses with the cervical artery. Middle hemorrhoidal arteries also anastomose with branches of the cervical artery. The obturator artery supplies the obturator muscle, ilium and hip joint, not the cervix.

35. **B** (1, 3) Page 64. The sympathetic and parasympathetic nerves make up the autonomic system. The parasympathetics originate in the cranial and sacral segments of the CNS and have ganglia near the visceral organs they serve. They generally cause vasodilation and muscle relaxation. The sympathetic fibers originate from the thoracic and lumbar portions of the spinal cord and cause constriction of the vessels and muscle contraction. Both

enter the pelvis through rather ill-defined plexuses, namely the superior hypogastric.

36. **B** (1, 3), Page 51. A small uterus is consistent with the state of menopause or other causes of ovarian failure such as persistent hypothalamic amenorrhea. You would expect that such a woman would be amenorrheic and not pregnant. Adenomyosis generally increases the uterine size. The uterus of a normal menstruating woman would be larger in all dimensions and weigh approximately 50–80 g. The upper limits of normal size would be approximately 110 g.

Chapter 4: Reproductive Endocrinology

DIRECTIONS: Select the one best answer or completion.

1. Tanycytes are cells in the third ventricle thought to be important in the transfer of
   A. GnRH.
   B. thyroxin.
   C. cortisone.
   D. FSH.
   E. estrogens.

2. β-Endorphin is found in the highest concentration in the
   A. arcuate nucleus.
   B. median eminence.
   C. pituitary.
   D. serum.
   E. ovary.

3. The reason gonadotrophin releasing hormone analogs can be used to inhibit FSH and LH is that:
   A. Receptors become refractory to binding.
   B. Receptors are all bound and therefore can no longer respond.
   C. Change in the ratio of bound to unbound receptors is needed to stimulate FSH and LH.
   D. The analogs are not the same as GnRH and therefore do not cause stimulation.
   E. Analogs do not bind the receptors but shield them from being bound by GnRH.

4. Delta 5 (Δ^5) steroid compounds have
   A. a double bond between carbon atoms 5 and 6.
   B. a double bond between carbon atoms 4 and 5.
   C. five carbon atoms in the A ring.
   D. a fifth benzene ring.
   E. none of the above.

5. Ovaries are unable to synthesize mineralocorticoids because they lack
   A. 3-betaoldehydrogenase.
   B. 17-hydroxylase.
   C. 21-hydroxylase.
   D. 11 β-hydroxylase.
   E. 19-hydroxylase.

6. Of the following, the hormone with the lowest concentration in the plasma is
   A. estrogen.
   B. progesterone.
   C. testosterone.
   D. androstenedione.
   E. dehydroepiandrosterone.

7. FSH has the same β subunit as
   A. LH.
   B. ACTH.
   C. TSH.
   D. HCG.
   E. none of the above.

8. The hormone most highly bound to steroid hormone binding globulin (SHBG) is
   A. progesterone.
   B. estrogen.
   C. testosterone.
   D. dehydroepiandrosterone.
   E. cortisol.

9. If the preovulatory plasma concentration of estradiol is 250 picograms per ml and the metabolic clearance rate is 1350 liters per day, what is the daily production rate of estradiol?
   A. .19 mg
   B. .338 mg
   C. 5.4 mg
   D. .338 g
   E. 5.4 g

10. Compared to a female of normal weight, a grossly obese woman will have an increased conversion of
    A. estradiol to estriol.
    B. testosterone to progesterone.
    C. progesterone to testosterone.
    D. estradiol to androstenedione.
    E. androstenedione to estrone.

11. The reason that the concentration of protein hormones in the blood is expressed in international units or milliinternational units per ml, rather than mg per dl is:
    A. Protein hormones metabolize so rapidly they cannot be measured by weight.
    B. Protein hormones are a combination of different molecules that constantly change.
    C. Protein hormones are hard to isolate in a pure form.
    D. Protein hormones exist in such small amounts that milligram weights would be meaningless.
    E. The measurement of protein hormones was developed by arbitrary convention, which is difficult to change.
12. The age at which a woman has the most primary oocytes is during
    A. organogenesis.
    B. mid to late fetal life.
    C. prepuberty.
    D. adolescence.
    E. mature young adulthood.
13. The structure of the ovum that prevents its fertilization by sperm of another species is the
    A. granulosa.
    B. theca interna.
    C. zona pellucida.
    D. vitelline membrane.
    E. theca externa.
14. Which of the following correlates directly with the increase of serum estrogen during an ovulatory cycle?
    A. Thickness of the theca externa.
    B. Size of the dominant follicle.
    C. Number of hilar cells in the ovary.
    D. Number of follicles in the ovary.
    E. Thickness of the ovarian cortex.
15. An ovulatory sequence is characterized by the following order of steps, starting with increased FSH secretion:
    A. Follicular growth
       Increased estradiol production
       LH surge
       Ovulation
       Increased estradiol and progesterone production
    B. Increased estradiol and estrogen production
       Follicular growth
       Increased progesterone production
       LH surge
       Ovulation
    C. Follicular growth
       Increased progesterone production
       LH surge
       Ovulation
       Increased estradiol production
    D. Increased progesterone production
       Follicular growth
       LH surge
       Increased estradiol production
       Ovulation
    E. LH surge
       Follicular growth
       Increased estradiol production
       Increased progesterone production
       Ovulation
16. While LH pulses are detected in serum, FSH pulses are not. Why?
    A. GnRH does not affect FSH secretion.
    B. FSH is not secreted in response to GnRH pulses but only in response to the steady state of GnRH.
    C. FSH has a longer half-life than LH.
    D. Inhibin decreases the amount of FSH secreted by the pulsatile GnRH.
    E. Estrogen interferes with the measurement of FSH in immunoassays.
17. The sensitivity of a laboratory test refers to
    A. the ability to measure only one substance.
    B. the least amount of substance that can be measured.
    C. the ability to measure the exact amount.
    D. the variation between intraassays and interassays.
    E. none of the above.

18. The sequence of events leading to menstruation is:
    A. Decrease in endometrial thickness
       Coiling of arteries
       Vasoconstriction
       Vasodilation
       Menses
    B. Coiling of arteries
       Vasodilation
       Decrease in endometrial thickness
       Vasoconstriction
       Menses
    C. Coiling of the arteries
       Vasoconstriction
       Vasodilation
       Decreased endometrial thickness
       Menses
    D. Vasoconstriction
       Coiling of the arteries
       Decrease in endometrial thickness
       Vasodilation
       Menses
    E. Vasodilation
       Decrease in endometrial thickness
       Coiling of arteries
       Vasoconstriction
       Menses

DIRECTIONS: For each numbered item, select the one heading most closely associated with it. Each lettered heading may be used once, more than once, or not at all.

19–21. Match the endometrium with the correct time of the cycle.
    (A) Menstrual
    (B) Early follicular
    (C) Late follicular
    (D) Early luteal
    (E) Midluteal
  19. Figure 4-1, Pseudostratified cells
  20. Figure 4-2, Subnuclear vacuoles
  21. Figure 4-3, Tortuous glands in edematous, vascular stroma

22–24. Match the times of the cycle with the appropriate serum level of hormone.
    (A) Early follicular phase
    (B) Late follicular phase
    (C) Ovulation
    (D) Midluteal phase
    (E) Late luteal phase

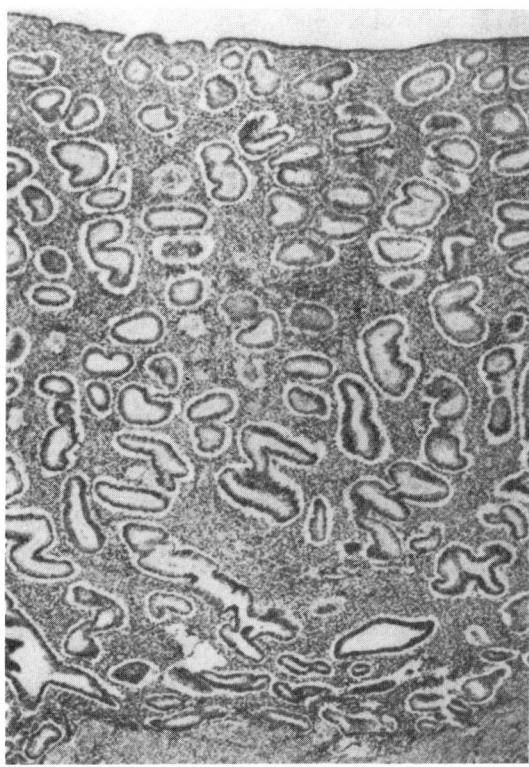

FIGURE 4-1.
(From Novak E, Novak ER, eds: Textbook of gynecology, 4th ed. Baltimore, Williams & Wilkins, 1952.)

  22. Estrogen from 100–150 picograms/ml, Progesterone 10–15 nanograms/ml.
  23. Estrogen greater than 200 picograms/ml, Progesterone 1–2 nanograms/ml.
  24. Estrogen less than 50 picograms/ml, Progesterone less than 1 nanogram/ml.

25–27. MATCH:
    (A) Steroid
    (B) Glycoprotein
    (C) Decapeptide
    (D) Catecholamine
    (E) Nucleotide
  25. GnRH (gonadotrophin releasing hormone)
  26. Dopamine
  27. Luteinizing hormone

24 Basic Sciences

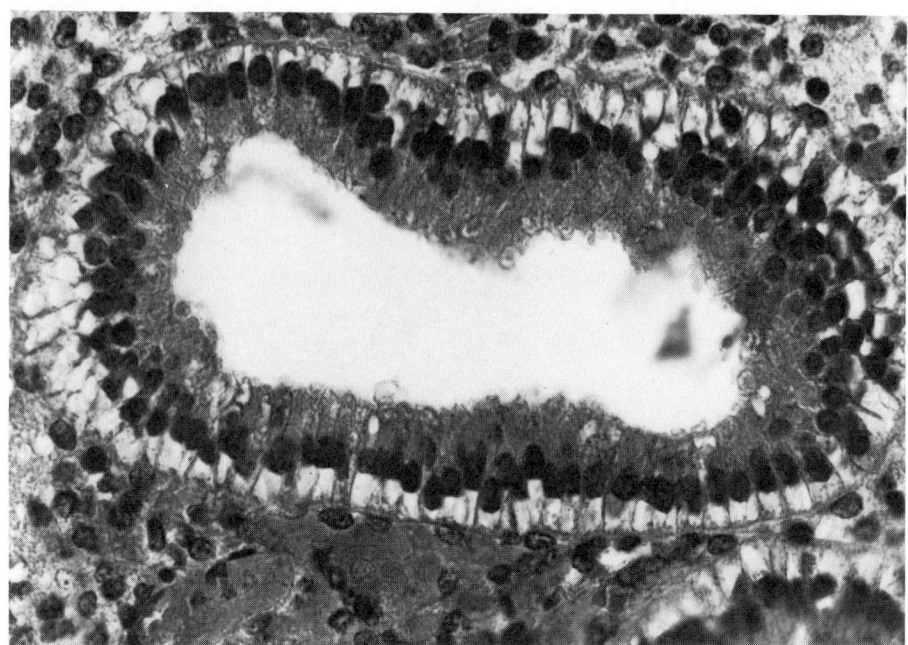

FIGURE 4-2.
(From March CM: The endometrium in the menstrual cycle. Reproduced with permission from Infertility, contraception and reproductive endocrinology, 2nd ed., edited by Daniel R. Mishell, Jr., M.D., and Val Davajan, M.D. Copyright ©1986 Medical Economics Books, Oradell, N.J. 07649. All rights reserved.)

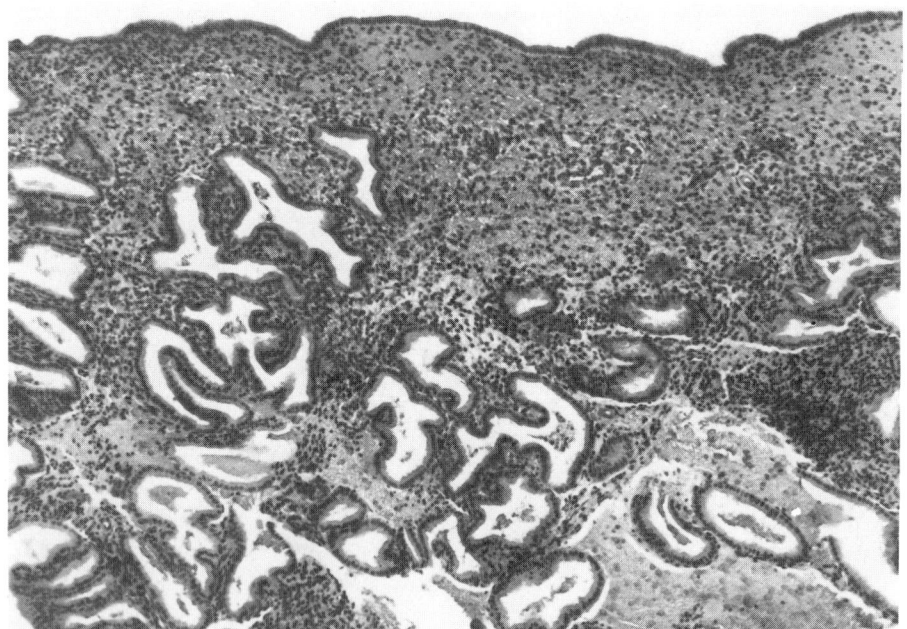

FIGURE 4-3.
(From March CM: The endometrium in the menstrual cycle. Reproduced with permission from Infertility, contraception and reproductive endocrinology, 2nd ed., edited by Daniel R. Mishell, Jr., M.D., and Val Davajan, M.D. Copyright ©1986 Medical Economics Books. Oradell, N.J. 07649. All rights reserved.)

DIRECTIONS: Each question contains four suggested answers of which one or more is correct. Choose the answer
- A if 1, 2, and 3 are correct
- B if 1 and 3 are correct
- C if 2 and 4 are correct
- D if 4 only is correct
- E if all are correct

28. True statements regarding steroid hormone receptors are:
    1. Steroid hormone receptors are intracellular.
    2. They bind a specific class of steroids.
    3. After binding with the steroid, the receptor complex enters the cell nucleus.
    4. The affinity of the receptor for a steroid does not correlate with the steroid's potency.

29. The amplitude and frequency of GnRH secretion is known to be modulated by
    1. ovarian steroids.
    2. gonadotrophins.
    3. catecholamines.
    4. serotonin.

30. Anovulation in a patient may be explained by
    1. altered pulse frequency of GnRH.
    2. decreased dopamine in the CNS.
    3. altered amplitude of GnRH secretion.
    4. low amounts of GnRH.

31. According to the two-cell hypothesis of ovarian estrogen production
    1. FSH stimulates theca cells to produce androgens.
    2. LH stimulates theca cells to produce androgens.
    3. LH stimulates granulosa cells to produce estrogens.
    4. FSH stimulates granulosa cells to produce estrogens.

32. Progestins decrease the effect of estrogens by
    1. inhibiting synthesis of estrogen receptors.
    2. binding on the estrogen receptors.
    3. Increasing synthesis of estrogen dehydrogenase.
    4. having an intrinsic androgenic effect.

33. During menstruation,
    1. the entire functional layer of endometrium is shed.
    2. the endometrium between muscle fibers is shed.
    3. enzymes destroy the myometrial matrix supporting the endometrium.
    4. endometrial regeneration is already beginning.

34. A 48-year-old woman asks you what her menstrual cycle will be like near menopause. You can accurately inform her that
    1. the mean age of menopause is approximately 51 years.
    2. periods are most apt to be irregular starting 3 years before actual cessation of flow.
    3. the time between periods normally increases near menopause.
    4. the mean duration of flow is 7 ± 2 days.

ANSWERS

1. **A**, Page 80. The tanycytes line the third ventricle and have microvilli which are postulated to absorb GnRH continuously and transport it into the portal system, thereby providing an alternative method for GnRH to reach the pituitary in contrast to the usual portal system transport.

2. **C**, Page 83. The reason for the high concentration in the pituitary is unknown. Infusion of β-endorphins decreases LH by causing an inhibitory effect on GnRH neurons in the hypothalamus. This action is theorized to contribute to anovulation in athletes who have high levels of β-endorphines.

3. **A**, Page 85. GnRH analogs function in a fashion similar to native GnRH; that is, they bind some of the target cell membrane receptors and stimulate them maximally. The unoccupied receptors become refractory to further binding and the occupied ones are saturated and not able to sustain the release of the second messenger, cyclic AMP, which maintains the activation of protein kinase. Protein kinase is needed to supply energy for the protein substrate that produces FSH and LH. The decreased FSH and LH results in anovulation.

4. **A**, Page 91; Figure 4-15 (from Droegemueller). Delta stands for a double bond between carbon atoms in the steroid molecule. When steroids are synthesized by the ovary, adrenal, or placenta, they follow specific pathways. Those with a double bond between carbon atoms 5 and 6 are called Δ^5 steroids. They have not yet been acted upon by the enzyme 4–5 isomerase, which changes the position of the double bond. This step is necessary to produce progesterone from pregnenolone and androsterone from dehydroepiandrosterone.

5. **C**, Page 91; Figure 4-16 (from Droegemueller). 21-hydroxylase is needed to hydroxylate carbon 21. This must be done before the steroids have significant mineralocorticoid effect. 11 β-hydroxylase is needed to confer the glucocorticoid effect by hydroxylation of the carbon in position 11.

6. **A,** Page 102. Although graphs often depict a higher curve for estrogen than for progesterone, the scales are different. The plasma levels of estrogens are measured in picograms, the progestins and androgens in nanograms, and conjugated dehydroepiandrosterone sulphate in micrograms. More important than concentration is the biological potency of a compound used to treat a specific deficit.

7. **E,** Page 87. FSH, LH, TSH, and HCG have the same α subunit but different β subunits. While also a pituitary hormone, ACTH has a different structure. Sensitive radioimmuno assay techniques utilize the β subunit to identify the specific compound.

8. **D,** Page 88. Dehydroepiandrosterone, testosterone, and estrogen are bound to SHBG in order of decreasing affinity. Cortisone and progesterone are bound to cortisone binding globulin. Steroids are also bound to albumin and approximately 5% of steroids are free. SHBG is increased by estrogen, obesity, and increased T4, and decreased by androgens and hypothyroidism. Therefore, thyroid dysfunction may change the concentration of SHBG and may cause changes in the amount of free estrogen, which in turn may cause abnormal uterine bleeding.

9. **B,** Page 93. Production rate equals the metabolic clearance rate times the concentration; therefore, 1350 liters per day times 250 picograms per ml times 1000 ml per liter equals 337,500,000 picograms per day, or approximately .338 mg per day. Preovulatory estrogen levels are higher than at any other phase of the cycle. The dose of replacement estrogen should have a pharmacologic effect similar to approximately .3 mg per day of estradiol after systemic absorption.

10. **E,** Page 92. Androstenedione is converted to estrone in fatty tissue. In obese women, regardless of age, a greater percentage (up to 7%) of androstenedione is converted to estrone than occurs in women of normal weight. This conversion can provide a constant pool of estrone, which inhibits ovulation and causes constant endometrial stimulation. This, in turn, can lead to the increased incidence of endometrial hyperplasia found in obese women.

11. **C,** Page 120. As most protein hormones are of high molecular weight and circulate attached to numerous other molecules, they are extremely difficult to isolate in pure form. Therefore, a reference standard is agreed upon and measurements are expressed in terms of that standard. If the standard is internationally agreed upon, the results will be expressed as international units or milliinternational units.

12. **B,** Pages 96–97, 99. Loss of human oocytes is tremendous, from seven to 10 million in mid to late fetal life. The number of oocytes decline rapidly, mainly because of atresia. Only 500–600 ovulatory cycles occur during the reproductive lifespan of a woman, with usually one or two eggs released at each ovulation. All the rest of the eggs degenerate. If the ovum is not surrounded by granulosa cells in the ovary, it degenerates. Ova surrounded by granulosa cells form follicles, most of which become atretic.

13. **C,** Page 99; Figure 4-21 (from Droegemueller). The zona pellucida is a mucopolysaccharide layer that allows only sperm of the same species to penetrate. When it is removed, as is done in a zona-free hamster egg penetration test, human sperm can penetrate the hamster egg. The sperm's ability, or inability, to penetrate the egg is used to determine fertilizing potential of the sperm. The theca interna and externa do not accompany the ovulated egg. The vitelline membrane blocks repeated penetration by sperm after one sperm has successfully entered the egg.

14. **B,** Page 99. The dominant follicle produces approximately 80% of the estrogen synthesized before ovulation. Its mean diameter is about 2 cm and its mean volume is approximately 3.8 ml. This increase in size, as monitored by ultrasound, is used when following women who are being stimulated for in vitro fertilization. This provides a criterion to identify maximum potential for ovulation.

15. **A,** Pages 97, 99. Knowledge of the normal sequence of events in the menstrual cycle enables you to evaluate abnormalities and prescribe rational therapy. The FSH stimulates the follicle, which in turn produces estradiol, which promotes the development of an LH-responsive dominant follicle and triggers the LH surge, resulting in ovulation. After ovulation the follicle develops into a corpus luteum, which produces both estrogen and progesterone. The progesterone causes secretion by an estrogen-stimulated endometrium preparing for the implantation of a fertilized ovum.

16. **C,** Page 105. GnRH does affect secretion and release of FSH, but because FSH has a half-life of approximately 4 hours, short bursts of its secretion are not apparent. LH has a half-life of 30 minutes, and the episodic nature of its secretion is apparent. Although inhibin, a nonsteroidal hormone produced in the granulosa cells, does inhibit FSH, it is only manifest when the granulosa is large, and therefore it is not a constant inhibitor of FSH. Estrogen does not interfere with the test used to measure FSH.

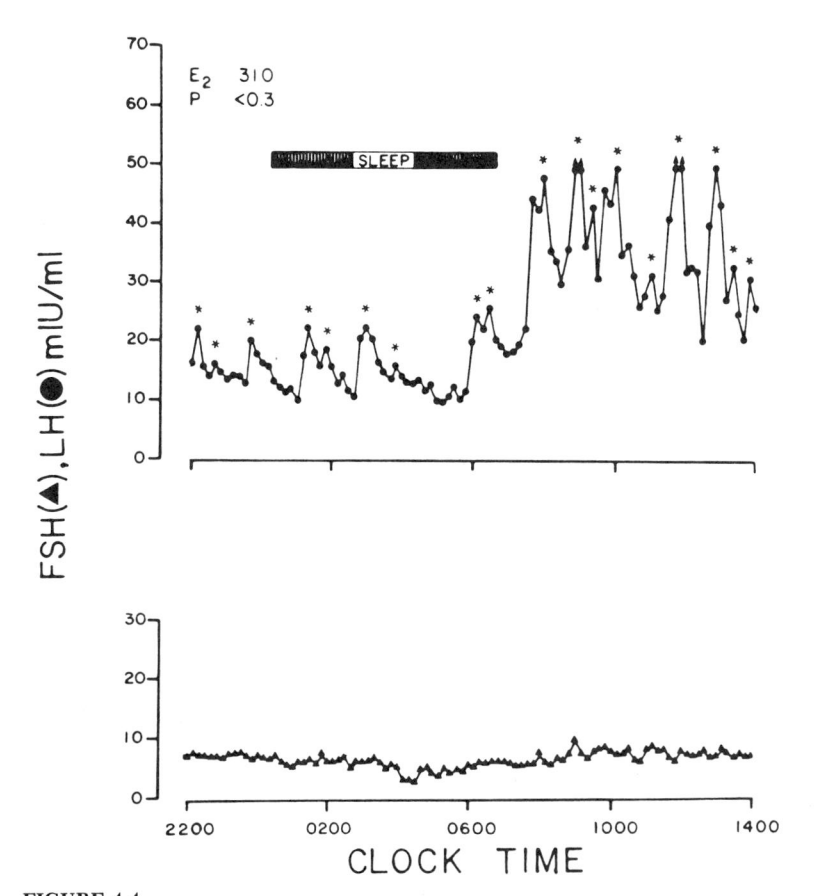

FIGURE 4-4.
(From Crowley WF, Filicori M, Spratt DI, et al: Recent Prog Horm Res 41:473, 1985.)

17. **B,** Page 119. The ability to measure only one substance is the specificity. The least amount of substance that can be measured is the sensitivity. The ability to measure the exact amount is accuracy. The variation between intraassays and interassays is the precision of a test.

18. **A,** Page 115. According to Markee's studies, first there is regression in the thickness of the endometrium with coiling of the spiral arteries and slowing of blood. This is followed by vasoconstriction, after which there is vasodilation, leading to escape of blood and menses. The initial decreased blood flow is thought to cause tissue ischemia, which releases lysosomal enzymes, which in turn break down the endometrium. This degraded tissue and bleeding from the coiled arteries of the functional layer of the endometrium make up the menstrual flow.

19–21. 19, **C;** 20, **D;** 21, **E;** Pages 112, 114. The endometrium undergoes specific, recognizable histologic changes during the menstrual cycle. These changes can be dated quite accurately to correlate with the days of the menstrual cycle. Endometrial biopsy and dating can be done to provide indirect evidence of ovulation.

22–24. 22, **D;** 23, **C;** 24, **A;** Pages 105, 108–109. Estrogen rises throughout the follicular phase and peaks just before the LH surge. Progesterone is low until after ovulation when it rises along with the secondary rise in estrogen. Both estrogen and progesterone fall just before menses. The 17-hydroxyprogesterone level rises slightly before the LH surge and falls again just before menses.

25. **C,** Page 82; Figure 4-1 (from Droegemueller). GnRH is a decapeptide produced in the hypothalamus, mainly by cells in the arcuate nucleus. It is then transported via neurons to the median eminence. The median eminence has capillaries that allow the GnRH molecules to pass into the pituitary portal blood supply and reach the gonadotrophin responsive cells in the pituitary, stimulating them to produce FSH and LH.

26. **D,** Page 82. Dopamine is a catecholamine produced from tyrosine in a sequence through dopa with further conversion to norepinephrine and later to epinephrine. It stimulates prolactin-inhibiting factor and appears to inhibit both GnRH and LH release. Bromocriptine is used to increase dopamine receptors, which in turn increases the stimulation of prolactin inhibiting factor and therefore decreases prolactin release.
27. **B,** Page 82. LH is a glycoprotein produced in the pituitary. Both its production and release are stimulated by GnRH. LH peaks about 30 minutes after an IV bolus of GnRH is given. If continuous GnRH is given, LH (and FSH) secretion is inhibited.
28. **A** (1, 2, 3), Page 95. Steroid hormone receptors are intracellular and bind a specific class of steroids after which the receptor steroid complex enters the cell nucleus. Estrogen receptors have the greatest affinity for estradiol, with less affinity for estrone and even less for estriol. Therefore, the affinity correlates with the observed potencies of these compounds. Once the hormone receptor complex is within the cell nucleus, messenger RNA is formed, which in turn enters the cytoplasm and translates its information to the ribosomes so that they will synthesize a new protein.
29. **A** (1, 2, 3), Page 80. Estrogen and progesterone are transmitted to the anterior and medial basal hypothalamus via the systemic circulation, whereas the gonadotrophins (LH and FSH) are returned via the portal system. Catecholamines (dopamine and norepinephrine) and serotonin arrive via neural pathways. Serotonin has not been shown to regulate GnRH release directly, but it does stimulate the release of prolactin.
30. **E** (All), Page 82. Several experimental systems in both primates and humans have shown that high or frequent GnRH pulsations are inhibitory to FSH and LH release, as is too little GnRH. Dopamine appears to act in the median eminence to inhibit the release of GnRH, and if too much dopamine is present, GnRH production drops, thereby decreasing FSH and LH. Without adequate FSH and LH, the usual sequence of follicle maturation, ovulation, and corpus luteum formation does not occur.
31. **C** (2, 4), Page 88. According to this hypothesis, LH acts on theca cell receptors to stimulate production of androgens, which are transported to the granulosa cells. Granulosa cells, under the influence of FSH, aromatize androgens to estrogens. FSH and estrogen stimulate LH receptors on the granulosa cells, allowing LH to be bound and cause luteinization.
32. **B** (1, 3), Page 95. Progesterone inhibits synthesis of estrogen receptors and increases synthesis of estrogen dehydrogenase, which converts the more potent estradiol to the less potent estrone. As estrogen receptors are quite specific, progestin does not bind to them. Also, progesterone has no intrinsic androgenic effect, although it may be converted to androgen if the appropriate enzymes are available.
33. **D** (4), Page 116. As there is no basement membrane between the myometrium and endometrium, the basal endometrium is interdigitated between the muscle fibers of the myometrium. This produces the gritty sensation felt on D&C. During menses, many of the endometrial cells remain in both the functional and basal layers. Regeneration of cells begins even as bleeding is continuing. Although enzymes may destroy endometrial cells, muscle cells are generally unaffected.
34. **A** (1, 2, 3), Page 110. The irregularity of periods that is common both at the beginning and the end of the menstrual years is more worrisome in the older woman, as the risk of endometrial carcinoma is much higher than in teenage years. A certain amount of irregularity is normal, with the normal pattern being a longer time between menses. The average age of menopause is 51 and the mean duration of flow during regular cycles is 4 ± 2 days.

PART TWO: APPROACH TO THE PATIENT

CHAPTER 5: History and Examination of the Patient

DIRECTIONS: Select the one best answer or completion.

1. Each of the following neoplasms can be screened during routine physical examination except
   A. carcinoma of the cervix.
   B. carcinoma of the breast.
   C. carcinoma of the ovary.
   D. carcinoma of the endometrium.
   E. carcinoma of the rectum.

2. Which of the following is *least* important in taking a menstrual history from a gynecologic patient?
   A. Symptoms associated with menstruation.
   B. Menstrual interval.
   C. Number of days of menses.
   D. Calculation of a numerical menstrual formula.
   E. Characteristics and amount of menstrual flow.

DIRECTIONS: For each numbered item, select the one heading most closely associated with it. Each lettered heading may be used once, more than once, or not at all.

3–6. Match the following diagnostic procedure with the *most* appropriate patient history listed below:
   (A) Mammography
   (B) Colposcopy
   (C) Hysteroscopy
   (D) Endometrial sampling
   (E) Pelvic ultrasonography
   (F) Vaginoscopy

3. 8-year-old girl with 2 month history of vaginal bleeding
4. 44-year-old nulligravid woman in clinic for annual exam
5. 44-year-old woman presenting with a problem of frequent "irregular periods"
6. 31-year-old patient with history of habitual abortion and unusually large cervical "erosion" (cockscomb-cervix)

DIRECTIONS: For each numbered item, indicate whether it is associated with

A only (A)
B only (B)
C both (A) and (B)
D neither (A) nor (B)

   (A) Cystocele
   (B) Rectocele
   (C) Both
   (D) Neither

7. Represents herniated peritoneal reflections
8. May present past the vaginal introitus
9. May be repaired vaginally
   (A) Bleeding manifestations of an ovulatory cycle
   (B) Bleeding manifestations of anovulatory cycle
   (C) Both
   (D) Neither
10. Consistent postcoital bleeding, regular menses
11. Intermenstrual spotting, regular menses
12. Consistently regular, painful menses
    (A) Bimanual exam, abdominal/vaginal
    (B) Bimanual exam, abdominal/rectovaginal
    (C) Both
    (D) Neither
13. Used to identify portio vaginalis
14. Used to appreciate uterosacral ligament nodules
15. Will identify a palpable postmenopausal ovary
    (A) Chlamydia
    (B) Gonorrhea
    (C) Both
    (D) Neither

16. Papanicolaou smear likely to identify cellular changes
17. Best identified by endocervical swab cultures
18. Culture attempts should follow cytologic sampling for pap smear

DIRECTIONS: Each question contains four suggested answers of which one or more is correct. Choose the answer
A if 1, 2, and 3 are correct
B if 1 and 3 are correct
C if 2 and 4 are correct
D if 4 only is correct
E if all are correct

19. Reproductive (pregnancy) history of a patient includes previous
    1. ectopic pregnancy.
    2. molar pregnancy.
    3. gestational diabetes.
    4. paternity.
20. Dermatologic findings of the vulvar and perineal skin of potential significance include
    1. hyperkeratosis.
    2. alopecia.
    3. pigmented nevus.
    4. cherry angioma.
21. Nonverbal clues given by patient behavior may be helpful in making which of the following clinical diagnoses?
    1. Endogenous depression
    2. Hidden anger
    3. Anxiety neurosis
    4. Seductiveness
22. Characteristics of the normal squamocolumnar junction (transformation zone) include:
    1. Areas of squamous metaplasia.
    2. Located at or near the portio vaginalis.
    3. May shift in location in response to infectious or hormonal influences.
    4. Contains glandular epithelium.
23. Historical points in sexual history that usually relate to the presence of organic gynecologic pathology include
    1. anorgasmia.
    2. dyspareunia.
    3. diminished libido.
    4. postcoital bleeding.
24. Nonverbal impressions gained from patient behaviors include
    1. anger.
    2. fear.
    3. apathy.
    4. sadness.
25. Papanicolaou testing should
    1. be performed yearly in all patients.
    2. first be performed regularly with onset of coitus.
    3. be done just prior to menstruation.
    4. contain an adequate sampling of endocervical cells.
26. Positive historical features that help to identify risks for endometrial neoplasia in a 43-year-old patient include
    1. chronic oligomenorrhea.
    2. prior short-term contraceptive use at age 40.
    3. nulligravidity.
    4. prior use of intrauterine device for 2 years.

ANSWERS

1. **D**, Pages 143, 809. Small endometrial tumors may not be appreciated by routine examination unless associated with a significant change in bleeding pattern. The others can be suspected by routine exam and/or diagnostic procedures such as pap smear and stool guaiac testing. Endometrial sampling is reserved for patients with abnormal menstrual histories, perimenopausal or postmenopausal bleeding, or it is advocated by some as routine in postmenopausal estrogen users.
2. **D**, Page 133. Calculation of a numerical menstrual formula (age of menarche × number of days of cycle × number of days of menstrual flow, e.g., 12 × 28 × 5 = 1680) is in itself of little value when used out of context of other more important information dealing with menstrual changes or associated symptoms. *Components* of the menstrual formula are more likely to relate to problems that may help in making a diagnosis. For example, if the age of menarche were 17 and the interval 42 days and the days of flow 7 (17 × 42 × 7 + 4998), this value in itself compared to the previous normal example (1680) is less helpful than identifying abnormalities in the specific components.
3–6. 3, **F**; 4, **A**; 5, **D**; 6, **B**; Pages 249–251, 343, 956, 359–363. A prepuberal girl with vaginal bleeding is at greatest risk for vaginal foreign body. A less likely source for this problem would be a functional ovarian neoplasm and thus, if vaginoscopy were unrevealing, a pelvic ultrasound might be helpful in ruling out this unusual cause.

Mammography is indicated as a routine screening exam in gynecologic perimenopausal patients, particularly patients with any risk factors.

Perimenopausal patients (over age 35) with change in bleeding (menstrual) patterns should be screened by office sampling of the endometrium at least. Further assessment of dilation and curettage or hysteroscopy should be dictated by other pertinent history or physical exam features.

Repetitive reproductive loss coupled with an unusual configuration of glandular cervical epithelium should alert the clinician to the possibility of previous material DES exposure and thus the necessity of performing an initial colposcopic evaluation and careful palpation of the vaginal fornices.

7–9. 7, **D**; 8, **C**; 9, **C**; Pages 138, 140. In the physical examination of the patients with pelvic relaxation, knowledge of potential herniations and loss of pelvic supporting structures is imperative. Cystocele and rectocele are usually apparent when present but not always symptomatic. Enterocele is a herniated peritoneal surface and is often more subtle, necessitating a thorough working knowledge of this defect. This is especially important with regard to planning surgical procedures designed to correct disorders of pelvic support.

10. **D**, Page 133. Postcoital bleeding usually occurs as a result of some inflammatory or neoplastic disorder of the cervix and/or endometrium rather than as a reflection of ovulatory or anovulatory endocrinologic milieu.

11. **C**, Page 133. Likewise, intermenstrual bleeding should be viewed as neoplastic or inflammatory until proven otherwise. Intermenstrual bleeding can also be associated with ovulation if it occurs near midcycle on a regular basis. This is due to the change in hormonal milieu at this time.

12. **A**, Page 133. Regular, painful menstruation is usually associated with ovulation, presumably because of the association of progesterone production with enhanced activity of prostaglandin on the smooth musculature of the uterus.

13–15. 13, **C**; 14, **B**; 15, **C**; Page 142. The portio vaginalis is usually a visual landmark of the cervix and is seen by speculum examination, but it also can be palpated during either of the above exams. Because the uterosacral ligaments insert onto the posterior cervicouterine junction and extend backwards to the hollow of the sacrum, they are best appreciated by the rectovaginal exam. An enlarged postmenopausal ovary is not necessarily better appreciated by either physical exam technique, depending on the anatomic relationships of the patient being examined. This finding suggests an ovarian neoplasm and needs further diagnostic assessment, regardless of how it is suspected.

16–18. 16, **D**; 17, **C**; 18, **C**; Pages 143–144. Neither chlamydia or gonorrhea can be specifically identified by the cytologic techniques used in Papanicolaou screening, whereas koilocytosis suggesting infection by human papilloma virus may be suspected by the pap smear. Both of the above organisms are endocervical culture.

Recent preliminary data suggest that cytologic screening for chlamydia may have promise, but this information is not yet generally accepted as a reliable, sensitive screen for this organism. (JAMA, February 14, 1985)

19. **E** (All), Page 133. Any pregnancy in the patient's history should be recorded, including nonviable and preterm pregnancies as well as metabolic pregnancy complications and paternity. These events may help the clinician in predicting future reproductive outcome and in offering a rationale for specific diagnostic or therapeutic measures such as ultrasonography, HCG testing, testing for carbohydrate intolerance, and identification of potential chromosomal problems.

20. **B** (1, 3), Page 137. Although skin findings such as hyperkeratosis and pigmented nevi may be normal variants, they warrant more careful follow-up and present the need for possible biopsy confirmation of underlying disorders such as intraepithelial neoplasias or atrophic dystrophies. Scattered cherry angiomata are not associated with more serious pathology when seen as an isolated incidental finding. Thinning of the pubic hair overlying the mons pubis may happen as women enter their later postmenopausal years.

21. **B** (1, 3), Page 132. Anger and seductiveness are not clinical diagnoses but may be *part of* another pathological process. Depression and anxiety are diagnoses (DM III) and may be detected in nonverbal patient behavior.

22. **E** (All), Page 142. The transformation zone, by definition, is the functional zone between squamous epithelium of the exocervix. It contains elements of both surfaces. This zone is dynamic and changes continually through the reproductive years in response to inflammation, trauma, pregnancy, and hormonal influences.

23. **C** (2, 4), Page 134. Whereas anorgasmia and vaginismus are usually related to psychological dysfunction, dyspareunia and postcoital bleeding are more likely to relate to potential nonsuppurative inflammation or neoplastic disorders. These historical findings warrant further assessment to rule out potential gynecologic pathology.

24. **E** (All), Pages 131–132. Nonverbal impressions gained from patient behaviors during preliminary assessment of the patient include clues that enhance the clinician's ability to extract useful information. This may be important in determining therapy at a later date.

25. **C** (2, 4), Page 143. American College of Obstetricians and Gynecologists guidelines suggest that papanicolaou testing begin at age 18 or when regular coital activity begins. In patients at higher risk—those with history of early coital activity and/or multiple partners or those with other risk factors such as prior herpes or condylomatous changes—this exam should occur *at least* annually. In patients with two successive negative smears and single sexual partners, intervals may safely be extended for up to 3 years.

26. **A** (1, 2, 3), Page 133. Aspects of the gynecologic history that place the patient at risk are factors relating to her chronic anovulation other than factors concerning her relatively short-term pharmacologic inhibition of ovulation or age alone in this example. Of course, more history is necessary, but as isolated fragments of information, oligomenorrhea and nulligravidity come to bear on the potential for problems with endometrial hyperplasia.

CHAPTER 6

Significant Symptoms and Signs in Different Age Groups

DIRECTIONS: For each numbered item, select the one heading most closely associated with it. Each lettered heading may be used once, more than once, or not at all.

(A) Malignant teratoma
(B) Serous cystadenocarcinoma
(C) Cystic teratoma
(D) Serous cystadenoma
(E) Granulosa cell tumor

1. Most common ovarian tumor in all age groups
2. Most common neoplasm of adolescence
3. Stromal cell tumor producing sex hormone

DIRECTIONS: For each numbered item, indicate whether it is associated with

A only (A)
B only (B)
C both (A) and (B)
D neither (A) nor (B)

(A) Menorrhagia
(B) Postmenopausal bleeding
(C) Both
(D) Neither

4. Adenocarcinoma of endometrium
5. Uterine myomata
6. Cervical cancer

(A) Molar pregnancy
(B) Twin pregnancy
(C) Both
(D) Neither

7. Size/dates discrepancy
8. Polyhydramnios
9. Quantitative HCG of greater than 110,000 MIU

(A) Chronic pelvic pain
(B) Retroversion of the uterus; nodularity of uterosacral ligaments
(C) Both
(D) Neither

10. Associated with abnormal findings at laparoscopy
11. Associated with dyspareunia

(A) Vaginal bleeding, positive HCG
(B) Missed period, positive HCG
(C) Both
(D) Neither

12. Formation of decidua in tubal pregnancy
13. Characteristic of unruptured tubal pregnancy
14. HCG stimulated production of progesterone by corpus luteum of pregnancy

(A) Uterine mass
(B) Adnexal mass
(C) Both
(D) Neither

15. Likely to be malignant when enlarging in the postmenopausal years
16. Commonly associated with ascites
17. Commonly associated with postmenopausal bleeding

(A) Perimenopausal dysfunctional bleeding
(B) Adolescent dysfunctional bleeding
(C) Both
(D) Neither

18. Associated with anovulation
19. Requires endometrial tissue evaluation
20. Caused by primary endometrial neoplasm

DIRECTIONS: Each question contains four suggested answers of which one or more is correct. Choose the answer

A if 1, 2, and 3 are correct
B if 1 and 3 are correct
C if 2 and 4 are correct
D if 4 only is correct
E if all are correct

21. Characteristics of dysfunctional uterine bleeding include
    1. perimenopausal age group.
    2. irregular menstrual interval.
    3. nonsecretory endometrium.
    4. postcoital bleeding.
22. Pain in an individual is
    1. unpleasant.
    2. subjective.
    3. emotional.
    4. quantifiable.

23. Causes of bleeding in the presence of human chorionic gonadotropin include
    1. tubal mole.
    2. incomplete spontaneous abortion.
    3. implantation bleeding.
    4. production of progesterone by the corpus luteum of pregnancy.
24. Mechanisms by which upper tract inflammatory changes contribute to abnormal vaginal bleeding include
    1. associated prostaglandin deficiency.
    2. the increase in capillary fragility.
    3. a deficiency of small vessel fibrinogen deposition.
    4. alteration in steroidogenesis from inflamed ovaries.
25. Characteristics of a missed abortion include
    1. size/discrepancy of the uterus.
    2. molar degeneration of the trophoblast.
    3. positive B-HCG determination.
    4. normal plasma progesterone determination for pregnancy.
26. Uterine leiomyomata
    1. are the most common bleeding source in postmenopausal women.
    2. are common in blacks.
    3. often progress to leimyosarcoma if untreated.
    4. may regress in size after menopause.
27. Most gynecologic processes presenting with acute abdominal pain
    1. have periumbilical origin.
    2. have rebound tenderness referable to the epigastrium.
    3. are associated with lower gastrointestinal symptoms.
    4. are most often limited to the pelvic peritoneum (right or left lower quadrants).
28. Risk factors increasing the likelihood of ectopic pregnancy include
    1. tubal reconstructive surgery.
    2. previous tubal pregnancy.
    3. previous gonococcal salpingitis.
    4. intrauterine contraceptive device.
29. Characteristics of patients with chronic pelvic pain include:
    1. A majority will have abnormal laparoscopic findings despite having "normal" pelvic exams.
    2. A high association with retrodisplacement of the uterus.
    3. A high percentage of positive laparoscopic findings in patients with complaints in the same areas for a minimum of 6 months.
    4. A predominance of patients with endogenous depressive disorders.

ANSWERS

1–3. 1, **D**; 2, **C**; 3, **E**; Pages 160–162; Tables 6-3, 6-4 (from Droegemueller). Bennington's cross-sectional study of a general gynecologic population revealed that serous cystadenoma is the most common true neoplasm of the ovary in all age groups combined. Of primary ovarian neoplasms seen in these age groups, serous cystadenocarcinoma is most often bilateral. In adolescents, cystic teratoma is most common and is important clinically because of the possibility of torsion or rupture.

The term *functioning*, when referring to true ovarian neoplasm, implies the production of a hormone, such as the production of estrogen from a granulosa cell tumor of the ovary, whereas the term *functional*, in reference to an ovarian cyst, implies a variant of normal reproductive ovarian anatomy.

4–6. 4, **B**; 5, **A**; 6, **B**; Pages 151–152; Table 6-1 (from Droegemueller). The occurrence of endometrial carcinoma is greatest in the postmenopausal age group and thus the usual bleeding manifestations of this tumor are not associated with true menstruation, but rather are manifested by irregular perimenopausal bleeding or postmenopausal bleeding. *Menorrhagia* is the occurrence of regular bleeding of greater than usual quantity for 10 days or more. *Metorrhagia* is the occurrence of significant intermenstrual bleeding one or more times.

7–9. 7, **C**; 8, **B**; 9, **A**; Pages 150–151. The rapidly enlarging uterus on clinical examination may be the result of multiple gestation or abnormal trophoblastic proliferation. Polyhydramnios may complicate multiple pregnancy but not gestational trophoblastic disease, whereas massively elevating HCG is the result of trophoblastic proliferation and not characteristic of otherwise normal multiple gestation.

10–11. 10, **A**; 11, **C**; Pages 157–158. Although a majority of patients with chronic pelvic pain may have associated abnormal findings at the time of laparoscopy, these findings represent nonspecific changes much of the time. Retrodisplacement of the uterus is a normal anatomic variant and, of itself, not a pathologic entity. When associated with infection or endometriosis, retroversion of the uterus may be associated with dyspareunia, as may be the case in the chronic pelvic pain patient. Neither entity, in itself, is associated with specific psychogenic origins.

12–14. 12, **C**; 13, **C**; 14, **B**; Page 150. Vaginal bleeding in tubal pregnancy is associated with decay of the decidualized endometrium as well as retrograde flow of blood from the fallopian tube. A missed menstrual period results from the early production of HCG, creating prolonged progestational support of the endometrium by the corpus luteum. An early unruptured tubal pregnancy will be associated with vaginal bleeding despite maintenance of viable trophoblast because of retrograde transport of blood through the tube.

15–17. 15, C; 16, B; 17, A; Page 163. Pelvic malignancy is to be suspected in either situation in the presence of an enlarging postmenopausal pelvic mass. Ascites is most often associated with epithelial cell malignant tumors of ovarian origin (serous cystadenocarcinoma) while uterine enlargements are more often associated with postmenopausal bleeding (adenocarcinoma of the endometrium).

18–20. 18, C; 19, A; 20, D; Page 151. Most dysfunctional uterine bleeding is anovulatory, regardless of age group. Because women over the age of 35 will have a greater likelihood of having endometrial atypia, it is mandatory to provide endometrial sampling in this group. When found, endometrial neoplasia removes the patient from the dysfunctional bleeding group by definition.

21. A (1, 2, 3), Page 151. Dysfunctional uterine bleeding implies irregular bleeding secondary to the lack of regular ovulation. This is most common at either end of the reproductive spectrum. Postcoital bleeding is more often associated with a cervical inflammatory or neoplastic lesion while consistent intermenstrual spotting is more often associated with hormonal changes associated with ovulation in the reproductive age group. The occasional patient with irregular intermenstrual bleeding may have a primary endometrial neoplasm, and this concern becomes more apparent in an older age group of patients.

22. A (1, 2, 3), Page 153. Pain, as a subjective response, cannot be quantified by external standards, and it is usually described as unpleasant, making pain an emotional experience. Pain is individualized through experience related to injury in early life. Thus, external standards cannot be used in an effort to quantify this sensory experience, even though studies attempt to do so.

23. A (1, 2, 3), Pages 148–149. Any condition associated with trophoblastic production of human chorionic gonadotropin may present with bleeding, including normal intrauterine pregnancy (implantation bleeding) and abnormal proliferation of gestational trophoblast. The corpus luteum of pregnancy nornormally secretes progesterone to help support an early gestation and, under normal conditions, it is not associated with bleeding in pregnancy.

24. C (2, 4), Pages 152–153. With severe inflammation of the upper genital tract, there can be endometrial inflammation with attendant small vessel and capillary oozing. Ovarian dysfunction may be encountered either because of severe inflammation altering steroid secretion or because of attendant lack of ovulation (progesterone production).

25. B (1, 3), Page 149. Missed abortion is generally associated with nonviable trophoblast without molar changes. The uterus is usually smaller than the gestational age and sensitive β-HCG testing will reflect low levels of this hormone. Although this entity is more common in pregnancies artificially supported by exogenous progesterone administration, endogenously secreted progesterone from the corpus luteum is at low levels for pregnancy.

26. C (2, 4), Page 162. Uterine leiomyomata are estimated to occur in as many as 40% of women by the age of 50 with a threefold higher occurrence in black women. They are only rarely (0.1% to 0.5%) associated with progression to malignant counterparts (leiomyosarcoma) and often will regress in size postmenopausally with diminishing amounts of endogenously produced estrogen.

27. D (4), Pages 154–155. Of the common acute gynecologic entities listed in Table 1, all share a common pattern of having right or left lower quadrant pain. Visceral pain from most gastrointestinal tract disorders is usually more specifically related to the part of the viscus involved, whereas urinary tract disease may present more diffuse pain, depending on the part of the tract involved.

28. A (1, 2, 3), Page 150. An antecedent problem that alters tubal physiology and/or anatomy contributes to an increase risk of ectopic gestation. Tubal distortion by infection or surgery is apparent. Increased risk incurred by IUD wearers is evident from the observation that, while protecting against *intrauterine* implantation of the trophoblast, the IUD does not prevent tubular implantation to the same extent.

TABLE 1 Conditions That May Cause Signs and Symptoms of Acute Abdomen and Abdominal Quadrants in Which They Most Often Occur

Condition	Right Upper	Right Lower	Left Upper	Left Lower
Salpingitis	−	+	−	+
Tubo–ovarian abscess	±	+	±	+
Ectopic pregnancy	−	+	−	+
Torsive adnexa	−	+	−	+
Ruptured ovarian cyst	−	+	−	+
Acute appendicitis	−	+	−	−
Mesenteric lymphadenitis	−	+	−	−
Crohn's disease	−	+	−	−
Acute cholecystitis	+	±	−	−
Perforated peptic ulcer	+	±	+	±
Acute pancreatitis	+	−	+	−
Acute pyelitis	+	±	+	±
Renal calculus	+	+	+	+
Splenic infarct	−	−	+	−
Splenic rupture	−	−	+	−
Acute diverticulitis	−	−	−	+

(From Droegemueller W, Herbst AL, Mishell DR, Steuchever MA: Comprehensive gynecology, St. Louis, 1987, C.V. Mosby Co.)

29. **B** (1, 3), Pages 156–158. In at least two large reviews, it has been shown that the occurrence of pelvic pain and abnormal laparoscopic findings are associated with "adhesions" and endometriosis heading the list of pathology. Most patients with retrodisplacement of the uterus do not have pain, as this finding exists in approximately 20% of women. While many chronic pelvic pain patients are experiencing stress, no specific cause and effect between chronic pelvic pain patients and organic depressive disorders has been shown.

CHAPTER 7

Counseling the Patient

DIRECTIONS: Select the one best answer or completion.

1. A 70-year-old male who has been married for 45 years is concerned because, since undergoing prostatic surgery, he is no longer capable of an erection. You should
   A. recommend estrogen for his wife.
   B. recommend a penile prosthesis.
   C. tell him that he should not be worried about this at his age.
   D. refer him for sexual counseling.
   E. none of the above.

2. A 21-year-old has been referred by her family physician who was unable to obtain a pap smear. Although the patient's history is entirely normal, she requests that you try to obtain the pap smear. The patient has been married for 2 years. You find that you are unable to insert a speculum; in fact, when you approach her, her levator muscles contract and she slides away from you on the examining table.
   From this information you can conclude that this woman
   A. has a phobic avoidance to the insertion of the speculum.
   B. has an unhappy marriage.
   C. has a vaginal septum or intact hymen.
   D. will never respond adequately to sexual stimulation.
   E. has never had intercourse.

3. Acceptance of the inevitability of death proceeds in the following stages:
   A. Denial
      Anger
      Bargaining
      Depression
      Acceptance
   B. Denial
      Bargaining
      Anger
      Depression
      Acceptance
   C. Denial
      Depression
      Anger
      Bargaining
      Acceptance
   D. Anger
      Denial
      Bargaining
      Depression
      Acceptance
   E. Anger
      Denial
      Depression
      Bargaining
      Acceptance

4. The G-spot
   A. is analogous to the seminal vesicle in a male.
   B. is another name for the clitoris.
   C. becomes exquisitely tender during sexual intercourse.
   D. may be stimulated to the point of ejaculation of fluid during orgasm.
   E. as the only source of orgasm indicates the individual has infantile sexuality, according to Freudian psychology.

DIRECTIONS: For each numbered item, select the one heading most closely associated with it. Each lettered heading may be used once, more than once, or not at all.

TABLE 2 Height and Weight Table for Women

Height		Weight in Pounds		
Feet	Inches	Small Frame	Medium Frame	Large Frame
4	10	102–111	109–121	118–131
4	11	103–113	111–123	120–134
5	0	104–115	113–126	122–137
5	1	106–118	115–129	125–140
5	2	108–121	118–132	128–143
5	3	111–124	121–135	131–147
5	4	114–127	124–138	134–151
5	5	117–130	127–141	137–155
5	6	120–133	130–144	140–159
5	7	123–136	133–147	143–163
5	8	126–139	136–150	146–167
5	9	129–142	139–153	149–170
5	10	132–145	142–156	152–173
5	11	135–148	145–159	155–176
6	0	138–151	148–162	158–179

A large-boned 27-year-old is overweight. You recommend dieting. In addition, you would suggest

(A) Weight Watchers
(B) Medically supervised behavior modification
(C) Pharmacologic therapy
(D) Gastric restriction operation
(E) None of the above

5. If she is 5 feet 9 inches tall and weighs 255 pounds
6. If she is 5 feet 0 inches tall and weighs 275 pounds
7. If she is 5 feet 11 inches tall and weighs 238 pounds

DIRECTIONS: For each numbered item, indicate whether it is associated with
A only (A)
B only (B)
C both (A) and (B)
D neither (A) nor (B)

Phases of Female Human Sexual Response
(A) Excitement
(B) Orgasm
(C) Both
(D) Neither

8. Can be affected by antihypertensive medication
9. Response due to stimulation of the parasympathetic nervous system
10. Development of the orgasmic platform

DIRECTIONS: Each question contains four suggested answers of which one or more is correct. Choose the answer
A if 1, 2, and 3 are correct
B if 1 and 3 are correct
C if 2 and 4 are correct
D if 4 only is correct
E if all are correct

11. A 25-year-old gravida 3, para 0, abortus 3 factory worker is seen 6 weeks postdelivery. Her last pregnancy ended at 20 weeks, and you feel that she has an incompetent cervix. Today she has multiple complaints, including tightness in the throat and chest, frequent sighing, and muscle weakness. You attribute this to a grief reaction. The patient continued to work during this last pregnancy despite your warning that this activity might lead to another pregnancy loss. Appropriate comments at this encounter include
    1. telling her that next time she must not only have surgery but also stop working.
    2. referring her to a self-help group.
    3. mentioning that she is still young and will have another chance.
    4. acknowledging her feelings of grief.
12. Organic problems associated with dyspareunia include
    1. urethritis.
    2. cystitis.
    3. trigonitis.
    4. endometriosis.
13. A young person has been picked up repeatedly for shoplifting. This individual has been seen by a police psychiatrist and you are told he has very antisocial behavior. The family history includes death of a parent by suicide following long-standing marital discord. Factors that often contribute to this outcome include:
    1. The parent died before this boy was 5 years old.
    2. The young person is an adolescent.
    3. The surviving parent is his mother.
    4. The surviving parent has remarried.
14. A woman on oral contraception who is anorgasmic during coitus should
    1. be allowed to masturbate during foreplay.
    2. use another form of contraception.
    3. discuss this with her husband.
    4. feel very abnormal.

15. Services included in a hospital-based hospice program are
    1. social work.
    2. postdeath follow-up.
    3. home care.
    4. support for ICU patients.
16. The amounts of alcohol are approximately the same in:
    1. 12 ounces of beer
    2. a wine glass of wine
    3. 30 ml of whiskey
    4. 30 ml of a liqueur
17. Childhood self-esteem is enhanced by
    1. praising.
    2. setting limits.
    3. touching.
    4. intimidation.

Questions 18, 19, and 20

18. A 15-year-old states that she began her menses at age 11 and that during her 13th year she had a regular 26 to 30-day cycle. She has not had a period in the last 6 months, and she has never had intercourse. The medical history is unremarkable except that she feels that she is 20 pounds overweight.

    Physical Examination
    BP: 100/70   T: 97.8   P: 55
    Ht: 5 ft 4 inches   Wt: 105 lbs
    Breast: Tanner Stage IV
    Abdomen: Unremarkable
    Pelvic:
    Escutcheon: Tanner Stage IV
    Outlet: Unremarkable
    Cervix: Unremarkable
    Corpus: Normal size, smooth, firm
    Adnexa: Unremarkable

    Given the most likely diagnosis, you would expect that she
    1. abuses laxatives.
    2. has an increased likelihood of having a relative with the same problem.
    3. vomits frequently.
    4. is an average student.
19. Several different approaches to the treatment of this young girl have met with success. These options include
    1. pergonal.
    2. insulin.
    3. psychoanalysis.
    4. cognitive therapy.
20. In discussing the prognosis of this patient with the family, you should mention that
    1. more than 50% recover completely.
    2. the mortality rate in those that do not respond is 3–18%
    3. there is a significant recurrence rate (>1%).
    4. there is an increased possibility of suicide.

Questions 21 and 22

21. A 35-year-old stockbroker was to be married for the first time 6 months ago, but her fiance was killed in an auto accident on the way to the church. When she saw your partner a week ago, your partner decided that she was severely depressed and prescribed an amitriptyline. She returns with a list of new symptoms, listed below. These symptoms are frightening to her, but they do not prevent her from functioning as a normal human being. Those that are secondary to the medication and not her basic problem include:
    1. a dry mouth.
    2. blurred vision.
    3. constipation.
    4. hesitancy of urination.
22. In addition to these symptoms, the woman is still depressed. You would now
    1. switch her to intramuscular administration.
    2. tell her to take a glass of wine at bedtime.
    3. add another antidepressive medication.
    4. offer her reassurance.

ANSWERS

1. **E**, Page 177. None of the answers is correct without more information. The next step is to discuss his concern with his wife. The patient and his wife need to decide how much of a problem his lack of an erection is. His concern may be that he can no longer satisfy his wife. A physician can be useful in helping a couple sort out their needs and desire for sexual compatibility at this stage of life.
2. **A**, Page 178. The question describes a woman who, according to Lamont's classification, has fourth-degree vaginismus, levator and perineal spasm, and retreat. This problem is generally based on a phobia to vaginal penetration based on a previous traumatic episode or a lack of appropriate learning about sex secondary to cultural or familial teaching that sex is evil, painful, or undesirable. Sexual dysfunction is not necessarily incompatible with a happy marriage. This couple could be very happy. The history did not suggest amenorrhea, so a septum or an intact hymen was ruled out. Treatment for this problem has a high success rate. Thus, one cannot assert that the woman will have an unhappy sex life. One cannot assert that she has never had intercourse. Traumatic intercourse, especially rape, could have been a precipitating factor.

3. **A**, Pages 186–187. The stages as suggested by Kübler-Ross are denial, anger, bargaining, depression, and acceptance. Unfortunately, many people die before all of these stages have been reconciled.
4. **D**, Pages 168, 176. The G-spot is an area on the anterior vaginal wall beneath the urethra believed to be analogous to the male prostate gland. During sexual arousal, it may be stimulated to the point of orgasm with ejaculation of fluid into the urethra. It was not mentioned by Freud, who felt that clitoral orgasm represented the hallmark of infantile sexuality.
5–7. 5, **B**; 6, **D**; 7, **A**; Pages 173–174, Table 2. All three patients have a large frame. Patient 5 is 50% overweight and therefore moderately obese. Patient 6 is 100% overweight and therefore severely obese. Patient 7 is 35% overweight or mildly obese. Mild obesity can be successfully managed by diet and behavior modification under lay supervision, whereas moderate obesity is best managed under medical supervision. Good results have been obtained in the severely obese who have had a gastric restriction operation. Additional studies are needed to verify good long-term results.
8–10. 8, **B**; 9, **A**; 10, **D**; Pages 175–176. The sympathetic portion of the autonomic nervous system influences the orgasmic phase. Medications, including the antihypertensive drugs reserpine and clonidine, may affect orgasmic response. Much of the response in the excitement phase is due to stimulation of the parasympathetic fibers of the autonomic nervous system. The plateau stage is associated with a marked degree of vasocongestion. This vasocongestion is marked in the lower third of the vagina and is known as the orgasmic platform.
11. **C** (2, 4), Pages 182–183. In the immediate grief period, the bereaved often feels guilt. Although you should acknowledge her shock, guilt, and grief, you should not add to it. It is counterproductive to talk to her about working during her recent pregnancy. Self-help groups have a great deal to offer patients who suffer a pregnancy loss. If the local group is appropriate for the needs of a given patient, a referral should be made. One investigator has found that grieving couples prefer to receive support and help in dealing with the reality of the loss rather than focus on other life events, such as the next pregnancy.
12. **E** (All), Page 178. Organic causes of dyspareunia include poor lubrication, urethritis, cystitis, trigonitis, a poorly healed vaginal laceration or episiotomy, pelvic inflammatory disease, and endometriosis.
13. **A** (1, 2, 3), Page 169–170. A serious threat to normal emotional development in childhood is the loss of a parent. The time period between the loss of a parent and the onset of the disorder is often quite long. The risk of developing a psychiatric disorder seems greatest if the child is under 5 years of age or an adolescent and if the child loses a parent of the same sex. Males seem more susceptible to the loss of a father than the loss of a mother. Delinquency is less likely to occur if there is a father substitute, a step-father, grandfather, or big brother, and more likely to occur with marital discord.
14. **B** (1, 3), Page 178. Couples should be encouraged to communicate their sexual needs to each other so that appropriate stimulation is offered during the arousal period and during intercourse. If the patient is anorgasmic during intercourse but has experienced orgasms, her partner may aid in bringing about an orgasm during intercourse by allowing her to stimulate her clitoral area or he may do so. Anorgasmia is not known to be secondary to oral contraceptive use. Furthermore, she would have to use a barrier method of contraception. As many as 10–15% of women have never experienced an orgasm through any form of sexual stimulation. The woman should not be made to feel abnormal. Sexuality is a question of pleasure or happiness, not of normalcy.
15. **E** (All), Page 187. Hospice organizations offer psychosocial support to patients and their families. The service includes postdeath follow-up. Hospital-based hospice teams may include physicians, nurses, social workers, chaplains, and volunteers who may minister to any patient in any bed. Home care programs are often available.
16. **E** (All), Page 179. Alcoholic strength is often denoted by the percent of alcohol present. Proof is twice the percent volume of alcohol. A 12 ounce can of beer, a glass of wine, and 30 ml of either whiskey or a liqueur have the same quantity of alcohol.
17. **A** (1, 2, 3), Page 169. Self-esteem begins to develop in early childhood and is the result of positive efforts. Touching, talking to the child in gentle ways, and praising the child's actions are reasonable steps in reinforcing the child's self-worth. Punishment should be limited to reinforcing the need for setting limits. Intimidation by verbal or physical means should be avoided.
18. **A** (1, 2, 3), Page 171. The occurrence of anorexia and bulimia is six times greater in first-degree relatives than in the general population. Vomiting and laxative abuse are common findings. These patients tend to be high achievers, usually A students.
19. **D** (4), Page 172. A number of medications have been tried in the treatment of anorexia nervosa with varying success. These medications have included insulin, lithium, tricyclics, and phenothiazides as well as high potency vitamins. In many cases they have not been found to be better than a placebo. Psychoanalysis is a long-term approach and anorexia nervosa requires

prompt intervention. Behavior modification and cognitive therapy have met with some success. Behavior modification is based on reward and punishment for a number of behaviors. Cognitive therapy is directed toward the specific thinking disorder rather than body image and food.

20. **E** (All), Page 172. Good to fair outcome has been observed in 88% of the anorexia nervosa patients treated as inpatients and 77% treated as outpatients. The mortality rate has been reported as high as 18% and the recurrence rate as high as 3%. Mortality is the result not only of starvation, but also of suicide.

21. **E** (All), Page 181. Most tricyclic drugs, including amitriptyline, have a parasympathomimetic effect. Dryness of the mouth, blurred vision, hesitancy of urination or dribbling, some menstrual disorders, and a decrease in sexual arousal are often complaints associated with their use.

22. **D** (4), Page 181. Although patients may note reduction of symptoms of depression after 1 or 2 weeks of drug use, real improvement may take as long as 1 month. It is unnecessary to add a second drug or switch to intramuscular medication at this time. A tricyclic may enhance the response to alcohol. This can increase the danger of a suicide attempt or overdosage. It would be best to reassure this patient and tell her it is too soon to expect improvement.

CHAPTER 8
Diagnostic Procedures

DIRECTIONS: Select the one best answer or completion.

1. A 22-year-old, 5 feet 6 inch, 125 lb., gravida 0 says that her last normal menstrual period was 8 weeks ago. Two hours ago she had the acute onset of severe RLQ pain. Two days ago she did notice vaginal spotting.
   On examination, the BP is found to be 90/60 and the pulse 110. The abdomen appears distended. Bowel sounds are not heard. A pelvic examination is difficult to interpret because the patient is so tender that she does not allow a reasonable evaluation. Your next step would be a
   A. β-HCG.
   B. pelvic ultrasound.
   C. culdocentesis.
   D. laparoscopic examination.
   E. laparotomy.

2. The optimal pressure in mm Hg for performing an adequate endometrial aspiration for an elective termination is
   A. 100–200.
   B. 201–300.
   C. 301–400.
   D. 401–500.
   E. 501–600.

3. On examination a patient has moderately severe cervical stenosis. She is about to have an endometrial biopsy as a part of an infertility investigation. The anesthesia of choice is a
   A. pudendal.
   B. paracervical.
   C. epidural.
   D. spinal.
   E. general.

4. The complications associated with hysteroscopy when the distending media is 5% dextrose and water include all of the following **EXCEPT**
   A. uterine perforation.
   B. bleeding.
   C. pelvic infection.
   D. circulatory overload.
   E. anaphylaxis.

5. The successful reversal of a previous sterilization procedure is most likely to follow a
   A. Pomeroy tubal ligation.
   B. Irving tubal ligation.
   C. laparoscopic tubal fulguration.
   D. laparoscopic tubal application of Silastic bands.
   E. laparoscopic tubal application of Hulka clips.

6. All of the following are recognized procedures performed through a laparoscope **EXCEPT**
   A. evaluation of a 25 cm intra-abdominal mass.
   B. laser ablation of an endometrial implant.
   C. ovarian biopsy for karyotype.
   D. lysis of adhesions.
   E. evacuation of a small ectopic pregnancy.

7. Ultrasound is useful in all of the following **EXCEPT**
   A. determining when to give HCG in ovulation induction.
   B. assisting in the laparoscopic egg retrieval process.
   C. assisting in the transvesical egg retrieval process.
   D. documenting when ovulation has occurred.
   E. preventing the hyperstimulation syndrome.

8. An infertility patient has a history of a 28-day cycle. She has an endometrial biopsy performed as part of the investigation 6 days after her basal body chart temperature rises. The narrative of the report states that one strip of endometrium is day 19 and the other proliferative. You conclude that the patient has
   A. a luteal phase defect.
   B. irregular shedding.
   C. a normal ovulatory response.
   D. an abnormal ovulatory response.
   E. an uninterpretable result resulting from a lab error.

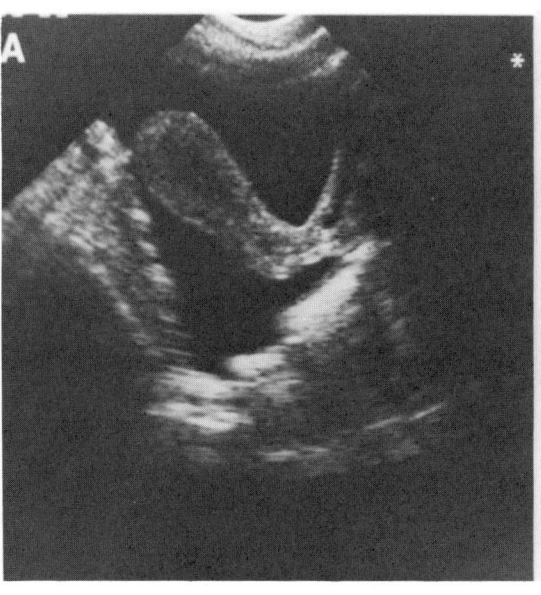

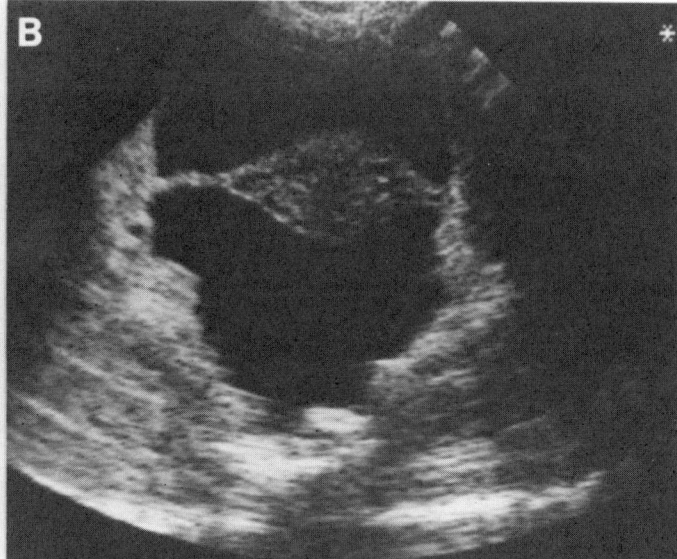

FIGURE 8-1.
(A) Longitudinal view of the pelvis. (B) Transverse view of the pelvis.

9. The patient depicted in Figure 8-1 was referred for pelvic ultrasound because of increasing girth. The diagnosis is
   A. an early intrauterine pregnancy.
   B. a molar pregnancy.
   C. a ruptured tubal pregnancy.
   D. ascites.
   E. ovarian carcinoma.

10. A 48-year-old woman who had an endometrial biopsy 6 months ago returns for a scheduled visit. The pathology report indicates a proliferative endometrium. Since her biopsy, this patient has bled every 2 weeks for 8–12 days. She uses 10–15 pads a day, but states this is not a problem. You advise
    A. a repeat visit in 6 months.
    B. an endometrial biopsy.
    C. endometrial cytological sampling.
    D. a dilation and curettage.
    E. a hysterectomy.

11. All of the following are recognized indications for hysteroscopy **EXCEPT**
    A. infertility.
    B. suspicion of uterine synechiae.
    C. repetitive abortions.
    D. irregular vaginal bleeding.
    E. oligomenorrhea.

12. The failure rate of laparoscopic tubal interruption procedures is around
    A. < 1/1000
    B. 1/1000
    C. 3/1000
    D. 6/1000
    E. > 6/1000

13. Which of the following modalities utilizes beam attenuation that results from different densities in adjacent tissues?
    A. Ultrasonography
    B. Magnetic resonance imaging
    C. Computed tomography
    D. Scintillation scan
    E. Tomography

14. The patient is a 22-year-old gravida 0. Until 9 weeks ago she was taking a low dose oral contraceptive. Since she stopped her oral contraceptive, she has not menstruated. Today, she developed RLQ pelvic pain of one day's duration, and you ordered the sonogram depicted in Figure 8-2. A β subunit HCG is positive. Vital signs are normal and stable.

    Proper management includes
    A. a quantitiative HCG.
    B. hysterosalpingogram.
    C. a repeat ultrasound in 48 hours.
    D. culdocentesis.
    E. an endometrial biopsy.

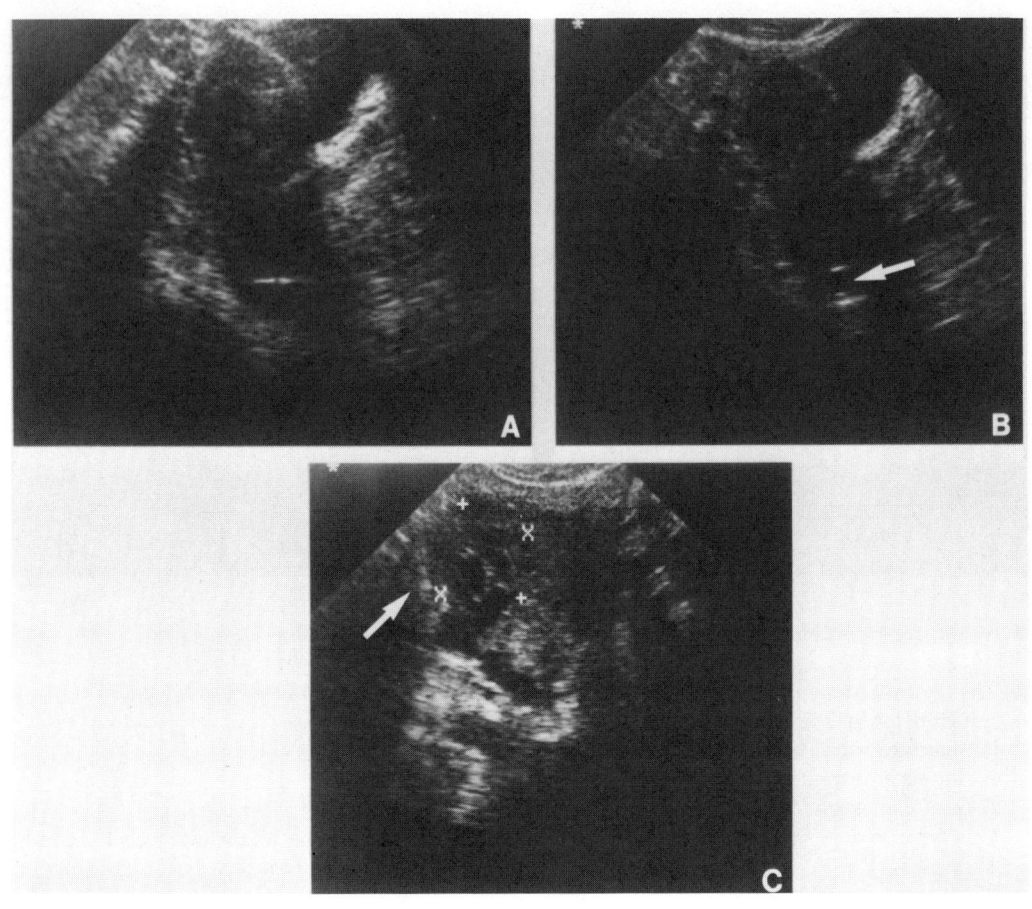

FIGURE 8-2.
(A) Longitudinal view to the left of midline. (B) Midline longitudinal view. (C) Longitudinal view to the right of midline.

DIRECTIONS: For each numbered item, select the one heading most closely associated with it. Each lettered heading may be used once, more than once, or not at all.

A woman who has had severe PID is eventually found to have a ruptured tubal pregnancy with 300 ml of blood in the peritoneal cavity.

Match the culdocentesis results:
- (A) 5 ml clotted blood, hematocrit 30%
- (B) 5 ml unclotted blood, hematocrit 17%
- (C) 5 ml unclotted blood, hematocrit 9%
- (D) 5 ml serosanguineous fluid, hematocrit 7%
- (E) No fluid after several attempts

15. Extensive adhesions in the cul-de-sac
16. True positive
17. Improper technique

Pick the procedure that is most useful in making the diagnosis:
- (A) Hysteroscopy with or without biopsy
- (B) Hysterosalpingogram
- (C) Dilation and curettage
- (D) Laparoscopy
- (E) Pelvic ultrasound

18. A submucous myoma
19. Peritubal adhesions
20. A tubal pregnancy

Assume that your hospital is capable of supporting all the procedures listed below. Choose the appropriate initial procedure after a complete history and physical:
- (A) Hysteroscopy
- (B) Laparoscopy
- (C) Computed tomography
- (D) Pelvic ultrasound
- (E) Magnetic resonance imaging

21. A 28-year-old gravida 0 who is 5 feet 6 inches tall and weighs 134 pounds has been trying to get pregnant for 3 years. Her husband has a normal semen analysis. She ovulates and has good midcycle mucus.
22. A 30-year-old mentally retarded gravida 0 who is 5 feet 1 inches tall and weighs 190 pounds complains of pelvic pain and is impossible to examine.

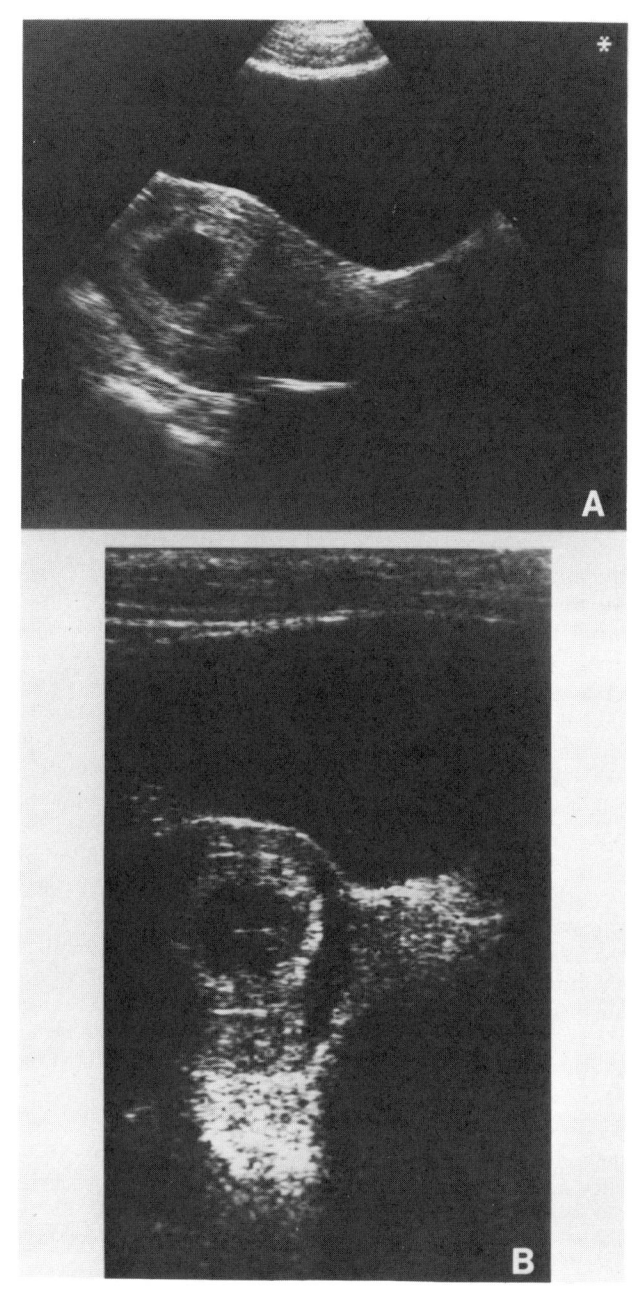

FIGURE 8-3

23. A 25-year-old gravida 2, para 1 ab 1, had an induced abortion 1 year ago. Since then she has had amenorrhea and intermittent pelvic pain.
24. A 30-year-old gravida 6, para 6 who is 5 feet 6 inches tall and weighs 130 pounds has a 5 cm cervical lesion. This is histologically a squamous cell carcinoma.

DIRECTIONS: For each numbered item, indicate whether it is associated with

A only (A)
B only (B)
C both (A) and (B)
D neither (A) nor (B)

    (A) Sonogram labeled A in Figure 8-3
    (B) Sonogram labeled B in Figure 8-3
    (C) Both sonograms
    (D) Neither sonogram

25. Linear array
26. Employs the piezoelectric effect
27. The transducer transmits 60% of the time and receives 40% of the time

DIRECTIONS: Each question contains four suggested answers of which one or more is correct. Choose the answer

A if 1, 2, and 3 are correct
B if 1 and 3 are correct
C if 2 and 4 are correct
D if 4 only is correct
E if all are correct

28. An endometrial biopsy is useful in the diagnosis of all of the following **EXCEPT**
    1. pelvic tuberculosis.
    2. luteal phase defect.
    3. adenomatous endometrial hyperplasia.
    4. adenomyosis.
29. Major complications attributed to laparoscopy include
    1. cardiac arrhythmias.
    2. gas embolism.
    3. laceration of the epigastric artery.
    4. intestinal perforation.
30. M.S. is a 25-year-old gravida 0. She has been trying to conceive for 5 years. Her past history includes menses every 28–30 days and flow for 3 days with moderate dysmenorrhea the first 2 days. She had an acute pelvic infection at age 22 for which she had to be hospitalized. She has not had a clinical recurrence or reinfection. Her gall bladder was removed at 20 for stones. She is allergic to shell fish. She smokes one pack of cigarettes a day and is a social drinker. Her physical examination, including a pelvic examination, is normal.

    This patient's investigation should include a(n)
    1. endometrial biopsy.
    2. pelvic ultrasound.
    3. chromopertubation at laparoscopy.
    4. hysterosalpingogram.
31. Complications following an endometrial biopsy include
    1. heavy bleeding.
    2. infection.
    3. perforation.
    4. hypotension.
32. Hysterosalpingography is useful in the diagnosis of
    1. an incompetent cervix.
    2. intermenstrual spotting (metrorrhagia).
    3. peritubal adhesions.
    4. acute endometritis.
33. Hysterosalpingography is useful in the diagnosis of
    1. submucous myoma.
    2. Asherman's syndrome (endometrial sclerosis).
    3. müllerian anomalies.
    4. accessory ostia of the fallopian tubes.
34. Procedures that can be performed through a hysteroscope include
    1. removal of a fragmented IUD.
    2. removal of a submucous myoma.
    3. laser ablation of the endometrium.
    4. cannulation of the ostia of the fallopian tubes.
35. Figure 8-4 is a CT scan of a patient who on exam is felt to have a pelvic mass. One is able to say that
    1. the bladder is markedly displaced by a large uterus.
    2. there are metastases.
    3. the patient is under 20 years of age.
    4. the mass is thin walled.
36. The patient pictured in Figure 8-5 is 25 years old and wishes to have children. You would recommend
    1. resection.
    2. insertion of a Foley catheter.
    3. premarin 7.5 mg per day.
    4. transabdominal metroplasty.
37. True statements about magnetic resonance imaging include:
    1. It utilizes nonionizing radiation.
    2. It penetrates air and bone.
    3. It can differentiate between normal and malignant tissue.
    4. Tomographic images are possible in coronal, sagittal, or transverse planes.
38. A 1984 Consensus Conference issued a *Statement of Caution* in the use of diagnostic ultrasound despite 20 years of clinical use with **NO** known adverse effects. The rationale was based on in vitro studies that demonstrated
    1. an increase in the immune response.
    2. changes in sister chromatid exchange frequency.
    3. formation of new macromolecules.
    4. cell death.
39. True statements about computed tomography include:
    1. The radiation dose to the midpelvis is 50% of the surface dose.
    2. It is useful in confirming the diagnosis of ovarian thrombophlebitis.
    3. The radiation dose is similar to a barium enema.
    4. It is more accurate in diagnosing intraperitoneal rather than retroperitoneal metastases.

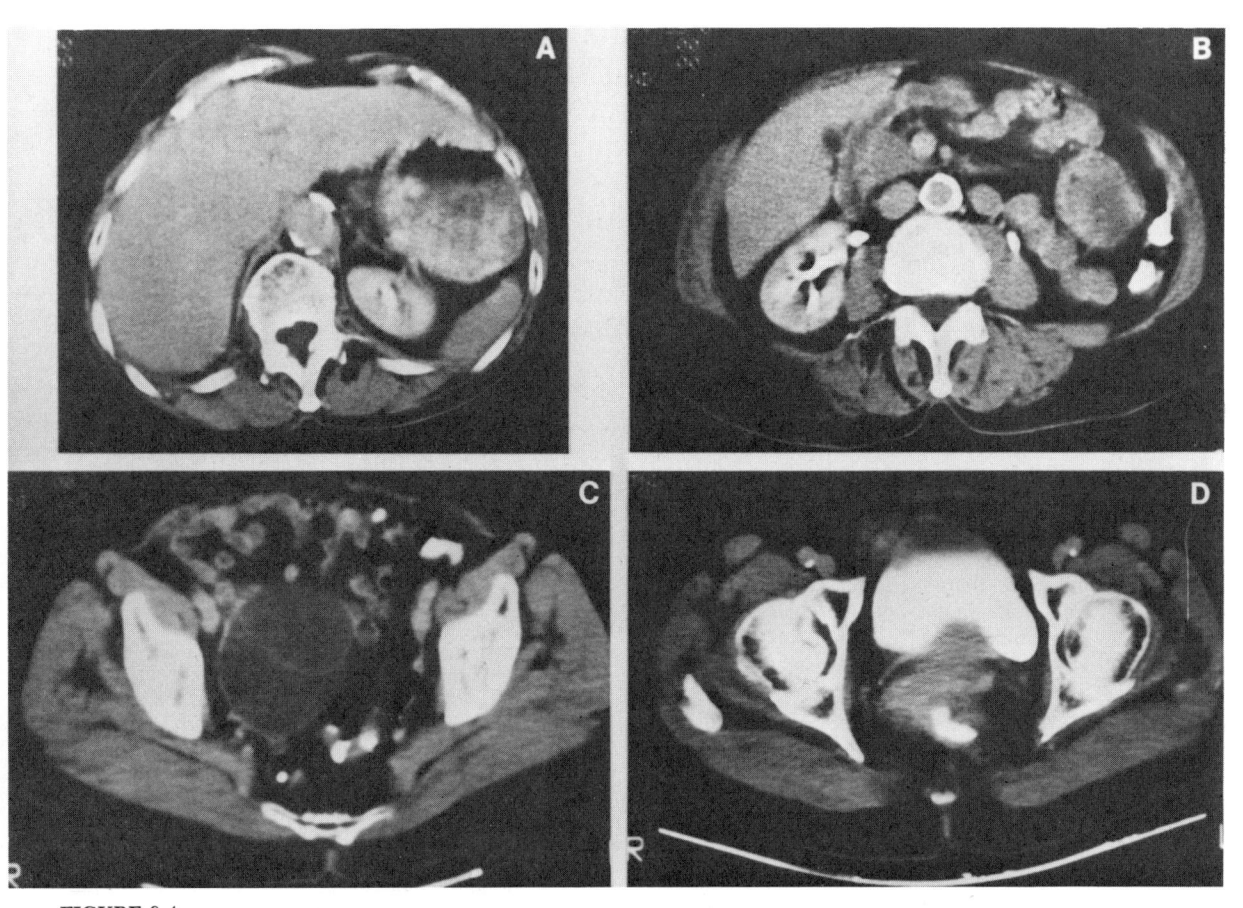

FIGURE 8-4.
(A) Computed tomography scan. (A), at the level of the liver; (B), below A; (C), above D; (D), at the level of the bladder.

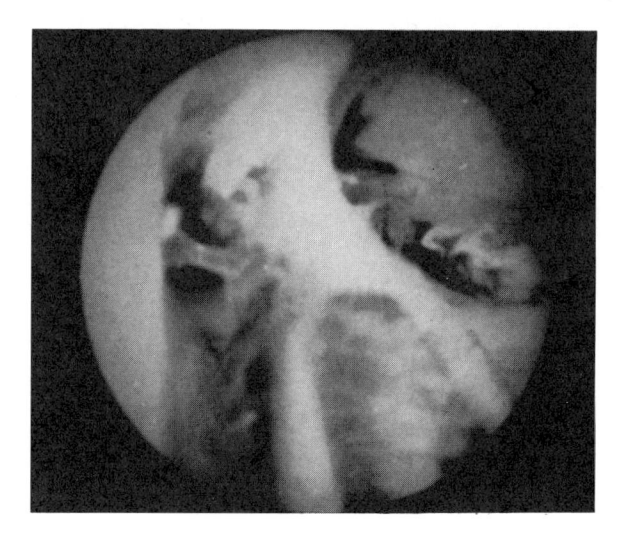

FIGURE 8-5.

Hysteroscopic view

(From Droegemueller W, Herbst AL, Mishell DR, Stenchever MA: Comprehensive Gynecology, St. Louis, 1987, The C. V. Mosby Co., p. 216.)

40. Endometrial cytological sampling
    1. is impractical for mass screening.
    2. should be placed in formalin.
    3. can not be performed in women over 70 years of age.
    4. has a false negative rate of 5% to 15%.
41. The use of high molecular weight dextran to expand the endometrial cavity during hysteroscopy is preferred because it is
    1. Nontoxic.
    2. Nonantigenic.
    3. Nonconductive.
    4. Miscible with blood.

ANSWERS

1. **C**, page 204–205. This patient is acutely ill. There is not time to get a β-HCG. Besides, a positive test won't differentiate an intrauterine from an extrauterine pregnancy. Likewise, there is no time for ultrasound. The patient might not have a full bladder. It might be nondiagnostic. Although invasive, a culdocentesis is likely to be helpful and it is inexpensive. A laparoscopy would be unnecessary, even contraindicated in the presence of a positive culdocentesis. It might be indicated if the culdocentesis were negative. A laparotomy is not in order until there is more evidence that the patient has a surgical abdomen.

2. **E**, Page 208. To denude the endometrium completely, the optimum pressure for aspiration is 500 to 600 mm Hg.

3. **B**, Page 207. An endometrial biopsy is usually performed without any anesthesia. In the presence of cervical stenosis, a paracervical will block transmission from fibers in the cervical ganglion.

4. **E**, Page 218. Complications of hysteroscopy include uterine perforation, pelvic infection, and bleeding. The potential complications of the distending media include circulatory overload with 5% dextrose and water. Anaphylaxis is a complication associated with the use of dextran.

5. **E**, Page 219. The spring-loaded clip causes necrosis of less than 1 cm of the tube and is the easiest sterilization procedure to reverse successfully.

6. **A**, Pages 222–224. An absolute contraindication to laparoscopy is a large intraperitoneal or pelvic mass. Laser ablation of an endometrial implant, ovarian biopsy, lysis of adhesions, and evacuation of a small ectopic pregnancy are recognized therapeutic laparoscopic procedures. Laser ablation may be a relative contraindication since there are reports of pulmonary problems occurring in the physician performing the procedures. This is believed to be the result of breathing the vapor, which may contain particles of carbon.

7. **B**, Page 195. When a dominant follicle has reached a size of 18 to 20 mm, one can give HCG to induce ovulation. Since the ovary is visible at laparoscopy, ultrasound would offer little or nothing to egg retrieval via the laparoscope. On the other hand, eggs have been successfully retrieved using a percutaneous transvesical, transurethral transvesical, or transvaginal approach under direct ultrasonic guidance. If the dominant mature follicle, seen a day or two prior, disappears, it is good presumptive evidence that ovulation has occurred. In most cases, the hyperstimulation syndrome can be avoided in non invitro fertilization patients if HCG is withheld when multiple follicles have reached a critical size, i.e., 16 mm or greater.

8. **C**, Page 207. The endometrium of the isthmus may be out of phase and give a false impression of lack of progesterone production. The description is that of a normal ovulatory response. If there is a luteal phase defect, the endometrium should be more than 48 hours less than the 20 days expected given in this patient's menstrual history. It should be noted, however, when doing an endometrial biopsy as a part of an infertility investigation, one should perform the biopsy later in the cycle in order to be in a position to make the diagnosis of a luteal phase defect. Irregular shedding should be diagnosed on the fifth or sixth day of bleeding.

9. **D**, Pages 194–196. Water, urine, and ascitic fluid are all extremely echolucent. Blood is usually more complex. In the longitudinal view there is no evidence of a gestational sac, blood, or tissue inside of the uterus. The ovaries are not seen in the transverse view. There is no mass in the pelvis. This is a woman with ascites due to cirrhosis.

10. **D**, Page 208. The diagnostic accuracy of endometrial biopsy is 90% to 98% when compared to subsequent findings at dilation and curettage or at hysterectomy. The gold standard is dilation and curettage. Therefore, if abnormal perimenopausal bleeding recurs following an endometrial biopsy, a dilation and curettage should be performed to rule out carcinoma.

11. **E**, Pages 214, 225. Indications for hysteroscopy include recurrent abnormal bleeding, repetitive abortion, uterine synechiae, abnormal hysterosalpingograms, and infertility. A patient with oligomenorrhea probably has a recycling problem that would not be diagnosed by hysteroscopy. Furthermore, the procedure should not be done if there is any chance of an existing intrauterine pregnancy.

12. **C**, Page 219. The failure rate of laparoscopic tubal sterilization is approximately 1 in 250 to 1 in 500 cases.
13. **C**, Page 197. Sonography utilizes sound waves that are reflected from interfaces back to the transducer.

    Magnetic resonance imaging uses radiofrequency radiation and a varying magnetic field.

    Prior to a scintillation scan, a radioisotope is injected. The liquid or crystal radiation detector "records" the X or gamma rays emitted from the subject.

    To perform tomography, objects out of the plane of interest are blurred during an x-ray study by simultaneously moving the x-ray tube and the recording plate.
14. **D**, Pages 194, 205. In this sonogram the arrow in Figure 8-2 (B) points to fluid in the cul-de-sac. The arrow in Figure 8-2 (C) and the pluses and Xs outline an adnexal mass. With an intrauterine pregnancy, a gestational sac should be present at 7 weeks. The cul-de-sac fluid suggests rupture. Thus, one should not delay in performing either a quantitative HCG or another ultrasound. One could go directly to laparoscopy, or do a culdocentesis first. The latter is most likely to be positive. If so, one would go directly to laparotomy rather than laparoscopy.
15–17. 15, **E**; 16, **B**; 17, **A**; Page 205. It is conceivable that in this patient who had a history of severe PID the cul-de-sac was obliterated and thus no fluid obtained. The diagnosis of a hemoperitoneum is made when 5 ml of unclotted blood with a hematocrit of > 15% is withdrawn. If the blood clots, usually a pelvic vein rather than the cul-de-sac has been aspirated.
18–20. 18, **A**; Page 216; 19, **D**; Page 211; 20, **D**; Pages 219, 423. Hysteroscopy is superior to hysterosalpingography in discovering and diagnosing intrauterine pathology. Comparative studies have documented that hysterosalpingography discovers only 50% of the peritubal disease diagnosed by direct visualization via the laparoscope. A pelvic ultrasound is often not diagnostic in the presence of a tubal pregnancy, although with a vaginal transducer tubal pathology can be seen more often. The question did not ask about the first procedure to be used but asked for the "most useful" procedure.
21. **B**, Page 218. In this hypothetical infertility patient, the male factor and cervical factor would appear to be normal. The patient is said to ovulate. As yet the tubal factor has not been evaluated. This could be done with a hysterosalpingogram or by laparoscopy. Authorities differ in approach. Another option that was not given was an endometrial biopsy to evaluate the luteal phase.
22. **D**, Page 195. The patient is a poor historian. She will not permit a pelvic examination. The least expensive, least invasive procedure possible should be attempted first. This young patient may or may not have pathology. In all likelihood she is difficult or impossible to examine. An ultrasound may demonstrate pathology. If there is pathology, a specific diagnosis may only be possible if a more invasive procedure is utilized. If no pathology is found, the best course to follow is observation, providing the history given above is complete and accurate. Another consideration is an examination under anesthesia if the ultrasound is negative.
23. **A**, Pages 214–215. It is likely that this patient developed intrauterine synechiae (Asherman's syndrome) following the therapeutic abortion. The intermittent pain that she has could be dysmenorrhea.
24. **C**, Page 200. This was a patient with cervical carcinoma. Often a CT scan will help in the initial evaluation of a pelvic neoplasm, particularly staging. This is not a standard protocol, although it is endorsed in some institutions.
25–27. 25, **B**; 26, **C**; 27, **D**; Pages 194–195. (Taylor KJW and Dyson, M.: Experimental insonation of animal tissues and fetuses. In Sanders, RC and James AE (eds.): The principles and practice of ultrasonography in obstetrics and gynecology, ed. 2, New York, 1980, Appleton-Century-Crofts, p. 15.) The picture obtained with a sector scan format is pie-shaped. Although the transducer is held stationary, incorporated within the transducer is a mechanical rocking motion Figure 8-3 (A). The format of a linear array is rectangular Figure 8-3 (B). The transducer of the sector scan is usually small, and thus it is easier to use to look at nonpregnant pelvic structures.

    The piezoelectric effect is the generation of an electric voltage when a crystal is compressed. The ultrasound transducer is made up of piezoelectric crystals. When the crystals receive an electric charge, they vibrate and emit acoustic pulses. Acoustic echoes return from the tissues being scanned and cause the piezoelectric crystals to vibrate again and release an electric charge. The electric charges from the various crystals are then integrated by a computer in the machine to display a two-dimensional image.

    The transducer emits sound only 0.01% of the time. Most of the time it is receiving, **NOT** sending, sound pulses.

28. **D** (4), Page 206. There are endometrial changes with pelvic tuberculosis and adenomatous endometrial hyperplasia. A timed biopsy is one of the principal methods used to establish a luteal phase defect. Adenomyosis is a disease of the myometrium, not the endometrium. The diagnosis cannot be made by endometrial biopsy; it is a clinical diagnosis confirmed only on microscopic evaluation of the myometrium.

29. **E** (All), Pages 222, 225. The three major complications of laparoscopy are laceration of vessels, intestinal injuries, and complications of the pneumoperitoneum, which include pneumothorax, diminished venous return, gas embolism, and cardiac arrhythmias.

30. **B** (1, 3), Page 213. The problem is this patient's previous infection and her allergy to fish. People who are allergic to shell fish often are allergic to iodine, which is found in the dye used for hysterosalpingography. Acute pelvic infection serious enough to require hospitalization develops in 0.3% to 3.1% of patients who have a hysterosalpingogram. This incidence of pelvic infection is directly related to the population studied, being more common in women with dilated tubes. Although the woman's history suggests that she is ovulating, this should be confirmed. This can be accomplished with an endometrial biopsy, which if properly timed will be helpful in ruling out a luteal phase defect as a cause of the couple's infertility. A pelvic sonogram is not indicated in the investigation of an infertility patient if the physical examination is normal.

31. **E** (All), Page 208. The major complication related to an endometrial biopsy is uterine perforation, which occurs in 1 or 2 cases per 1000. Infection and postoperative bleeding are rare. Some women develop a severe vasovagal reflex.

32. **A** (1, 2, 3), Pages 211–212. Although the anatomical changes in the diameter of the internal os in the nonpregnant state may have little predictive value for future competency in pregnancy, hysterosalpingography measurements are used by some to make the presumptive diagnosis. The metrorrhagia might be secondary to endometrial polyps or submucous myoma, both of which can be seen on hysterosalpingogram. Heavy acute abnormal uterine bleeding and acute pelvic infection are contraindications to the procedure. Hysterosalpingography discovers only 50% of peritubal disease diagnosed by direct visualization via the laparoscope.

33. **E** (All), Pages 211–213. Asherman's syndrome (endometrial sclerosis) can be identified by slowly injecting a water-soluble medium under fluoroscopic control. Tubal anomalies, including diverticula and accessory ostia, can be diagnosed by hysterosalpingography.

34. **E** (All), Page 214. Procedures performed under hysteroscopic guidance include location and removal of intact or fragmented IUDs, resection of submucous myomas, lysis of synechiae, incision of uterine septa, removal of endometrial polyps, laser ablation of the endometrium, and placement of silicone plugs into the tubes for sterilization.

35. **D** (4), Pages 200, 202. The scan depicted in Figure 8-4 D is that of a bladder filled with contrast medium, indented by a uterus that appears normal in this view. In Figure 8-4 A there is a scan of a normal liver. None of the scans suggests lymph node involvement. The patient is probably older than 20, since her aorta is calcified (Figure 8-4 B). Figure 8-4 C shows a thin-walled pelvic mass, probably benign, probably ovarian.

36. **A** (1, 2, 3), Pages 216–217. Figure 8-5 depicts uterine synechiae which can be cut with a pair of microscissors. Then a large Foley catheter is placed in the cavity as a splint. For the next two months the patient should receive 7.5 mg of conjugated estrogen per day. This procedure and postoperative therapy avoids a transabdominal metroplasty.

37. **E** (All), Pages 203, 224. Magnetic resonance imaging utilizes nonionizing radiation. Because it can penetrate both bone and air, it allows identification of soft tissue pathology inaccessible to other imaging techniques. It has the capacity to differentiate between normal and malignant tissue. Images are tomographic and may be visualized in coronal, sagittal, or transverse planes.

38. **C** (2, 4), Page 195. The National Institutes of Health has recently reviewed the potential harmful effects of ultrasound studied in laboratory experiments. They discovered reduction in immune response, changes in sister chromatid exchange frequency, cell death, changes in function of cell membranes, and degradation of macromolecules. Greater attention has been directed toward the safety of ultrasonic equipment. The 1981 AIUM/NEMA *Safety Standard for Diagnostic Ultrasound Equipment* (J. Ultrasound Med., 2:S1–S49, April, 1983) was revised in late 1986. The current recommendation for clinical obstetrical ultrasound equipment is an intensity of energy waves of less than 100 mW/cm^2 of tissue being exposed.

39. **A** (1, 2, 3), Pages 197, 200, 202. The radiation dose of computed tomography to the midpelvis is approximately 50% of the 2 to 10 rad surface dose. This modality is more accurate in diagnosing retroperitoneal metastases than intraperitoneal ones. A CT scan is able to identify a node when it reaches a diameter of 1.5 to 2 cm, and it is an excellent tech-

nique for confirming the diagnosis of ovarian vein thrombophlebitis.

40. **D** (4), Page 208. To preserve cytonuclear detail, the cellular material from endometrial cytological sampling should be placed in Bouin's solution rather than in formalin. The false negative rate is between 5% and 15% when compared to material from dilation and curettage or hysterectomy. This is identical to the false negative rate of cytological screening associated with invasive carcinoma of the cervix. Patient acceptance appears to be high so that mass screening appears realistic. Although endometrial cytological sampling can be difficult in older women, age is not the limiting factor. Sampling success is determined by the status of the endocervical and endometrial canal. Women in this age group who are not on estrogen replacement therapy often have a pinpoint os.

41. **B** (1, 3), Pages 214–215, 225. High molecular weight dextran is biodegradable, nontoxic, nonconductive, and *immiscible* with blood. It is antigenic, sometimes causing anaphylaxis.

PART THREE GENERAL GYNECOLOGY

CHAPTER 9 Congenital Abnormalities

DIRECTIONS: Select the one best answer or completion.

1. A 25-year-old female treated by another physician for congenital adrenal hyperplasia (CAH) presents for a premarital examination. The patient is expected
   A. to be infertile.
   B. to be grossly overweight.
   C. to transmit the disease to only their male children.
   D. to require cortisol replacement therapy.
   E. to have uterine anomalies.

2. Laparoscopy may be useful during the surgical management of patients with
   A. Rokitansky-Küster-Hauser syndrome.
   B. hematocolpos.
   C. uterine septum.
   D. longitudinal vaginal septum.
   E. congenital adrenal hyperplasia.

3. An infant is born with ambiguous genitalia. The physician should
   A. assign male sex and later change if needed.
   B. assign female sex and later change if needed.
   C. delay gender role assignment until investigation is complete.
   D. assign male sex with no subsequent change.
   E. assign female sex with no subsequent change.

4. A newborn is seen in the nursery with an enlarged clitoris, hypertension, and fusion of the labia. An older sister was diagnosed as having congenital adrenal hyperplasia. The most likely enzyme deficiency is
   A. 5-α-reductase.
   B. 21-α-hydroxylase.
   C. 11-β-hydroxylase.
   D. 20,22 desmolase.
   E. 3-β-ol dehydrogenase.

5. A supernumerary ovary is
   A. the presence of a third ovary separated from the normally situated ovaries.
   B. the presence of one large ovary in the midline.
   C. the presence of two ovaries, one normal size and the other much larger, both situated on one side.
   D. the presence of an ovary in a male with two testes.
   E. the presence of excess ovarian tissue near a normally placed ovary and connected to it.

6. In patients with Rokitansky-Küster-Hauser syndrome, vaginal reconstruction should be performed
   A. when the patient is well motivated.
   B. as soon as the condition is diagnosed.
   C. in childhood.
   D. only after marriage.
   E. after coital attempts have been unsuccessful.

DIRECTIONS: Each question contains four suggested answers, of which one or more is correct. Choose the answer
   A. if 1, 2, and 3 are correct
   B. if 1 and 3 are correct
   C. if 2 and 4 are correct
   D. if 4 only is correct
   E. if all are correct

7. Enlargement of the clitoris is often the result of
   1. masturbation.
   2. müllerian duct defect.
   3. estrogen deficiency.
   4. androgen stimulation.

8. True statements concerning congenital adrenal hyperplasia (CAH) include:
   1. CAH is an autosomal recessive disorder.
   2. The most common form is a deficiency of 21-α-hydroxylase.
   3. The gene for this enzyme is coded on chromosome 6.
   4. Affected children will have elevated levels of ACTH.

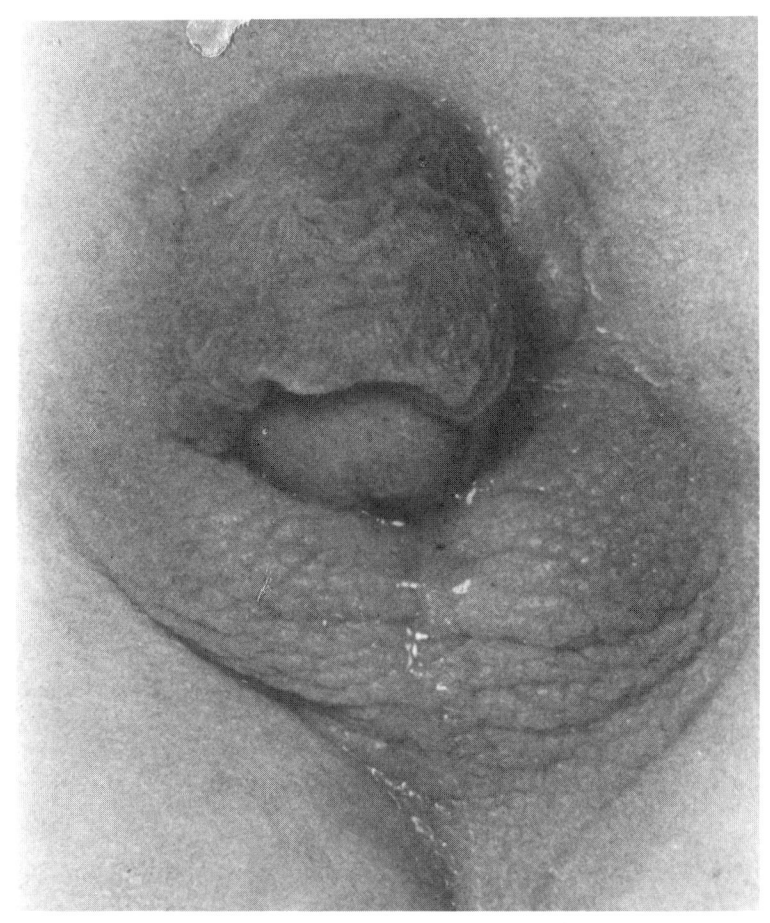

FIGURE 9-1.

9. A newborn is found to have the findings seen in Figure 9-1. Explanations for this finding include
   1. in utero exposure to 19 nor-progestins.
   2. congenital adrenal hyperplasia.
   3. the child is a true hermaphrodite.
   4. prematurity.
10. Guidelines for treatment of children losing salt due to congenital adrenal hyperplasia include
    1. serial measurements of 17-α-hydroxy progesterone.
    2. frequent determination of blood electrolytes.
    3. maintenance of growth chart.
    4. serial measurements of plasma FSH.
11. Obstructive lesions of the vagina in a 15-year-old girl may result in
    1. amenorrhea.
    2. hematocolpos.
    3. abdominal pain.
    4. mucocolpos.
12. If untreated, an imperforate hymen may cause
    1. endometriosis.
    2. urinary obstruction.
    3. abdominal pain.
    4. obstipation.
13. A significant number of patient with Rokitansky-Küster-Hauser syndrome often have
    1. primary amenorrhea.
    2. ovarian failure.
    3. urinary tract malformation.
    4. abnormal karyotype.
14. A short blind vagina is a clinical finding in patients with
    1. Rokitansky syndrome.
    2. congenital adrenal hyperplasia.
    3. androgen insensitivity.
    4. in utero exposure to DES.

15. A 16-year-old girl with primary amenorrhea is seen in the clinic. On examination she is found to have a short blind vagina and no uterus. Proper management of a patient with vaginal agenesis includes
    1. karyotype.
    2. vaginoplasty.
    3. IVP.
    4. gonadectomy before puberty.
16. Vaginal reconstruction can be achieved by
    1. creating a coital pouch (Williams vulvo-vaginoplasty).
    2. McIndoe-Reed reconstruction.
    3. graduated dilatation (Frank's method).
    4. diversion of a bowel loop.
17. True statements concerning transverse vaginal septum include:
    1. The diagnosis is easily made in children.
    2. Lower vaginal septa are more likely to be complete.
    3. Having menstrual periods excludes the possibility of a transverse vaginal septum.
    4. Upper vaginal septa are more likely to be incomplete.
18. Failure of lateral fusion of the müllerian duct may result in
    1. uterus didelphys.
    2. transverse vaginal septum.
    3. longitudinal vaginal septum.
    4. absence of uterus.
19. A longitudinal vaginal septum is commonly associated with
    1. dysmenorrhea.
    2. recurrent vaginal infections.
    3. irregular menses.
    4. uterus didelphys.
20. Pregnancy in a rudimentary uterine horn is associated with
    1. fetal death.
    2. missed abortion.
    3. uterine rupture.
    4. hyperemesis gravidarum.
21. True statements concerning a noncommunicating rudimentary uterine horn include:
    1. It needs to be removed as soon as the diagnosis is made.
    2. It often is associated with dysmenorrhea.
    3. If not removed, it increases the risk of ectopic pregnancy and uterine rupture.
    4. Endometriosis is a common finding in these patients.
22. Anomalies that should be surgically corrected include
    1. an imperforate hymen.
    2. uterus didelphys.
    3. rudimentary uterine horn.
    4. an arcuate uterus.
23. Septate uterus can be unified by using which of the following procedures?
    1. Hysteroscopic division of the septum
    2. Strassman procedure
    3. Tompkins procedure
    4. Jones procedure
24. Findings helpful in determining whether a child with ambiguous genitalia is a male or female include
    1. palpation of gonads in the labia or inguinal canal.
    2. presence of cardiac anomalies.
    3. palpation of a uterus on rectal examination.
    4. observing passage of meconium from a patent anal canal.
25. A patient 15 years of age presents with complaints of abdominal pain, a palpable abdominal mass, and primary amenorrhea. Which diagnoses should be considered?
    1. Imperforate hymen
    2. Precocious puberty
    3. Transverse vaginal septum
    4. Congenital adrenal hyperplasia
26. In order to make the correct diagnosis of the complaint in #25, the physician may gain valuable information by performing
    1. pelvic exam.
    2. ultrasound.
    3. visualization of the uterine cervix.
    4. Measurement of 17-α-hydroxy progesterone.
27. Conditions that tend to be diagnosed prior to puberty or adolescence include
    1. congenital adrenal hyperplasia.
    2. septate uterus.
    3. imperforated anus.
    4. rudimentary uterine horn.
28. A patient with five repetitive first trimester abortions underwent a hysterosalpingogram that showed a uterine septum. Proper additional diagnostic studies include
    1. semen analysis.
    2. endometrial biopsy.
    3. laparoscopy.
    4. genetic studies on both partners.
29. Absence of the uterus may be found in female patients with
    1. androgen insensitivity syndrome.
    2. hematocolpos.
    3. Rokitansky-Küster-Hauser syndrome.
    4. congenital adrenal hyperplasia.
30. Impairment of sexual activity is expected in patients with
    1. vaginal agenesis.
    2. arcuate uterus.
    3. transverse vaginal septum.
    4. supernumerary ovary.

ANSWERS

1. **D**, Pages 233–234. Patients with congenital adrenal hyperplasia have accelerated growth during childhood, but the epiphyseal plates close prematurely, reducing final adult height. When adequately replaced, growth pattern is expected to be normal. As with all autosomal recessive disorders, when both parents are affected, all children are expected to suffer from the disease. Infertility is not a predominant feature of the disorder, since ovarian function is expected to be normal in patients who are adequately treated. However, some studies have shown that these patients suffer from relative infertility.

2. **C**, Pages 241–242. Hysteroscopic division of a uterine septum is the preferred method of surgical management. It is monitored by laparoscopy to ensure that the incision does not extend through the myometrium. Laparoscopy is not indicated for patients with Rokitansky syndrome, in whom the diagnosis is made clinically, and supported by a pelvic sonogram. Similarly, it has no role in the care of patients with hematocolpos or with a longitudinal vaginal septum.

3. **C**, Page 232. An infant born with ambiguous genitalia presents a neonatal emergency. The majority of the virilized females have CAH. Some are salt losers, and unless treated with cortisol, they may die of an Addisonian crisis. In order to avoid future change in gender assignment, it is recommended that the decision regarding the newborn's sex be deferred until the investigation is complete.

4. **C**, Page 232. The newborn described has ambiguous genitalia. Most female infants with ambiguous genitalia suffer from CAH. In addition, this child has an older sister with CAH, which is an autosomal recessive disorder. Congenital adrenal hyperplasia is not associated with 5-α-reductase. The remaining three enzymes are essential steps in the production of cortisol. Deficiency of 20,22 desmolase, which converts cholesterol to pregnenolone, often is incompatible with life. Since the child has an older sister, this enzyme is not likely to be affected. The most commonly affected enzyme in patients with CAH is 21-α-hydroxylase, and 11-β-hydroxylase is the second most common, accounting for about 5% of all patients, and is associated with hypertension. Therefore, the most likely diagnosis is 11-β-hydroxylase deficiency.

5. **A**, Page 244. Supernumerary ovary is defined as the presence of a third ovary separated from the normally situated ovaries, while an accessory ovary is defined as the presence of excess ovarian tissue near a normally placed ovary and connected to it.

6. **A**, Page 237. Patients with vaginal agenesis require vaginal reconstruction. Graduated dilation is probably the preferred method, and should be delayed until the patient is motivated and therefore cooperative. It should be performed after puberty, when the adolescent girl is contemplating sexual activity or marriage. Since sexual activity may commence prior to marriage, marriage should not be a precondition for vaginal reconstruction.

7. **D** (4), Page 232. Clitoral enlargement often is the result of excess androgenic stimulation. Estrogen deficiency states or müllerian duct defects do not cause clitoral enlargement. Masturbation, although it may cause clitoral erection, is not associated with an increase in clitoral size. The genital tubercle, from which the clitoris develops, is very sensitive to androgenic stimulation in utero. With age, the sensitivity diminishes, but even late in adult life, prolonged exposure to androgens causes clitoral enlargement.

8. **E** (All), Pages 233–234. Congenital adrenal hyperplasia is an autosomal recessive disorder caused by an enzyme deficiency in the pathway of cortisol production. As a result, cortisol levels are low, thus increasing ACTH production. Accumulation of precursors occurs. These are converted to androgens that virilize the female infant. In 90–95% of patients with CAH, the deficient enzyme is 21-α-hydroxylase, the gene for which is coded on chromosome 6.

9. **A** (1, 2, 3), Page 232. An infant with ambiguous genitalia may be a virilized female, an undervirilized male, or a true hermaphrodite. Female infants may virilize in utero when exposed to androgens ingested by the mother (i.e., 19 norprogestins in oral contraceptive pills, Provera, etc.), or androgens produced by the infants (congenital adrenal hyperplasia, etc.). Premature infants do not have ambiguous genitalia on the basis of prematurity alone.

10. **A** (1, 2, 3), Pages 233–234. 17-α-hydroxy progesterone is the best indicator of adequate cortisol replacement. A less sensitive method is determination of growth pattern. Overreplacement of cortisol retards growth whereas underreplacement accelerates growth. In addition, in patients who are salt losers like this patient, frequent determinations of electrolytes are necessary to monitor replacement therapy. Measurement of FSH has no role in monitoring cortisol replacement therapy.

11. **A** (1, 2, 3), Pages 234, 235, 237. Obstructive lesions of the vagina cause the accumulation of fluid or blood behind the obstructive membrane. Initially, the accumulation is in the vagina, forming a mucocolpos in a child or hematocolpos in a postmenarcheal girl. As the fluid accumulates, it backs up into the uterus, causing hematometra and retrograde menstruation through the tubes. This results in abdominal pain and the development of endometriosis. The obstruction prevents the egress of blood from the vagina, and primary amenorrhea is one of the diagnostic features of obstructive lesions of the vagina.

12. **A** (1, 2, 3), Pages 234–235. Patients with imperforated hymen accumulate blood behind the obstructive membrane. As the blood accumu-

lates, the pressure within the vagina increases, and urethral obstruction may occur causing urinary retention. As the blood flows from the uterus through the tubes into the peritoneal cavity, abdominal pain is a frequent symptom. As a result, endometriosis may develop. Obstipation is not a feature of imperforated hymen.

13. **B** (1,3), Pages 235, 237. Patients with Rokitansky-Küster-Hauser syndrome suffer from vaginal agenesis and, in most cases, absence of the uterus. They often present with primary amenorrhea. In over 50% of the patients, urinary tract malformation coexists. An IVP is indicated on all patients who are diagnosed as having vaginal agenesis. Development of the ovaries is normal in these patients, and secondary sexual development is expected to be normal. Patients with Rokitansky-Küster-Hauser syndrome usually have a normal (46,XX) karyotype.

14. **B** (1,3), Page 235. A short blind vagina indicates either vaginal absence, or a transverse septum which shortens the vagina and prevents one from seeing the cervix. Vaginal absence is found in patients with Rokitansky syndrome or androgen insensitivity in whom the vagina does not develop. Women who were exposed to DES in utero may have vaginal adenosis, but the vagina is of normal length. Patients with congenital adrenal hyperplasia may have a narrow introitus, but the vagina is of normal length and the cervix is visible.

15. **A** (1, 2, 3), Pages 235, 237. A patient with vaginal agenesis requires vaginoplasty to create a functional vagina, an IVP to rule out the presence of a urinary tract anomaly, and a karyotype to identify those in whom the vagina did not develop because of müllerian inhibiting factor produced by a testis. Gonadectomy is not indicated in patients with Rokitansky syndrome in whom the karyotype is normal (46,XX).

16. **E** (All), Page 237. There is a potential space filled with loose areolar tissue between the bladder and the rectum, which can be developed to reconstruct a vagina. This can be achieved by graduated dilation (Frank's method). In this method, graduated dilators are pressed against the location in which the vagina should be present, and with time, as they are pushed in, a vagina is created. It requires a well-motivated patient and can be successful in about 60% of them. Alternatively, this space can be created surgically and lined with a split thickness skin graft or amnion graft (McIndoe-Reed). Under unusual circumstances, it may be necessary to utilize a loop of bowel to line the space. If such a space cannot be created, a coital pouch is created from the labia minor and perineal skin (Williams vulvo-vaginoplasty).

17. **C** (2,4), Page 237. A transverse vaginal septum occludes the vagina beyond the hymenal opening. On genital inspection the hymen appears open and thus diagnosis is not made in young children unless a large amount of fluid accumulates in the vagina (mucocolpos, hydrocolpos). Rectal examination may reveal a cystic mass, which is a vagina filled with fluid. Transverse vaginal septa may be complete, obstructing the vagina, or incomplete, allowing menstrual flow to egress through a central opening. Vaginal septa located in the upper vagina are often incomplete, while those in the lower vagina are often complete.

18. **B**, (1, 3), Pages 241–242. The uterus and vagina are formed from paired müllerian ducts that fuse in the midline. When fusion fails to occur in the distal portion, the patient has a longitudinal vaginal septum. When fusion fails to occur in the proximal portion, bicornuate uterus is found. Complete failure of lateral (longitudinal) fusion results in genital tract duplication: a longitudinal vaginal septum and uterus didelphys. Transverse vaginal septum is an example of failure of vertical fusion. Complete failure of müllerian duct development leads to uterine and vaginal agenesis.

19. **D** (4), Pages 241–242. Longitudinal vaginal septum is an example of failure of lateral fusion and is associated with uterus didelphys. The presence of a septum may interfere with sexual function, and the patient may complain of dyspareunia. Vaginal infections and irregular menses are unrelated to the presence of a longitudinal vaginal septum.

20. **A** (1, 2, 3), Page 240. Pregnancy in a rudimentary uterine horn is often associated with a missed abortion or fetal death. The blood supply to a rudimentary horn is often compromised and insufficient to support a pregnancy. On occasion, when the blood supply is adequate, as the fetus grows, rupture of the horn occurs. The prevalence of hyperemesis gravidarum is not increased in these patients when compared with other pregnant women.

21. **E** (All), Page 240. The cavity of a rudimentary uterine horn is lined with endometrium. When it sheds, it escapes through the tube into the peritoneal cavity, causing abdominal pain. Such retrograde menstruation is considered by some to cause endometriosis. These women often complain of dysmenorrhea. Pregnancy in a noncommunicating uterine horn is considered to be an ectopic gestation. Pregnancy in a rudimentary horn often results in missed abortion, fetal death, and uterine rupture. When rupture occurs, if often causes a massive intraperitoneal hemorrhage. Unless the bleeding is controlled, it may lead to maternal death. It is therefore recommended that a noncommunicating rudimentary uterine horn be removed as soon as the diagnosis is made.

22. **B** (1, 3), Pages 234, 240. A rudimentary uterine horn exposes the patient to the risks of ectopic gestation, uterine rupture, endometriosis, and infertility. It needs to be removed as soon as the diagnosis is made. Imperforate hymen leads to obstruction of the vagina, and should be incised. Arcuate uterus and uterus didelphys require no surgical treatment.

23. **E** (All), Pages 242, 244. A uterine septum should be removed if the patient is having repetitive fetal losses. It is assumed that the septum provides an unfavorable area for implantation and leads to abortion. There are many techniques for the removal of a uterine septum: Strassman procedure, in which a coronal incision is made through the fundus and the septum is excised; Tompkins procedure, in which a sagittal incision is made through the fundus and the septum is excised; and Jones procedure, in which the fundus is excised on both sides of the septum and the septum is incised. In all these methods, a laparotomy is performed and the uterine fundus is removed. The preferred method uses an operative hysteroscope, which is inserted through the cervical os. The procedure is monitored by laparoscopy. The advantages of this procedure are: 1) it does not require a laparotomy, 2) risks of pelvic adhesions are reduced, and 3) the risk of future uterine rupture is less.

24. **B** (1, 3), Page 232. Certain physical findings may support an initial impression of the true sex of a newborn with ambiguous genitalia. When gonads are palpable in the labia or the inguinal canal, the infant is likely to be a male. Palpation of a uterus on rectal examination suggests the newborn is a female. The presence or absence of cardiac and anal anomalies is not helpful in sex determination.

25. **B** (1,3), Page 234. The patient complains of primary amenorrhea, abdominal pain, and a palpable mass—a triad suggestive of vaginal obstruction. The diagnoses to be considered in this particular instance are imperforate hymen or a complete vaginal septum.

26. **A** (1, 2, 3), Pages 234–235. The patient presented has an obstructed vagina trapping menstrual blood. Pelvic examination may reveal a large cystic mass. A sonogram may show the level of obstruction and provide useful information prior to surgical correction. When the uterine cervix is seen, the diagnoses of imperforate hymen or complete transverse vaginal septum are excluded. Measurement of 17-α-hydroxy progesterone levels is not helpful in the workup of patients with outflow tract obstruction.

27. **B** (1,3), Pages 232–233, 240. Genital anomalies of the upper genital tract are often not diagnosed until late in life when they interfere with menstruation or with fertility. The diagnosis of septate uterus or rudimentary uterine horn is rarely made in childhood. The diagnosis of imperforated anus should be made immediately following delivery if the infant does not pass meconium. Digital examination of the anal canal confirms the diagnosis. Congenital adrenal hyperplasia, with its increased androgen production, is often diagnosed at birth in the virilized female. The male infant, even if not virilized at birth, may be diagnosed if he is a salt loser or when he virilizes during childhood.

28. **D** (4), Pages 240–241. Presented is a patient with five repetitive first trimester abortions who during her infertility workup was found to have a septate uterus. Division of the septum, which represents an unfavorable site for implantation, is indicated. A complete workup of both parents is indicated to exclude other causes for fetal wastage. It is recommended that a karyotype of both parents be done to identify chromosome abnormalities. Endometrial biopsy, laparoscopy, and semen analysis, though important steps in the evaluation of the infertile couple, are not required in the patient presented. The patient has no difficulties in conception, but suffers from recurrent abortions.

29. **B** (1, 3), Pages 235, 237. Absence of the uterus is caused by failure of the müllerian ducts to form properly, as in patients with Rokitansky-Küster-Hauser syndrome. Patients with testicular tissue (androgen insensitivity) produce müllerian-inhibiting factor, which causes regression of the müllerian ducts, and these individuals are born without a uterus. Patients with hematocolpos or congenital adrenal hyperplasia have a normal uterus.

30. **B** (1,3), Pages 235, 237. Sexual activity is impaired in patients with vaginal anomalies which make the vagina either too short or too narrow. Patients with vaginal agenesis often have difficulties during intercourse. Most of them have only a short vagina; they require vaginal reconstruction. A transverse septum, particularly if situated in the lower vagina, prevents adequate penetration. A supernumerary ovary and arcuate uterus have no effect on sexual activity.

CHAPTER 10
Pediatric Gynecology

DIRECTIONS: Select the one best answer or completion.

1. All of the following are typical characteristics of a patient with true precocious puberty **except**
    A. normal menopausal age.
    B. normal intellectual development.
    C. normal uterine size.
    D. normal interpersonal relationships.
    E. normal reproductive capacity.

2. Which is **not** a component of a complete gynecologic examination of a pediatric patient?
    A. History
    B. Visualization of cervix
    C. Cultures of the vagina
    D. Bimanual rectal-vaginal examination
    E. Bimanual rectal-abdominal examination

3. A 4-year-old child is seen with symptoms of dysuria and bloody discharge. Inspection of the external genitalia reveals a small hemorrhagic mass with a central aperture situated in the midline above the anterior aspect of the vaginal opening. (See Figure 10-1.) The most likely diagnosis is
    A. endometrial polyp.
    B. sarcoma botryoides.
    C. urethral prolapse.
    D. vaginal polyp.
    E. sacro-coccygeal tumor.

4. The ovarian tumor that most commonly causes incomplete precocious puberty is
    A. thecoma.
    B. granulosa cell.
    C. luteoma.
    D. Sertoli-Leydig cell.
    E. teratoma.

5. In a child, the neutral pH of the vagina is the result of
    A. higher than usual vaginal salt content.
    B. the presence of a predominance of anaerobic bacteria.
    C. a lack of glycogen in the epithelial cells.
    D. poor perineal hygiene.
    E. contamination of the vagina with urine.

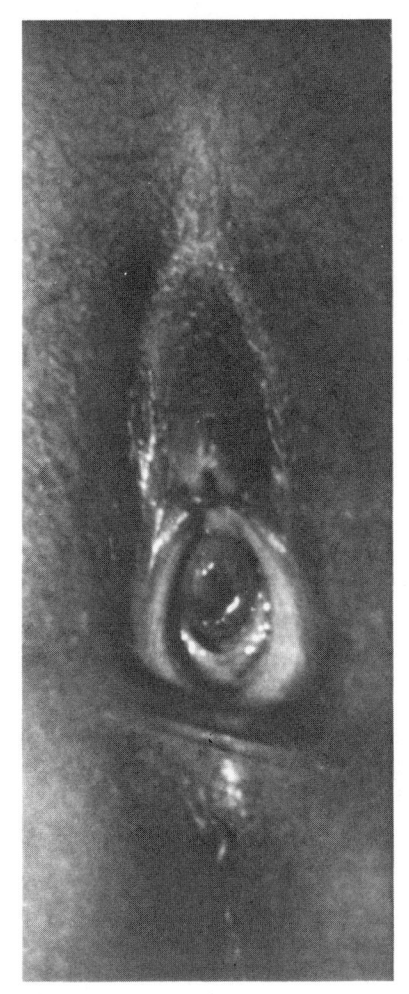

FIGURE 10-1.

DIRECTIONS: For each numbered item, indicate whether it is associated with
  A only (A)
  B only (B)
  C both (A) and (B)
  D neither (A) nor (B)

(A) Vaginoscopy
(B) Bimanual rectal-abdominal examination
(C) Both
(D) Neither

6. Suspicion of foreign body
7. Pelvic pain
8. Recurrent vulvovaginitis
9. Abnormal bleeding
   (A) Complete precocious puberty
   (B) Incomplete precocious puberty
   (C) Both
   (D) Neither
10. Ovulation
11. Uterine bleeding
12. Related to central nervous system disease

DIRECTIONS: Each question contains four suggested answers, of which one or more is correct. Choose the answer
A if 1, 2, and 3 are correct
B if 1 and 3 are correct
C if 2 and 4 are correct
D if 4 only is correct
E if all are correct

13. Normal findings in a pediatric gynecologic examination include
    1. nonpalpable ovaries.
    2. palpable uterine corpus.
    3. thin vaginal epithelium.
    4. pale vaginal epithelium.

14. Physiological vaginal discharge in a perimenarcheal girl
    1. is caused by the increase in estrogen level.
    2. requires periodic acid douches.
    3. usually is not symptomatic.
    4. should be evaluated with serum estradiol.

15. A 5-year-old girl presents to the office with a history of a small amount of bloody discharge that occurred 3 days ago. The discharge subsided and now the girl is free of symptoms. General physical examination and inspection of the external genitalia is normal. Proper management includes
    1. obtaining pelvic ultrasound.
    2. obtaining blood for WBC and differential.
    3. performing examination under anesthesia.
    4. obtaining urine for urine analysis and culture.

16. The assessment of a prepubertal child differs in what ways from that of an adult?
    1. Time needed to establish rapport
    2. Implications for subsequent health care
    3. Focus on a specific problem
    4. Emphasis of medical rather than surgical therapy

17. Which statements regarding ovarian tumors in children are true?
    1. They account for about 1% of childhood malignancies.
    2. Abdominal pain is the most common presenting complaint.
    3. Teratomas account for the majority of these neoplasms.
    4. Over half of ovarian tumors in children are malignant.

18. In young girls, which of the following conditions may result in precocious puberty?
    1. McCune-Albright syndrome
    2. Hypothyroidism
    3. Granulosa cell tumor
    4. Diabetes

19. Which statements about the gynecologic evaluation of a 3-year-old child are true?
    1. Most gynecologic symptoms are of very short duration when the patient is first seen by the physician.
    2. Draping the patient is a recommended procedure.
    3. If necessary, moderate restraint of an uncooperative patient should be used in order to avoid use of sedation.
    4. The knee-chest position allows visualization of the cervix without instruments.

20. Recurrent or persistent vulvovaginitis may be the result of
    1. foreign body.
    2. sexual abuse.
    3. ectopic ureter.
    4. pinworms.

21. Which statements about the management of pinworms are true?
    1. Mebendazole (Vermox) is safe during pregnancy.
    2. Mebendazole (Vermox) is the drug of choice.
    3. Adjunctive topical estrogen treatment is needed in pediatric patients.
    4. The treatment of all family members over 2 years of age is recommended.

22. A 9-year-old girl is brought to the ER following a straddle injury on a bicycle bar. A large, nonexpanding vulvar hematoma is noted. One should
    1. send the child home with appropriate analgesics.
    2. obtain an I.V.P.
    3. incise and drain the hematoma.
    4. prescribe an ice pack and observe the child.

23. Which drugs used to treat true precocious puberty will slow advancement of bone age?
 1. Danazol (Danocrine)
 2. Depo-Provera (Medroxyprogesterone acetate)
 3. Cyproterone acetate
 4. GnRH agonist
24. Which of the following organisms in a child with premenarcheal vulvovaginitis may be indicative of sexual molestation?
 1. *Neisseria gonorrhoeae*
 2. *Chlamydia trachomatis*
 3. *Trichomonas vaginalis*
 4. *Shigella flexneri*
25. True statements concerning pinworms include:
 1. The adult worm lays eggs on the perineal skin.
 2. The adult worm resides in the vagina.
 3. Itching occurs mainly at night.
 4. The diagnosis is made by identifying antibodies in the blood.
26. True statements concerning adhesive vulvitis include:
 1. The condition may mimic congenital absence of the vagina.
 2. It is most common in girls under 2 years of age.
 3. The pathognomonic sign is a translucent vertical line.
 4. Agglutination initially occurs anteriorly.
27. Figure 10-2 shows a 7-year-old girl. True statements concerning the patient's condition include:
 1. In North America, it is defined as "sexual maturation before the age of 8."
 2. The eventual adult height is shorter than normal.
 3. Complete precocious puberty is more common than incomplete precocious puberty.
 4. Heterosexual precocious puberty is usually caused by adrenal androgens.
28. A child is more susceptible than an adult to vulvovaginitis because children
 1. often maintain poor perineal hygiene.
 2. have vaginal mucosa that lacks the protective effect of estrogen.
 3. have a vagina with neutral pH.
 4. are more likely to be malnourished.
29. A 7-year-old girl presents with accelerated growth and breast enlargement. Appropriate initial studies include

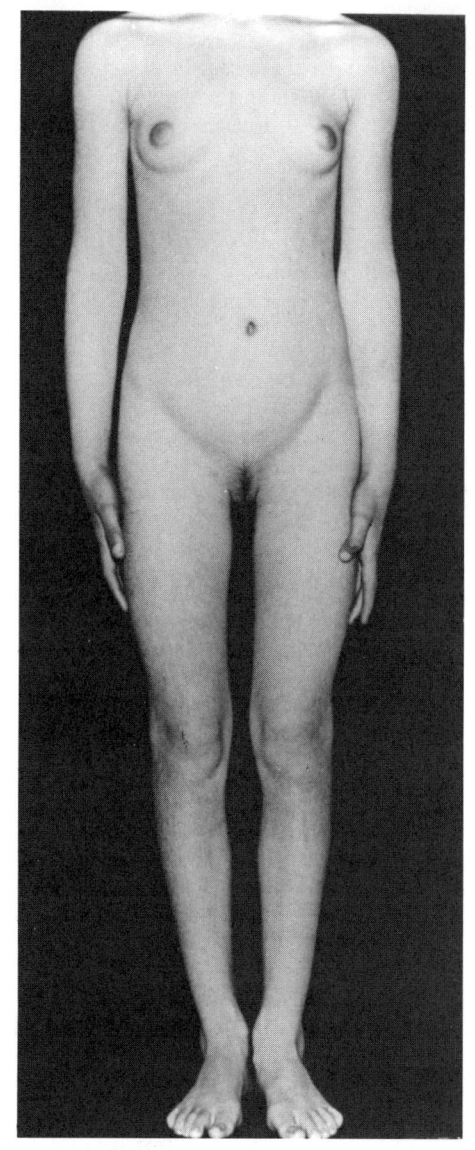

FIGURE 10-2.

 1. bone age.
 2. pelvic ultrasound.
 3. FSH, LH.
 4. DHEAS.
30. True statements concerning the use of topical estrogen in childhood vulvovaginitis include:
 1. Topical estrogen is the mainstay of therapy.
 2. The cream should be applied to the vulva, not inserted into the vagina.
 3. Systemic absorption is of little concern.
 4. Most nonspecific infections respond to a combination of estrogen cream and oral broad-spectrum antibiotics.

31. True statements concerning vaginal foreign bodies include:
    1. The most common foreign body is a small piece of toilet paper.
    2. The girl usually denies the possibility that a foreign body is in the vagina.
    3. Foul smelling bloody discharge is common.
    4. Pelvic X-ray can identify a foreign body in almost half the instances.

ANSWERS

1. **D**, Page 260. The cause of premature maturation of the hypothalmic-pituitary-ovarian axis is unknown. Idiopathic (constitutional) development accounts for 85% of the cases of complete precocious puberty. Emotional problems in these young girls arise from the fact that they are put under extreme social pressures. The child may be exposed to sexual exploitation and ridiculed by her peers. The child needs extensive sex education and help in anticipating such difficulties. Most of these patients are shy and withdrawn from their peers.
2. **D**, Page 248. The successful gynecologic examination of a child requires a slow pace with ample time taken to show gentleness and patience on the part of both the physician and staff. A bimanual rectal-vaginal examination is not recommended. Instead, a rectal examination should be performed if the patient has vaginal bleeding or abdominal or pelvic pain. It is even sometimes best to defer the pelvic examination to a second visit in order to allay the child's anxiety. It should be noted, however, that in the area of pediatric gynecology, clinical errors tend to be those of omission rather than commission.
3. **C**, Page 255. A bloody vaginal discharge can be caused by rare conditions such as urethral prolapse, precocious puberty, and carcinoma. Careful physical examination will aid in making this differential diagnosis.
4. **B**, Pages 262–263. Granulosa cell tumors account for 60% of cases. They are usually quite large when associated with precocious puberty, and with approximately 80% can be palpated abdominally. Thecomas and luteomas are much smaller and usually cannot be palpated abdominally. Overall, only 5% of granulosa cell tumors and 1% of thecomas occur prior to puberty.
5. **C**, Page 252. The thin vaginal epithelium of a prepubertal child has a neutral pH, thus providing a better medium for bacterial growth than a woman of reproductive age. This higher pH is due to a paucity of lactobacillus that produces acid from glycogen in reproductive age women.
6–9. 6, **C**; 7, **B**; 8, **A**; 9, **C**; Pages 249–250. Both vaginoscopy and bimanual rectal-abdominal examination provide important information in evaluating various problems in the child. Depending on the child's symptoms, different evaluation techniques must be utilized.
10–12. 10, **A**; 11, **C**; 12, **A**; Page 259. The various types of precocious puberty are definitions that are only of clinical value after the final diagnosis has been established. Prolonged follow-up is sometimes necessary to rule out subtle, slow-growing lesions of the adrenal gland, brain, or ovary.
13. **B** (1, 3), Pages 249–250. Normal findings in a prepubertal child differ from that of an adult. These findings include a vaginal wall that appears redder and thinner than the vagina of an adult. The cervix appears as a transverse ridge that is redder than the vagina. Neither uterine corpus nor ovaries should be palpable. In addition, the vagina is narrower, thinner, and lacking in the distensibility of the vagina of a woman of reproductive age.
14. **B** (1, 3), Page 253. In the 6 to 12 months prior to menarche, a grayish-white, nonirritating discharge may be seen. This leukorrhea contains sheets of vaginal epithelial cells. The mother and child should be reassured that this is a normal physiological process that will diminish with time.
15. **D** (4), Page 254. Both urinary and vaginal etiologies for this type of complaint must be followed up on the first episode. Therefore, vaginal inspection and evaluation of the urinary tract should be done initially in cases of bloody discharge.
16. **E** (All), Page 247. The outpatient visit for a child should be structured differently from a visit by a woman of reproductive age. More time is needed to gain the child's confidence. That child's long-term relationship with physicians will be affected if her initial encounter is a negative one. A child's visit to the gynecologist typically focuses on a specific, perceived medical problem rather than on preventive health care. Typically, children's gynecologic problems are treated by medical rather than surgical means. The physician and the nursing staff should be prepared to approach a child's visit with these important considerations in mind.
17. **A** (1,2,3), Pages 257–258. Ovarian neoplasia must be considered in the differential diagnosis whenever a child complains of persistent or recurrent abdominal pain. Ovarian tumors account for 1% of childhood malignancies and most commonly present with abdominal pain. Often in these patients, ovaries are abdominal organs. Ultrasound and computerized tomography are most useful in establishing a diagnosis. Acute complications of adnexal masses include torsion, hem-

orrhage, and rupture. These complications occur in children more frequently than in adult patients with similar ovarian tumors. Approximately 75% of ovarian neoplasms in premenarcheal females are benign teratomas, and approximately 25% are malignant tumors.

18. **A** (1, 2, 3), Page 262. Early sexual development is found in patients with McCune-Albright syndrome, hypothyroidism, and estrogen-producing ovarian neoplasms such as granulosa cell tumor. Diabetes is not a cause for early sexual development.

19. **D** (4), Pages 248–249. Unlike the adult patient, gynecologic histories in children are not easily obtained either from the patient or from the family. As a result, most gynecologic symptoms are chronic when first seen by a physician. Draping the patient often produces more anxiety than it relieves; as a result, draping is not recommended. A combination of meperidine, chlorpromazine hydrochloride, and promethazine hydrochloride may be used to relieve some of the anxiety in carefully selected children. A child should never be restrained for an examination. The knee-chest position usually allows visualization of the vagina and cervix of a child after the age of 2 without instrumentation. This is attributed to the filling of the vaginal canal with air as the abdominal wall is relaxed and deep inspirations are taken.

20. **E** (All), Pages 250, 252. In addition to these diagnoses, a primary vulvar skin disease should be considered if vulvovaginitis is persistent. A foul, bloody vaginal discharge strongly suggests a foreign body, but a discharge associated with a foreign body is not necessarily either bloody or foul smelling.

21. **C** (2,4), Pages 252, 254. Vermox is given as one chewable tablet for each *nonpregnant* family member over the age of 2 years. Approximately 20% of female children who are infected with pinworms then develop vulvovaginitis.

22. **D** (4), Pages 255–256. The usual causes of genital trauma during childhood are accidental falls, the majority of which involve straddle injuries. If a sharp object is involved, a laceration with potential deep damage may occur. In most cases, the hematoma will stop growing when the pressure from the expanding hematoma exceeds venous pressure. If an artery has been traumatized, bleeding may continue until the artery is surgically ligated. The treatment of a nonexpanding vulvar hematoma is the use of an ice pack. Only rarely is surgical evacuation and ligation of bleeding vessels necessary. Extensive lacerations require general anesthesia for diagnosis and management. Children with vulvar trauma should have a booster injection of tetanus toxoid if the last immunization was more than 5 years prior to the event.

23. **D** (4), Page 264. The present drug of choice for true precocious puberty is one of the potent agonists or analogues of gonadotrophin releasing hormone. The agonists bind to the pituitary's GnRH receptors and remain attached for a prolonged period, rendering the pituitary incapable of response to endogenous GnRH. Such a mechanism is called *down regulation*. The other medications suppress menstruation and inhibit further breast development but have no effect on growth rate.

24. **A** (1,2,3), Page 250. Vulvovaginitis is the most common gynecologic problem in the premenarcheal patient. Approximately 80% to 90% of visits of children to gynecologists involve introital irritation and discharge. When cultures of the vagina are taken, it must be remembered that the normal vagina is colonized by an average of nine different species of bacteria. There are specific pathogens, however, that might indicate sexual molestation.

25. **B** (1, 3), Page 252. At night the pin-sized adult worms migrate from the rectum to the skin of the vulva to deposit eggs. They may be detected by using a flashlight or by dabbing the vulvar skin with clear cellophane adhesive tape, then examining the tape under the microscope.

26. **B** (1,3), Page 255. Adhesive vulvitis is a self-limiting consequence of chronic vulvitis. Denuded epithelium agglutinates and occurs most commonly in young girls between 2 and 6 years of age. Most infants are asymptomatic. Early stages of the process reveal posterior agglutination. In more advanced cases, fusion over both the urethral and vaginal orifices may occur. No treatment is necessary unless the child has difficulty in voiding. Topical estrogen cream will result in spontaneous separation within 2 to 4 weeks.

27. **E** (All), Pages 258–259. Precocious puberty is arbitrarily defined as the appearance of any signs of secondary sexual maturation at an age more than 2.5 standard deviations below the mean. The mean age in North America for menarche in recent years is 12.5 years and onset of breast development usually commences 2 years earlier. Secondary sexual development—i.e. breasts and pubic hair—prior to age 8 is considered precocious. Similarly, the onset of menses prior to age 10 merits investigation. Isosexual precocity denotes early sexual development which corresponds to the sex of the individual; that is, a girl who notices breast development. Heterosexual precocity denotes secondary sexual development which does not correspond to the individual's sex; that is, virilization of a girl at puberty. The principal concerns of parents of these children are the social stigma and the diminished height

caused by premature closure of epiphyseal growth centers. Without therapy, approximately 50% of patients will be under five feet tall. Both complete and incomplete precocious puberty are rare; however, complete precocious puberty is five times more common than incomplete precocious puberty.

28. **A** (1, 2, 3), Page 252. There are both physiologic and behavioral reasons why a child is more susceptible to vulvar and vaginal infections than a reproductive age woman. In addition to lacking estrogen's protective effect, the vagina at this age lacks glycogen, lactobacilli, and an adequate level of antibodies to fight infection.

29. **E** (All), Page 263. The initial evaluation of patients with possible precocious puberty places an emphasis on the exclusion of neoplasms of the central nervous system, ovaries, or adrenal glands. Hand-wrist films are typically repeated at 6-month intervals to evaluate the rate of skeletal maturation and the necessity for active treatment. Advancement of bone age more than 95% of the norm for the child's chronological age documents a peripheral estrogen effect.

30. **C** (2,4), Pages 253–254. The foundation of treating childhood vulvovaginitis is the improvement of local perineal hygiene. Approximately one in four cases is cured by improved local hygiene alone. Most cases respond to a combination of topical estrogen cream and oral antibiotics given for 10 to 14 days. The estrogen cream is to be applied to the vulvar area at night. The cream should not be used longer than 3 or 4 weeks because of systemic absorption.

31. **A** (1, 2, 3), Pages 254–255. Symptoms related to a vaginal foreign body constitute 4% of all pediatric gynecologic outpatient visits. Neither the mother nor the child typically remembers the insertion of a foreign body, most often pieces of toilet paper. Large objects may be removed by bayonet forceps, and small objects such as sand may be washed out by irrigation. The differential diagnosis of a bloody vaginal discharge should also include the possibility of shigella and group A beta-hemolytic streptococcus. The latter usually occurs 7 to 10 days after a sore throat and upper respiratory infection.

Chapter 11: Contraception, Sterilization, and Pregnancy Termination

DIRECTIONS: Select the one best answer or completion.

1. All of the following statements regarding depomedroxyprogesterone acetate (DM-PA) are true except:
   A. Contraceptive doses lower secretion of gonadotrophins.
   B. Estradiol levels are lowered to levels similar to early follicular phase.
   C. There is an increase in body weight among users.
   D. There are changes in lipid metabolism similar to those seen with oral estrogen gestagen users.
   E. Number of patients with amenorrhea increases in proportion to the time the patient has received the drug.

DIRECTIONS: For each numbered item, select the one heading most closely associated with it. Each lettered heading may be used once, more than once, or not at all.

(A) Sterilization
(B) Oral contraceptive
(C) Diaphragm
(D) Condom

2. Most widely used contraceptive in women aged 25–29
3. Most commonly used method for women over 35
4. Overall most popular method of birth control
5. Method that has the highest continuation rate

DIRECTIONS: For each numbered item, indicate whether it is associated with
A only (A)
B only (B)
C both (A) and (B)
D neither (A) nor (B)

(A) Method effectiveness
(B) Use effectiveness
(C) Both
(D) Neither

6. Highest for oral contraceptives
7. Nonactuarial method of calculating failure rates (Pearl index)

8. Pregnancy after tubal sterilization
   (A) Cooper 7
   (B) Lippes loop
   (C) Both
   (D) Neither

9. Increase in mean blood loss in each menstrual cycle
10. Increased vascular permeability in areas not in direct contact with the IUD
11. Blood loss significantly reduced by use of protaglandin synthetase inhibitors
    (A) Estrogenic OCP component
    (B) Gestagen OCP component
    (C) Both
    (D) Neither

12. Responsible for direct inhibitory effect on both hypothalamus and pituitary gland
13. Responsible for depression
14. Responsible for amenorrhea
    (A) 19-nortestosterone gestagens
    (B) C-21 gestagens
    (C) Both
    (D) Neither

15. Contained in all oral contraceptives manufactured in the United States
16. Have greater potency per unit weight than natural steroids
17. Associated with the development of breast cancer in experimental models
    (A) Ethinyl estradiol
    (B) 19-norgestagens
    (C) Both
    (D) Neither

18. Increase in globulin factor precursors of angiotensinogen responsible for blood pressure elevations
19. Increase in Factors VII and X associated with hypercoagulability
20. Component in oral contraceptives responsible for increased incidence of breast cancer in users
    (A) Ethinyl estradiol
    (B) Mestranol
    (C) Both
    (D) Neither

21. Synthetic estrogen found in U.S. manufactured oral contraceptives
22. Binds to estrogen cytosol receptors

23. Enzymatic conversion necessary to render biologically active in humans

DIRECTIONS: Each question contains four suggested answers of which one or more is correct. Choose the answer
A if 1, 2, and 3 are correct
B if 1 and 3 are correct
C if 2 and 4 are correct
D if 4 only is correct
E if all are correct

24. Characteristics describing the mechanism of action of contraceptives containing estrogen/progesterone include
    1. alteration of cervical mucus.
    2. alteration of tubal mobility.
    3. diminished endometrial glandular productions of glycogen.
    4. abolition of gonadotrophin production and ovarian steroidogenesis.
25. Mechanisms of action of the intrauterine device include
    1. alteration of sperm transport to oviduct.
    2. luteolysis secondary to increased prostaglandin release.
    3. endometrial inflammatory response.
    4. ovulatory inhibition associated with delayed follicular maturation.
26. Which statements explaining the relatively high failure rate associated with the rhythm method are true?
    1. The human ovum is capable of being fertilized for more than 24 hours following ovulation.
    2. Sperm are capable of fertilization for more than 48 hours after intercourse.
    3. Ovulation occurs 12–16 days after the onset of subsequent menstruation.
    4. The fertile period cannot be calculated accurately.
27. The noncontraceptive health benefits of oral contraceptives include
    1. lowering of incidence of iron deficiency anemia.
    2. a reduction in the number of breast fibroadenomas.
    3. a decreased risk of developing ovarian cancer.
    4. less clinical salpingitis in women infected with gonorrhea.
28. Which statements regarding the performance of elective abortion in the United States are true?
    1. Most pregnancy terminations occur with gestations of greater than 12 weeks menstrual age.
    2. Twenty-five percent of abortions are obtained by married women.
    3. Complication rates are similar for first and second trimester pregnancy terminations.
    4. It is the least safe of all methods of birth control.
29. Problems related to successful contraception for the male include
    1. difficulty in separating suppression of major testicular functions.
    2. the long lag period from initiation of treatment until elimination of sperm from the ejaculate.
    3. variability in the time required for return of fertility.
    4. an expected high degree of impotence in male users of hormonal contraception.
30. Which statements are true regarding the risk of developing cardiovascular disease in oral contraceptive users?
    1. Long-term users have a higher incidence of atherosclerosis.
    2. Relative risk increases significantly in smokers in each age group over 35.
    3. Death rates from myocardial infarction have increased in the past 15 years in women age 20–45.
    4. Relative risk increases significantly for women with preexisting vascular disease.
31. IUD users have an increased incidence of
    1. ectopic pregnancy (when pregnancy occurs at all).
    2. spontaneous abortion.
    3. salpingitis.
    4. abnormal embryogenesis.
32. Which statements are true regarding the contraceptive use of intrauterine devices?
    1. Pregnancy rates decline with increasing age over 35.
    2. Expulsion rates decline with increasing age over age 25.
    3. Removal rates are highest in women under the age of 25.
    4. Woman-months of use are greatest in the age group 35–49.
33. Factors related to adverse bleeding events in IUD wearers include
    1. delay in follicular maturation.
    2. delay in ovulatory events associated with a late midcycle LH surge.
    3. disruption of corpus luteum function.
    4. increased rate of prostaglandin release.

ANSWERS

1. **D**, Pages 294–296. Depometroxyprogesterone acetate (DMPA) has mechanisms of action similar to oral combination contraceptives. This includes suppression of midcycle LH surge, thus preventing ovulation, as well as suppression of estradiol levels comparable to early follicular phase levels. Unlike orally administered combination contraceptives, there are no changes in liver function or lipid metabolism because of the bypass of hepatic circulation. Because of the anabolic effect of DMPA, users experience a modest weight gain with increased duration of use. There is complete disruption of the menstrual cycle so that bleeding is unpredictable and a number of patients experience amenorrhea.

2–5. 2, **B**; 3, **A**; 4, **A**; 5, **C**; Pages 271–272; Tables 11-2 and 11-4 (from Droegemueller). Oral contraceptives are by far the most popular contraceptive method in women under the age of 30 with almost 50% of women who practice contraception using this method in the 20–24 age group. The use of OCPs markedly declines after the age of 30.

For women over the age of 35 the condom is the most commonly used *nonsurgical* method of contraception, although for all age groups taken together, surgical sterilization is the most widely practiced method of fertility regulation. This is due largely to extremely high rates of sterilization among women between the ages of 35 and 44.

Although used much less frequently, when used, the IUD carries the highest continuation rate for more than 1 year with this method favored by roughly equal percentages in all age groups. IUD supplies are currently limited due to manufacturers' concerns regarding product liability, and this will further decrease its use in the near future.

To estimate continuation rates, only method stoppage techniques can be used, thereby excluding tubal ligation.

6–8. 6, **C**; 7, **C**; 8, **A**; Pages 269, 271. The terms *method effectiveness* and *use effectiveness* have been used to differentiate whether conception occurred while a contraceptive was used *properly* or improperly. Failure rates in both categories are lowest for oral contraceptives. Overall value of a method as used by a couple (correctly or incorrectly) is determined by calculation of actual effectiveness as well as the continuation rate. These rates can be estimated by either actuarial or nonactuarial methods such as the Pearl index.

An example of a *method failure* would be tubal sterilization, provided that the procedure had been done properly and provided that the patient was not pregnant at the time of the procedure.

9–11. 9, **C**; 10, **C**; 11, **C**; Pages 301–302. Recent evidence indicates that mean blood loss in all IUD wearers is greater than in nonwearers. This ranges from an approximate twofold increase in loop wearers to a 50%–60% increase in wearers of a copper-coated device. Vascular erosions in areas remote from the device occur in IUD wearers of both types. Evidence for excess local prostaglandin production exists and can be modified by use of prostaglandin synthetase inhibitors, thereby decreasing the amount of blood loss with each menses.

The IUD has limited availability with few manufacturers willing to continue production. Product liability seems to have dictated this, despite the fact that the IUD is a safe, reliable form of contraception for many women.

12–14. 12, **C**; 13, **A**; 14, **B**; Pages 278, 280–281. Both components of OCPs are responsible for suppression of both pituitary (gonadotrophins) and hypothalamus (GnRH) factors involved with initiating ovulation and seem to be estrogen dose related.

Estrogen alters the pathway for tryptophan metabolism from the brain to the liver so that the end product, serotonin, is decreased in the central nervous system, producing various mood changes, including depression.

Amenorrhea occurs primarily because of decreased endometrial growth in response to the gestagen's effect on estrogen receptors. With decrease in estrogen receptors in the endometrial glandular tissue, there is decreased cellular proliferation and diminished endometrial slough.

15–17. 15, **A**; 16, **C**; 17, **B**; Page 295. Because high doses of the C-21 gestagens have been associated with the development of breast cancer in female beagles, these gestagens are not found in oral contraceptives sold in the United States. Depomedroxyprogesterone acetate (C-21 gestagen) is widely used as a contraceptive in other countries. Only the 19-nortestosterone derivatives are used in OC formulations marketed in this country.

All synthetic steroids (including all 19-nortestosterone gestagens and all C-21 gestagens) are more potent per unit weight than their natural counterparts.

18–20. 18, **A**; 19, **A**; 20, **D**; Pages 282–283; Tables 11-6 and 11-7 (from Droegemueller). Synthetic estrogens have been associated with increase in globulins of which one, angiotensinogen, may cause increased angiotensin II, resulting in hypertension, while other globulins such as Factor VII and Factor X may be associated with the development of hypercoagulable states. This may lead to the development of thrombosis in certain OC users.

No long-term study documents an increased breast cancer rate in OC users since the gestagen component of the pill counteracts the stimulatory action of estrogen on target tissues. For this reason, OC users have a lower incidence of nonmalignant breast disease.

21–23. 21, C; 22, A; 23, B; Page 276. Both of the above synthetic estrogens are present in oral contraceptives, although compounds containing mestranol require conversion to ethinyl estradiol to become biologically active. This is because human estrogen cytosol receptors do not bind to mestranol. Therefore, human endometrial response and the effect on liver corticosteroid-binding globulin (biologic end points) differ with these two estrogens, and when mestranol is used, they are dependent on the rate of conversion to ethinyl estradiol.

24. A (1, 2, 3), Pages 277–278. Although combination oral contraceptives consistently inhibit the midcycle gonadotrophin surge, thereby suppressing ovulation, there remain residual low levels of gonadotrophin production and ovarian steroidogenesis. The altered hormonal milieu also alters cervical mucus and affects tubal mobility so the ova and sperm are not transported effectively. Endometrial histology is likewise changed to render blastocyst implantation unlikely.

25. B (1, 3), Pages 297–298. The intrauterine device produces a localized sterile inflammatory response which is associated with a marked leukocytosis. Tissue breakdown products of these leukocytes are toxic to both sperm and blastocyst. Although there may be excessive prostaglandin production in some IUD users, no evidence exists for luteolytic effect of alteration of ovulatory mechanisms.

26. E (All), Page 274. All of the assumptions stated above can contribute to rhythm method failures. Cycle irregularity is especially important since it is likely to be more prevalent at either extremes in the reproductive years (adolescence and perimenopause) during a time in life when a higher proportion of pregnancies are unwanted. Actual survival of fertilizing sperm is quite variable and ovum fertilizability may well exceed 24 hours after ovulation.

27. E (All), Pages 291–293. The noncontraceptive benefits stated above have all been documented in extensive collaborative studies. By decreasing endometrial glandular proliferation (diminished estrogen receptors), menstrual blood loss at the time of shedding is reduced. Similarly, with decreased estrogen receptors in breast tissue (gestagen effect), there is a significant reduction in proliferative breast disease. Oral contraceptive users can expect protection against ovarian cancer similar to that associated with childbearing, which may relate to "quiescence" of ovarian surface epithelium as a result of ovulation inhibition. Although the number of patients with positive gonococcal cultures of the cervix may not differ from non OCP users, the rate of clinical upper tract disease is lower, presumably because of decreased menstrual flow and/or alteration of cervical mucus.

28. C (2, 4), Pages 310, 312. Most elective pregnancy terminations (90%) are performed at 8 weeks' gestation or less by vaginal evacuation. This procedure can be carried out safely through 20 weeks of gestation.

Complication rates are higher for second trimester termination, especially those related to uterine perforation and excessive bleeding.

One quarter of all patients seeking pregnancy termination are married, although approximately one third of all abortion patients are under the age of 20. Abortion is the *least safe* method of birth control, although it is safer than actual childbirth or ectopic pregnancy.

29. A (1, 2, 3), Pages 270, 309. Despite research in hormonal male contraception, problems encountered include the lack of *selective* suppression of the major testicular functions, spermatogenesis and androgen production. Another disadvantage is the lag time preceding sperm-free ejaculation. It is thought that approximately 15–20 ejaculates are necessary to produce sperm-free ejaculates, since the testicle can store large numbers of mature sperm. With hormonal suppression of testicular function, the time for return to fertile status is variable, as are the number of normal sperm initially produced after the contraceptive interval.

No data exists as to whether male sexual function would be altered by hormonal contraception, although male contraceptive compliance will likely be limited because he is not the partner who becomes pregnant.

30. C (2, 4), Pages 285–287. Currently, it has been found that only OC users over the age of 35 who smoke or who have a preexisting vascular disease are at risk for developing cardiovascular disease. There is no evidence that long-term users have a higher incidence of atherosclerosis, despite some evidence that certain OC formulations lower HDL-cholesterol and raise LDL-cholesterol.

Death rates from myocardial infarction have, in fact, decreased during the past 15 years for women aged 20–45, despite the fact that OC use has increased dramatically.

31. A (1, 2, 3), Pages 303, 304, 306. The relative risk of ectopic pregnancy increases in IUD users because although the rate of tubal pregnancy is unchanged, the rate of intrauterine pregnancy is greatly reduced. With conception, the chance of an extrauterine pregnancy is increased tenfold.

Although there is no increase in congenital abnormalities or abnormal embryogenesis with IUD pregnancies, the spontaneous abortion rate is approximately tripled.

The occurrence of salpingitis in IUD users is less clear. Although overall rates are increased, this increase is most likely due to high rates during the first 4 months after insertion. Salpingitis beginning after this time is mostly likely caused by a sexually transmitted disease and not by the IUD itself.

32. **A** (1, 2, 3), Page 297; Table 11-13 (from Droegemueller). The incidence of all major adverse events with IUDs, including removal and expulsion, decreases with increasing age, and women over 35 have pregnancy rates less than 2% in the first 2 years of using the loop. Continuation rates are highest in older subgroups; younger women (under age 25) have the highest removal rate. Because many more are inserted for the first time in this age group (2753 vs. 1187), the overall woman-months of use is greater in the 15–24 age group than in the 35–49 age group.

33. **D** (4), Pages 300–301. The IUD does not affect ovulatory events, including those factors related to gonadotrophin production or endogenous ovarian production of sex steroids. The IUD does create a localized inflammatory response associated with increased local prostaglandin production, causing onset of menses to be slightly early, as well as an increase in the amount of menstrual blood lost.

CHAPTER 12

Rape, Incest, and Abuse

DIRECTIONS: Select the one best answer or completion.

1. A young woman was seen 2 weeks ago in the emergency room after a rape that occurred in her apartment. She was not injured physically. She now complains of difficulty sleeping, fear of being alone in her apartment, and withdrawal from her usual personal contacts. This behavior is
   A. paranoid and delusional.
   B. part of the rape-trauma syndrome.
   C. a manifestation of preexisting psychoses.
   D. an unusual response in the absence of physical injury.
   E. rapidly resolved by moving from her apartment.

2. You see a 22-year-old woman who has come alone to the emergency room after an alleged rape. Examination reveals no physical injury, and though there is evidence of recent coital exposure, she is calm, well-organized, and answers all questions regarding the incident. She states she is fine and wants to return to her apartment after all the information and appropriate tests are obtained. Of the following choices, which is the most appropriate action?
   A. Discharge her to return to the health care facility in 2 weeks.
   B. Give her an appointment to a qualified social worker in the next week.
   C. Have her see a qualified social worker before she leaves.
   D. Refer her to a local minister for counseling if she needs it.
   E. Ask her to call a friend to take her home.

3. You see an apparently healthy 28-year-old woman, who gives a history of recent loss of interest in men and demonstrates increasing anxiety as you question her about her feelings. She states she has become fearful and has a loss of self-esteem. She has numerous minor physical complaints that include pelvic pain, but there are no objective findings. Of the following, the most likely etiologic factor is
   A. recent loss of a loved family member.
   B. low grade pelvic inflammatory disease.
   C. drug reaction.
   D. AIDS-related complex.
   E. a recent history of sexual assault.

4. A 14-year-old is referred to you from a youth center. Her school grades have suddenly dropped, and she has run away from home and become involved in prostitution. She appears intelligent and healthy. Of the following, the most plausible explanation for her behavior is
   A. the excitement of street life.
   B. nymphomania.
   C. psychoses.
   D. incest.
   E. disenchantment with school.

5. A victim of a sexual assault sustained no injuries, did not acquire any STD, and did not become pregnant. She feels very guilty, however, and has lost self-esteem and confidence. Of the following, which is the most appropriate action?
   A. Assure her that over time all will be well.
   B. Reevaluate her for sexually transmitted diseases and normalcy of her pelvis to assure her that everything is all right.
   C. Provide professional counseling that attaches no blame to her.
   D. Point out that rape happens to a lot of women and they usually do well.
   E. Tell her that most women who are raped are asking for it and she should feel guilty.

6. A victim of an alleged rape is examined. The incident occurred approximately 8 hours ago. She states only vaginal penetration occurred. She is calm, has no injury, and has no motile sperm in her cervical mucus on examination. You should record
   A. that no recent intercourse took place.
   B. that no rape occurred.
   C. that the assailant probably wore a condom or had a vasectomy.
   D. that sperm "die" in 4 to 6 hours.
   E. the findings as you discovered them.

7. Studies of individuals who have had long-term incestual relationships in childhood have found that:
   A. Only a small percent (less than 10%) of them have abnormal psychosocial sexual development.
   B. Anxiety and psychosomatic complaints tend to get worse with time.
   C. Incestual relationships with siblings is more damaging than with parents.
   D. The closer the family member, the more damaging the incestual relationship.
   E. Most incestual relationships continue for years.
8. Which of the following history or physical finding would constitute sufficient evidence for you to make a diagnosis of rape on the patient's record when seeing her in the emergency room?
   A. Vaginal laceration
   B. Patient's statement that she was sexually assaulted
   C. Motile sperm in the vagina
   D. All of the above
   E. None of the above
9. When seeing an injured female in the office or emergency department, one should remember that many such patients are there as a result of domestic violence. What percentage of injured women seen in the emergency department are victims of battering?
   A. 1%
   B. 5%
   C. 10%
   D. 25%
   E. 40%
10. When you discover a case of marital, family, or elderly abuse, what is the most appropriate action?
    A. Notify the police.
    B. Have a stern talk with the abuser.
    C. Involve community social resources.
    D. Ignore the incident, as it will probably be resolved by the participants.
    E. Refer to a psychiatrist.
11. Which of the following has the highest annual rate?
    A. Child abuse
    B. Rape
    C. Abuse of the elderly
    D. Wife battering
12. Sperm will survive for the longest time in which anatomic site?
    A. Rectum
    B. Vulva
    C. Pharynx
    D. Vagina
    E. Endocervix
13. Forensic evidence in a case of possible rape should be
    A. submitted to the general hospital lab.
    B. given to the ER nurse.
    C. left in the emergency room "out" basket for routine collection.
    D. sent to the county police lab.
    E. handled according to a strict protocol that insures security.
14. The risk of pregnancy from a single random, unprotected coital exposure is approximately what ratio?
    A. 1 in 5
    B. 1 in 15
    C. 1 in 30
    D. 1 in 60
    E. 1 in 100
15. The legal definition of rape varies from state to state and must include which of the following?
    A. Force or threat of force
    B. Lack of mutual consent
    C. Penile penetration
    D. Presence of semen
    E. None of the above
16. How long does the reorganization phase of the rape/trauma syndrome usually last?
    A. A few hours
    B. A few days
    C. A few weeks
    D. A few months
    E. Many months
17. Cases of forcible rape resulting in injury requiring surgery and/or hospitalization occur in what percentage of victims?
    A. 1%
    B. 5%
    C. 20%
    D. 40%
    E. Greater than 50%
18. What is the recommended prophylactic treatment for sexually transmitted diseases after a rape?
    A. Benzathine penicillin
    B. Ampicillin
    C. Ampicillin and probenicid
    D. Penicillin with probenicid, followed by tetracycline
    E. Gentamicin and clindamycin

19. Prophylaxis against an unwanted pregnancy after rape is best achieved by
    A. performing a D&C
    B. inserting a progestasert IUD
    C. using DES, 25 mg b.i.d. for 5 days
    D. using ethinyl estradiol, 2.5 mg b.i.d. for 5 days
    E. using Ovral, 2 tabs every 12 hours times 2
20. Who is the most likely abuser of an elderly woman living with her family?
    A. An adult son or daughter
    B. A husband
    C. A sibling
    D. A social case worker
    E. A stranger who enters the home

DIRECTIONS: For each numbered item, select the one heading most closely associated with it. Each lettered heading may be used once, more than once, or not at all.

21–23. You see a suspected rape victim who is worried about several sexually transmitted diseases. Match the disease with the best method of its detection.
    (A) Culture on living cells
    (B) Serology
    (C) Culture in agar
    (D) Saline preparation
    (E) None of the above
21. Chlamydia
22. Syphilis
23. Hepatitis

DIRECTIONS: Each question contains four suggested answers of which one or more is correct. Choose the answer
    A if 1, 2, and 3 are correct
    B if 1 and 3 are correct
    C if 2 and 4 are correct
    D if 4 only is correct
    E if all are correct

24. The described phases of the rape trauma syndrome are divided into short-term and long-term. Manifestations of the short-term phase include
    1. physical symptoms.
    2. fear of normal situations.
    3. loss of emotional control.
    4. lifestyle changes.
25. You have been asked to give an inservice talk on sexual assault to the ER nursing staff. You can correctly inform them:
    1. Rape victims are basically promiscuous.
    2. Perpetrators of rape are commonly known to the victim.
    3. More than half of all rapes are reported.
    4. The very young, the handicapped, and the very old are especially at risk for sexual assault.
26. During an examination for alleged rape, no sperm are found on a vaginal wet mount. Which of the following exams are in order?
    1. Sample of the cervical mucus for sperm.
    2. Pap smear.
    3. Acid phosphatase concentration of the vaginal content.
    4. ABO typing of vaginal secretions.
27. Initial evaluation of a sexual assault victim who is seen in the emergency room should include
    1. general physical for serious or preexisting conditions.
    2. specific tests for common sexually transmitted diseases.
    3. examination for the possibility for existing pregnancy.
    4. collection of evidence for medical-legal purposes.
28. When seeing a woman with bizarre injuries, you suspect marital abuse. If that is true, sympathetic questioning may reveal that abuse is occurring. What else might be revealed?
    1. The woman is afraid that she will not be able to support herself if she leaves the marriage.
    2. The woman does not recognize the abnormal nature of her husband's behavior.
    3. The abuse has been repetitive over a long period of time.
    4. More than one member of the family is regularly abused.
29. An 82-year-old woman, apparently healthy, is seen with multiple circular sores on both her lower legs, which do not correspond to any physiologic pattern. You discover that she lives with her daughter and son-in-law and has recently become unable to control her urine. She seems confused and somewhat frightened in the strange emergency room surroundings. The differential diagnosis includes
    1. diabetic ulcers.
    2. bed sores.
    3. herpes zoster.
    4. domestic violence.

ANSWERS

1. **B**, Page 320. The rape-trauma syndrome is common in victims of rape, even in individuals who are in good mental health. It may take a long time to resolve the fear and distrust engendered by the rape event, even if no significant physical injury occurred.

2. **C**, Page 323. Although some rape victims will be extremely calm and controlled after the assault, they should always have the benefit of a knowledgeable person for counseling and support. Regardless of the victim's apparent calmness and control of the situation, they should not leave the health care facility without having a known and accessible support system available.

3. **E**, Page 320. The story is very suggestive of the silent rape reaction, manifested by a victim of sexual assault who has been psychologically traumatized, but who has not admitted, or resolved, the episode and is unwilling to tell you about it. She would probably tell you of a recent loss of a loved one, as such an occurrence carries no social stigma. Pelvic inflammatory disease should not be diagnosed without some objective confirmation. AIDS-related complex is a rare diagnosis in a low risk, apparently healthy woman in whom drug reaction is also unlikely. The latter can usually be resolved by history.

4. **D**, Pages 324–325. One should consider rape, incest, or drug abuse whenever you encounter a sudden change in behavior pattern in a teenager. Obviously many other factors could be responsible, but you should always ask straightforward questions about rape, incest, or drug abuse without moralizing.

5. **C**, Page 323. Many rape victims struggle with feelings that they are to blame and somehow caused the episode. They should be supported and counseled that they are the victim and are not responsible for the attackers behavior. Many of the victims need time and consistent support to overcome the feelings of guilt and self-blame.

6. **E**, Pages 322–323. In alleged rape cases it is important to record the findings and not make judgments either for or against rape. The patient's record is a medical-legal one and speculation has no place—including speculation on the possibility that the assailant used a condom or was azospermic. Sperm can "live" in midcycle cervical mucus for 3 to 5 days, although they usually "die" rapidly in vaginal secretions. Therefore it is important to get specimens from the cervical mucus.

7. **D**, Pages 324–325. Most incestual contacts appear to be of short duration, with only about 27% lasting more than a year. Approximately one third of the children who have an incestual experience feel it was detrimental. An equal number feel that it was neither positive or neutral. Generally, the more trusted the family member with whom it occurred, the more damaging the experience, but in most cases the impact fades with time. In any individual case, however, the effect is difficult to predict.

8. **E**, Pages 322–323. When examining a patient for alleged rape, the facts should be entered in the record, but the diagnosis of rape is a legal term, rather than a medical term, that should be decided in the courts.

9. **D**, Page 325. Studies have documented that up to 25% of injured women seen in ERs are victims of domestic violence. Interestingly, physicians treating these injured women made a diagnosis of domestic battering in only 3% of cases. They were often treated with pain medications or psychiatric referrals only.

10. **C**, Page 326. The physician not only should arrange for appropriate involvement of the community resources, but also should follow the family to be sure that appropriate action is and continues to be taken.

11. **C**, Page 326. There are an estimated 500,000 to 2.5 million cases of elderly abuse each year. This exceeds the number estimated, or reported, for the other forms of violence against the unprotected. One must anticipate that this will be an increasing problem with the rapidly rising number of elderly people. Accurate statistics are difficult to obtain because a large proportion of episodes are never reported or discovered. One must be aware of the possibility when interviewing elderly patients with strange behaviors and apparently irrational fears.

12. **E**, Page 322; Table 12–1 (from Droegemueller). The presence of motile or nonmotile sperm documents ejaculation. If motile sperm are found in the vagina, the ejaculation occurred within hours. Motile sperm may survive for several days in the endocervix.

13. **E**, Page 323. To be accepted in a court without question, a verifiable trail of responsible and secure transmission of forensic evidence is desirable. Such material should not be left unattended in an accessible area. Receipts for delivery should be obtained. Many emergency departments have a protocol for the transmission of such material, and one should follow the specified procedures. If there is no protocol, it would be wise to suggest that one be developed after consulting the statutes of the state in which you reside.

14. **C**, Page 322. A single random, unprotected coital exposure by a healthy woman will result in a 2% to 4% pregnancy rate. A major factor influencing the rate is the time of exposure during the menstrual cycle. Still, most women will not accept even a small possibility of pregnancy and wish to have prophylaxis to protect themselves from becoming pregnant.

15. **E**, Page 319. Rape is legally defined by the states, so you should be familiar with the specific definition in your locale. However, it generally is defined as sexual intimacy without consent, with or without penetration, and with or without

force. The inability to give appropriate consent by virtue of age or mental condition is deemed to be lack of appropriate consent. The presence of semen is not necessary.

16. **E**, Page 320. If a rape victim has the rape-trauma syndrome, the resolution phase involves long-term adjustment and reorganization of her (or his) life. This usually takes several months, and if not adequately addressed, it can persist for years. It should be considered when patients manifest unexplained anxieties, particularly in sexual areas.

17. **A**, Page 320. Although up to 40% of rape victims will have minor bruises, only a small number will have serious injury. However, it is important to document any bruising, even though it is minor, as this evidence is fleeting and may not be present at a revisit in 1 or 2 weeks. To painlessly outline epithelial injury that is not easily noted otherwise, one can apply gentian violet to the vulva and remove the excess with K-Y jelly. Fissures or breaks in the epithelium will retain the dye and become easily visible. This application and removal does not cause pain.

18. **D**, Pages 321–322. Prophylactic antibiotic treatment is given after a rape in an attempt to avoid infection with gonorrhea, chlamydia, or treponema pallidum. According to the 1985 STD treatment guidelines, the prophylactic treatment recommended after rape is tetracycline, 500 mg 4 times a day, or doxycycline, 100 mg b.i.d. for 7 days. Ampicillin, 3.5 g and 1 g of probenicid can be given to patients allergic to tetracycline or to pregnant women. Either regime may result in some antibiotic side effects. Often an antifungal preparation is beneficial in preventing vaginal yeast infection. Benzathine penicillin should not be used. Injections of antibiotics can be given, but they add to the patients' trauma and are generally best avoided.

19. **E**, Page 296, 322. Women worry greatly about pregnancy and sexually transmitted diseases after a rape. The efficacy of "morning after" therapy for pregnancy prevention is well known. The side effects are least from the Ovral, 2 tablets 12 hours apart for 2 doses. This treatment has a high rate of efficacy. Ethinyl estradiol and DES cause a lot of nausea. DES has a known teratogenic effect if a pregnancy does occur and is not interrupted. There is no reasons to further traumatize a rape victim by IUD insertion or a D&C. Another consideration is that progestasert IUDs are not readily available.

20. **A**, Page 326. Abuse of aging adults is becoming increasingly common and may be either physical or emotional abuse. The most common abuser is an adult child with whom the elderly person lives. If such a situation is suspected, community resources should be involved to remove the victim and counsel the abuser.

21. **A**, Page 321. Chlamydia is an obligate intracellular bacteria that must be grown on cell culture. It lacks the energy systems to survive on its own.

22. **B**, Page 321. Syphilis can be diagnosed by serology or dark field examination. Immediately after rape neither will be positive as it takes more than 10 days to develop a lesion that will yield treponema, which can be seen in dark field examination. Positive serology develops in 4 to 6 weeks. However, it is best to document that the victim has a negative serology at the time of the incident. Serology should be repeated 6 to 12 weeks later.

23. **B**, Page 321. Hepatitis screening is done to document seronegativity. The development of positive serology takes 1 to 3 months.

24. **A** (1, 2, 3), Page 320. Burgess and Holstrom (1974) described the rape-trauma syndrome. Their report was based on the response of 92 victims of forcible rape. Reactions were divided into two phases. The first is acute, or immediate, and last for hours or days. It is associated with disorganization of usual behavior patterns as well as emotional and somatic symptoms. Fear is common in both phases. The second phase is one of reorganization with a general decrease in symptoms and a return toward a normal function. During this phase, nightmares and fears of normal situations are common and may be difficult to resolve. Major lifestyle changes may be instituted, such as change of job or residence.

25. **C** (2, 4), Pages 319–320. Rape is done primarily to assert power, rather than to fulfill a sexual urge. People who are relatively helpless are therefore at higher risk. Rape occurs regardless of any provocation or inducement on the part of the victim. Although (and perhaps because) many victims know their assailants, rapes often are not reported, due to shame, guilt, fear of reprisal, or uncertainty as to how to proceed.

26. **E** (All), Pages 322–323. Sperm die and disintegrate rapidly in vaginal secretions. Therefore, cervical mucus sampling should always be done. Also, review of wet mounts may miss sperm that are present. Careful scrutiny of a pap smear gives one another chance to reveal the sperm if any are present. Men with vasectomy will not deposit sperm, but will ejaculate acid phosphatase secretions from the prostate and seminal vesicles. ABO typing may be useful if an ABO type is found that is other than the victim's. It would prove exposure to a different antigen, and may also be useful in determining identity of the assailant.

27. **E** (All), Pages 320–323. A general history and physical examination should always be done as it may reveal serious injury (in approximately 1% of rapes) and minor injuries (in up to 40% of rapes). Preexisting conditions should be sought and documented. Obtain cultures, serologic test for syphilis, and HCG to exclude the possibility of preexisting pregnancy or syphilis. Review of evidence for coitus will be important if the victim intends to prosecute the perpetrator. Recognition of trauma is also valuable.

28. **E** (All), Page 326. Marital abuse is more common than generally recognized. It frequently involves many family members, especially if it has gone on for a long time. Often the woman stays in the relationship because she does not recognize how abnormal it is, and she is more afraid of being alone than remaining in the relationship.

29. **D** (4), Page 326. If the sores are bizarre and not on pressure points or over areas of decreased blood supply or dermatomes, one should think of self-inflicted trauma or domestic violence. In this setting she may be receiving punishment for urinary soiling.

CHAPTER 13

Breast Diseases

DIRECTIONS: Select the one best answer or completion.

1. Which factor associated with benign breast disease is most closely associated with an increased risk of developing breast cancer?
   A. The degree of pain.
   B. The amount of nipple discharge.
   C. The size of the mass.
   D. The degree of epithelial hyperplasia seen microscopically on a biopsy specimen.
   E. The presence of a palpable axillary node.

2. The most commonly encountered cancer of the breast is
   A. lobular carcinoma in situ.
   B. ductal carcinoma in situ.
   C. lobular infiltrating carcinoma.
   D. ductal infiltrating carcinoma.
   E. inflammatory carcinoma.

3. Which of the following represents the clearest indication for open breast biopsy in a woman with known fibrocystic breast disease?
   A. A persistent, dominant three-dimensional mass on breast examination.
   B. Blood-tinged fluid on cyst aspiration.
   C. Lack of pain relief to premenstrual diuretic therapy.
   D. Spontaneous, unilateral nipple discharge.
   E. Multiple cystic areas seen on breast ultrasound.

4. A 52-year-old woman presents with persistent, unilateral, spontaneous bloody nipple discharge and a cluster of microcalcifications by xeroradiography 3 cm deep under the nipple of the left breast. What is the next step in her management?
   A. Needle aspiration under ultrasound guidance.
   B. Repeat mammography in 3 months.
   C. Submission of the bloody discharge for cytologic examination.
   D. Open biopsy of the left breast as an outpatient.
   E. CT examination of the breast and ipsilateral axillary nodes.

5. The drug showing the most efficacy in treating severe symptomatic fibrocystic disease is
   A. tamoxifen.
   B. danazol.
   C. bromocriptine.
   D. hydrochlorothiazide.
   E. medroxyprogesterone acetate.

6. All of the following are important variables in treatment selection of invasive breast cancer **except:**
   A. Microscopic assessment of axillary nodes.
   B. Histologic aggressiveness.
   C. Receptor status.
   D. Patient age.
   E. Extent of disease on mammography.

DIRECTIONS: For each numbered item, select the one heading most closely associated with it. Each lettered heading may be used once, more than once, or not at all.

7–10. (A) Digital radiography
   (B) Ultrasound
   (C) Thermography
   (D) Computed tomography
   (E) Magnetic resonance imaging

7. Best used in differentiating a cystic breast mass from a solid mass.

8. Can best differentiate benign from malignant tissue.

9. Radiation exposure one tenth that of conventional mammographic equipment.

10. Published clinical studies suggest low sensitivity and poor specificity.

11–13. (A) Fibrocystic breast disease
   (B) Fibroadenoma
   (C) Cystosarcoma phyllodes
   (D) Intraductal papilloma

11. Rapidly growing breast tumor occurring primarily in the fifth decade accounting for 1% of breast malignancies.

12. Predominant symptom is spontaneous, unilateral nipple discharge in perimenopausal women.

13. Most common breast tumor in adolescents.

14–16. (A) Hyperplastic phase of fibrocystic breast disease
(B) Mazoplastic phase of fibrocystic breast disease
(C) Adenosis phase of fibrocystic breast disease
(D) Cystic phase of fibrocystic breast disease

14. Usually occurs in women in their 40s and includes cysts of up to 5 cm in size.
15. Usually occurs in women in their 20s and characterized by pain in axillary tails.
16. Usually occurs in women in their 30s with a histologic picture showing marked ductal hyperplasia.

DIRECTIONS: For each numbered item, indicate whether it is associated with
A only (A)
B only (B)
C both (A) and (B)
D neither (A) nor (B)

17–19. (A) Radical Mastectomy
(B) Conservative surgery plus radiation
(C) Both
(D) Neither

17. Five year disease-free survival approximately 85% for stage I disease.
18. Treatment that enables bypass of primary chemotherapy if axillary nodes are tumor-free.
19. Additional chemotherapeutic or surgical castration indicated if this operation is performed.

20–22. (A) Xeromammography
(B) Screen film mammography
(C) Both
(D) Neither

20. Radiation dose to the breast is between 0.1 and 0.8 rad for two views.
21. Edge enhancement to see microcalcifications
22. Vigorous breast compression helps separate dense breast tissue for better detail.

DIRECTIONS: Each question contains four suggested answers of which one or more is correct. Choose the answer
A if 1, 2, and 3 are correct
B if 1 and 3 are correct
C if 2 and 4 are correct
D if 4 only is correct
E if all are correct

23. On palpation you find a 3 cm cystic mass in the upper outer quadrant of the left breast of a 38-year-old woman. Your plan is to aspirate this "cyst" in the office. What else should you do?
   1. Perform aspiration on newly detected breast masses before mammography.
   2. Tell the patient there is a probably malignancy if the fluid is bloody.
   3. Routinely submit the fluid for cytologic examination.
   4. Do nothing more if the fluid is clear and mass disappears after aspiration.

24. A 2 cm lesion is found by a woman of 54 who has been doing self breast examination (SBE) at monthly intervals for the past 4 years. Assuming the presence of breast cancer, true statements regarding this tumor include:
   1. It was not present at the age of 50 when she began SBE.
   2. It takes 6 to 8 years to reach the size of 1 cm.
   3. The average breast cancer will double in diameter every 6 months.
   4. There is a greater than 35% chance that this represents a clinical stage I cancer.

25. What are characteristics of fibrocystic breast disease?
   1. Clinical evidence can be found in approximately one third of all premenopausal women.
   2. There is cyclic enlargement of the axillary nodes.
   3. It represents an exaggerated response to cyclic ovarian hormones.
   4. It is found primarily in women with elevated serum prolactin levels.

26. In trying to implicate estrogen as a causative factor in the development of breast cancer, what facts have been noted about the risk of breast cancer?
   1. It becomes more common with advancing age.
   2. Higher risk occurs in obese women in the postmenopausal years.
   3. The risk is lower in women with bilateral oophorectomy before the age of 35.
   4. There is an increase in breast cancer rates of women who use postmenopausal replacement therapy.

27. In discussing the results of a mammogram (xeroradiography) in which an area of calcification has been identified, what would you tell the patient?
    1. Microcalcific clusters are more likely to be associated with breast cancer than with benign breast disease.
    2. Microcalcific cluster is better seen by xerography than by the screen film technique.
    3. You would order an ultrasound to confirm these findings.
    4. You would schedule a breast biopsy.
28. A 35-year-old has just learned that her mother has breast cancer. She is both concerned about her mother and at the same time worried about the possibility that she will develop the disease. What should you tell this woman?
    1. Because of the short latency, you will be able to give her more specific information in 3 years.
    2. Risk factors are additive.
    3. A specific pattern of genetic inheritance has been worked out.
    4. Risk factors identify only 25% of women who will eventually develop breast cancer.
29. What are the American Cancer Society guidelines regarding mammograms?
    1. Baseline mammogram for all women 35 to 40 years of age.
    2. Mammogram at 1 or 2 year intervals from 40 to 49 years.
    3. Annual mammogram for women 50 years or older.
    4. Mammogram twice annually for women with first-degree relatives with breast cancer.
30. Cyclic changes in breast tissue include
    1. parenchymal ductal proliferation.
    2. increase in breast volume.
    3. differentiation of alveolar cells into secretory cells.
    4. acinar prolactin production.

ANSWERS

1. **D**, Page 333. Symptomatology and physical findings may be similar in both benign breast disease and in breast cancer. Pain and tenderness, a mass, and nipple discharge are characteristics of both. Numerous epidemiologic studies have found that the risk of developing breast cancer is increased in women with benign breast disease with associated epithelial hyperplasia.
   Although the presence of a palpable axillary node in a patient with breast cancer worsens the prognosis, this finding alone, with no known malignant disease of the breast, does not indicate an increased risk for the future development of breast cancer.
2. **D**, Pages 348–349; Table 13-3 (from Droegemueller). There are numerous classifications of breast cancer that contain both clinical and pathologic subgroups. In general, this tumor is similar to other adenocarcinomas found in other female reproductive organs. It originates most often in the epithelium of the collecting ducts and less often in the terminal lobular ducts. Ductal infiltrating carcinoma is by far the most common cancer (80%) with infiltrating lobular carcinoma occurring in approximately 9%. Ductal carcinoma in situ is limited to the surface of the ductal epithelium with invasive cancer developing from this disease within 10 years of diagnosis in 35% of patients.
   Both variants of lobular carcinoma occur in a young age group, are less virulent, and have a longer latency period.
   Inflammatory carcinomas comprise approximately 2% of breast cancers. This type is recognized clinically as a rapidly growing, highly malignant carcinoma. Infiltration of malignant cells into the lymphatics of the skin produces a clinical picture that simulates a skin infection. There is not a specific histologic type.
3. **A**, Page 334. Although most symptomatic patients with fibrocystic breast disease respond to medical treatment, the presence of a dominant, three-dimensional mass that does not change mandates biopsy. When blood-tinged fluid is aspirated, it should be sent for histologic analysis. Biopsy is indicated if the histology is positive or if the mass does not disappear with aspiration. The approach would be similar for cysts seen on breast ultrasound. Spontaneous discharge alone does not necessarily warrant biopsy until further diagnostic assessments (such as mammography) are made. Lack of response to symptomatic treatment of symptoms likewise does not in itself warrant biopsy.
4. **D**, Pages 347–348. This patient has two indications for open breast biopsy—the presence of a spontaneous bloody nipple discharge and the presence of microcalcifications (cluster) on xeroradiography. The cluster itself creates approximately a 25% chance of cancer that needs to be diagnosed by thorough tissue evaluation. A positive needle biopsy alone is accepted in certain centers, but open biopsy is still required in most centers in the U.S. because needle biopsy shows a *false negative* rate of approximately 20%. Further imaging studies would not be useful in this patient prior to histologic evaluation.
5. **B**, Page 335. Danazol relieves breast symptoms *and* reduces nodularity in approxi-

mately 90% of patients. Depending on the age of the patients, this effect may last for several months following discontinuation of danazol, although symptoms eventually reappear. Tamoxifen, synthetic progestins, or bromocriptine may be beneficial in patients not responding to danazol. Diuretic therapy is often used for symptomatic treatment of women with mild to moderate premenstrual complaints associated with water retention. Some data indicate efficacy when using tamoxifen as adjunctive treatment for breast cancer. This medication may be used in situations where positive estrogen receptors are identified in malignant breast tissue.

6. E, Pages 349, 351–353. The three most important variables in treatment selection are the inherent histologic aggressiveness of the tumor, the presence of histologically positive nodes, and the receptor status (as another indicator of cell maturation). Microscopic metastatic disease occurs early via both hematogenous and lymphatic routes with approximately one third of women having positive histologic involvement of the nodes without gross adenopathy. It should be understood that breast cancer is to be considered a systemic disease at the time of diagnosis regardless of initial clinical presentation. In general, hormone receptor positive tumors are better differentiated and exhibit less aggressive clinical behavior with a 60% to 80% response rate to adjunctive hormonal manipulation when both estrogen and progesterone receptors are positive.

Because breast cancer should be considered a systemic disease, findings on mammography generally do not predict the type of treatment that patients should receive. This technique does not identify involvement of disease outside of the involved breast.

7–10. 7, **B**; 8, **E**; 9, **A**; 10, **C**; Pages 345–346. Certain characteristics of numerous screening and diagnostic tests available limit their usefulness and/or application to large-scale use.

Ultrasound may be useful when there is a need to differentiate a cystic mass from a solid mass, especially when an attempt to aspirate the mass has failed. However, it is limited by not being able to reliably identify microcalcifications or lesions smaller than 2 mm.

Thermography is both insensitive *and* nonspecific, so it is not recommended.

Digital radiography is the technique by which X-ray photons are detected after passing through the breast tissue. It will probably be the screening modality of the future, for it reduces radiation exposure to one tenth that of other radiographic techniques.

Magnetic resonance imaging is too cumbersome to be considered an effective screening measure, but it can differentiate benign from malignant tissue. It may prove effective as a diagnostic test in certain cases, such as predicting the extent of disease and recurrence.

11–13. 11, **C**; 12, **D**; 13, **B**; Pages 335–336. Cystosarcoma phyllodes are fibroepithelial tumors that usually arise from fibroadenomas. They are rare, but as they are malignant approximately 25% of the time, they constitute the most common type of breast sarcoma. This is in contrast to fibroadenoma of the breast, which is often found in teenagers as an isolated painless lump. The treatment of fibroadenoma is simple excision.

Intraductal papilloma is usually small (<2 mm) and often presents as spontaneous unilateral discharge in perimenopausal women. Further treatment is not necessary if malignancy has been ruled out by excisional biopsy.

14–16. 14, **D**; 15, **B**; 16, **C**; Page 334. The three phases of clinical fibrocystic breast disease are mazoplasia, adenosis, and cystic, and they correlate well with changes found in women in their third, fourth, and fifth decades of life. Each stage has associated histologic characteristics and symptomatology.

The histology of fibrocystic breast disease in general is characterized by proliferation and hyperplasia of the lobular, ductal, and acinar epithelium with accompanying fibrous tissue proliferation.

17–19. 17, **C**; 18, **C**; 19, **D**; Pages 352–353. Until 20 years ago, radical mastectomy was considered the standard operation for breast cancer because it enabled en bloc removal of the breast, contiguous tissue, and lymphatic drainage system. More recently, less mutilating operations have been advocated as a result of controlled studies which suggest similar disease-free survival rates of approximately 85% for patients treated by either radical or conservative surgical approaches for stage I disease.

The receptor status of a breast cancer will generally predict its response to hormonal manipulation during adjunctive treatment rather than dictate the type of *primary* surgical treatment. If axillary nodes are free of microscopic disease, either surgical treatment will suffice as the only primary treatment, although medical or surgical castration may be warranted as additional treatment depending on the receptor status of the tumor.

Current multicenter protocols for adjunct chemotherapy are being used to study the efficacy of chemotherapy when lesions beyond stage I are encountered, regardless of initial surgical approach.

20–22. 20, C; 21, A; 22, C; Pages 344, 345, 347. Xerograms are obtained by photoelectric image enhancement of selenium-coated aluminum plates. Two advantages of this technique are *wide recording latitude*, which emphasizes subtle differences in density of breast tissues, and *edge enhancement*, which improves visualization of microcalcifications. Both techniques use very low dose (0.1 to 0.8 rad) radiation for two views. It is estimated that this low dose will result in one excess breast cancer per year per one million women. Vigorous breast compression is used in both techniques so that there is maximal spreading of the dense breast tissue; this helps to identify microcalcifications and "hidden carcinomas."

23. D (4), Pages 346–347. Needle aspiration of breast pathology is a useful test intermediate between palpation of the breast and open biopsy. Although in young women (<35 years), needle aspiration of cysts may be done without mammography, in women over the age of 35, mammography should be performed first because needle aspiration might cause hematoma formation that would obscure mammographic detail. Aspirated fluid need not be sent for cytology if it is clear. In this event, the aspiration completes the work-up if the mass concomitantly disappears. Bloody fluid most often indicates a traumatic aspiration rather than the rare cystic carcinoma.

24. C (2, 4), Pages 339–340. The kinetics of growth in breast carcinoma suggest that it doubles in volume every 3 months and doubles in diameter every year. It usually takes 6 to 8 years before reaching a diameter of 1 cm. It takes another year before reaching 2 cm, which is the mean diameter of a breast cancer found through regular monthly SBE. When found by this technique, the cancer will be clinical Stage I 38% of the time.

25. B (1, 3), Pages 333–334. Fibrocystic breast changes represent an exaggerated response of the breast tissue to cyclic ovarian hormone production, and clinical evidence of this entity can be found in approximately one third of American women. Characteristic findings in these patients do not include demonstrable cyclic changes in the axillary nodes, although some women complain of pain radiating toward the axilla along the axillary tail of Spence.

Some have postulated that fibrocystic changes occur in the response to increased daily prolactic production, although there is no documentation that fibrocystic change occurs more commonly in women with elevated serum prolactin levels.

26. A (1, 2, 3), Pages 338–339. Many clinical studies suggest that the risk of developing breast cancer is related to the intensity and the duration of exposure to unopposed endogenous estrogen. This accounts for the increased incidence with age as well as the observation that if oophorectomy is performed before the age of 35, there is a reduction by 70% in the development of breast cancer. The relationship to obesity is less clear, although it is appreciated that the obese woman peripherally converts androgenic precursors into estrone at an increased rate; in addition, there are decreasing levels of sex hormone binding globulin.

Most studies of exogenously administered estrogens of any type fail to show an increased risk of developing breast cancer.

27. C (2, 4), Pages 344–345. The presence of five calcifications within the volume of one cubic centimeter is termed a *cluster*. Subsequent breast biopsies will find 25% of these to be associated with cancer and 75% with benign disease. Because of these observations, this finding should be more vigorously pursued by tissue confirmation. Because of better *edge enhancement* using xeromammography, microcalcifications are generally better seen using this technique. Microcalcifications are not seen well with ultrasound due to poor resolution of masses less than 2 mm.

28. C (2, 4), Page 337. Although there are a number of known risk factors for the development of breast cancer, the long latency period of the disease prior to clinical presentation makes the importance of identifying risk factors less helpful. At best, knowledge of risk factors identifies only 25% of women who get the disease. In the United States approximately one in 11, or 9%, of women can be expected to develop breast cancer.

Although familiar tendencies have been noted, no specific genetic inheritance pattern has been identified. A twofold to fourfold risk extends from the mother to first-degree relatives (daughters and sisters).

29. A (1, 2, 3), Page 343; Table 13–2 (from Droegemueller). Based on large-scale studies regarding the efficacy of mammographic screening programs (Health Insurance Plan of New York; Breast Cancer Detection Demonstration Project), and the development of sensitive low dose radiation techniques, the American Cancer Society suggests a baseline mammographic examination between ages 35 and 40; mammography at least every other year between the ages of 40 and 50; annual mammography for women age 50 and older. No specific guidelines were made for more frequent mammographic exam with available techniques because analysis of rate of tumor growth vs. sensitivity of current techniques did not support such recommendations.

30. **A** (1, 2, 3), Pages 332–333. Breast tissue responds to the cyclic hormonal changes of estrogen and progesterone production. During the follicular phase, there is parenchymal proliferation of the ducts, followed by dilation of the ductal system and differentiation of the alveolar cells into secretory cells during the luteal phase. Premenstrual breast symptoms are thought to be secondary to increased blood flow, vascular engorgement, and water retention resulting in increased breast volume. Although the breast secretory cells are sensitive to prolactin, none is thought to be produced locally in the breast tissue.

CHAPTER 14: Problems of Prenatal DES Exposure

DIRECTIONS: Select the one best answer or completion.

1. Clear cell adenocarcinoma appears to originate in a specific cell type within vaginal adenosis. This cell type is the
   A. endocervical cell.
   B. tuboendometrial cell.
   C. reserve cell.
   D. underlying stroma cell.

2. The origin of vaginal adenosis is thought to be columnar epithelium derived from the
   A. metanephros.
   B. yolk sac.
   C. wolffian ducts.
   D. vaginal plate.
   E. müllerian ducts.

3. A woman is known to have had an in utero exposure to DES. A cervical biopsy is taken from the most abnormal portion of the cervix as determined by colposcopic evaluation. Histologically this does not appear to be invasive. Analysis of the DNA content of the lesion indicates aneuploidy. What does this mean?
   A. Chromosomal content is double the haploid number, and the tissue is consistent with CIN I.
   B. Chromosomal content is abnormal, not an exact multiple of the diploid number, and the tissue is consistent with CIN III.
   C. Chromosomal content is double the haploid number, and the tissue is consistent with metaplasia.
   D. Chromosomal content is abnormal, being less than the haploid number, and the tissue is consistent with CIN II.
   E. Tissue is frankly malignant.

4. Assuming a normal initial pelvic examination in a DES-exposed woman, when should follow-up examinations be scheduled?
   A. Every month for a year, then every 3 months for a year, then every 6 months.
   B. Every 3 months for 2 years, then every 6 months.
   C. Every 6 months for 2 years, then every year.
   D. Every 6 months.
   E. Every year.

5. When should the initial pelvic examination for a DES-exposed woman be performed?
   A. After menarche or by the age of 12.
   B. After menarche or by the age of 14.
   C. After menarche or by the age of 16.
   D. After 18 years of age.
   E. When the individual becomes sexually active.

6. What are the cervicovaginal abnormalities, such as vaginal adenosis, associated with DES-exposure likely to do over time?
   A. Remain stable
   B. Become dysplastic
   C. Develop into a squamous carcinoma
   D. Develop into a clear cell adenocarcinoma
   E. Regress

7. Diethylstilbestrol-associated clear cell adenocarcinoma is a time-limited disease since this medication can no longer be used during pregnancy. When were FDA limitations placed on DES?
   A. 1941
   B. 1951
   C. 1961
   D. 1971
   E. 1981

8. A 30-year-old, whom you have been following with vaginal adenosis associated with in utero DES exposure, is planning to get pregnant. What should she have before becoming pregnant?
   A. A cerclage
   B. A hysterosalpingogram
   C. The adenosis ablated
   D. A laparoscopic examination
   E. None of the above

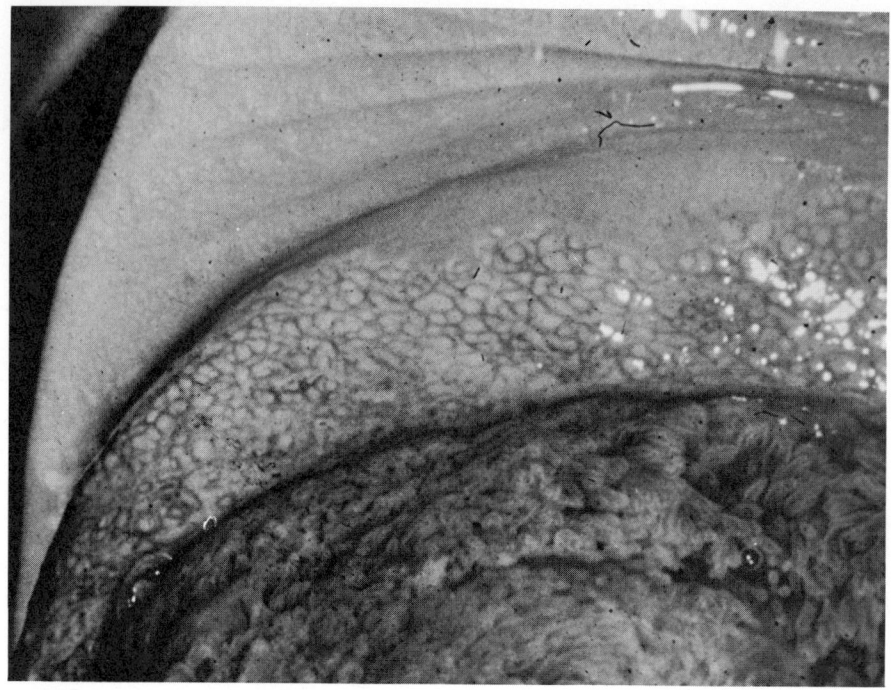

FIGURE 14-1.

9. What is the risk of developing a clear cell adenocarcinoma of the vagina and cervix in DES-exposed women?
   A. > 1/100
   B. 1/200
   C. 1/400
   D. < 1/500
   E. < 1/1000

10. The patient is a 32-year-old gravida 0 whom you saw for the first time 4 weeks ago. Because of the appearance of her cervix, you asked her to find out whether her mother had taken DES while "carrying her." The mother's physician forwarded his records. They indicate that he had prescribed 50 mg of DES per day from the 10th to the 20th week of pregnancy because your patient's mother had vaginal bleeding during early pregnancy.

    The pap smear that you obtained 4 weeks ago is negative (Class I). The patient states that she has had a pap every year for more than 5 years, and she has never had an abnormal one. Today, you use a colposcope and see the cervix as pictured in Figure 14-1.

    You would recommend

    A. a hysterectomy.
    B. a cold knife conization.
    C. a laser conization.
    D. four quadrant biopsies.
    E. that the patient return in a year.

11. The formula for Diethylstilbestrol is seen in
    A. Figure 14-2 A.
    B. Figure 14-2 B.
    C. Figure 14-2 C.
    D. Figure 14-2 D.
    E. Figure 14-2 E.

12. There is a strong statistical correlation between in utero DES exposure and
    A. oligomenorrhea.
    B. hypomenorrhea.
    C. female infertility.
    D. all of the above.
    E. none of the above.

13. Clear cell adenocarcinomas of the vagina and cervix associated with DES exposure are most likely to be diagnosed in patients in the
    A. group under 9 years of age.
    B. 9 to 14 year age group.
    C. 15 to 21 year age group.
    D. 22 to 28 year age group.
    E. group over 29 years of age.

FIGURE 14-2.

14. A 25-year-old gravida 0 DES-exposed female has a pap and biopsy diagnosis of CIN II of the cervix. The biopsies were obtained under colposcopic direction. Colposcopy was satisfactory. The appearance of the cervix is depicted in Figure 14-3.

   Acceptable care of this patient should include
   A. laser vaporization.
   B. cryotherapy.
   C. cold knife conization.
   D. trachelectomy.
   E. observation.

DIRECTIONS: For each numbered item, indicate whether it is associated with
A. only (A)
B. only (B)
C. both (A) and (B)
D. neither (A) nor (B)

   (A) Steroidal estrogen
   (B) Stilbene-type estrogen
   (C) Both
   (D) Neither

15. Constriction rings near the entrance of the fallopian tube
16. Cervical collar
17. Neural tube defect

   (A) DES exposure at 25 weeks
   (B) DES exposure at 10 weeks
   (C) Both
   (D) Neither

18. Duplication of a ureter
19. Smaller than normal endometrial cavity
20. T-shaped uterus

DIRECTIONS: Each question contains four suggested answers of which one or more is correct. Choose the answer
   A. if 1, 2, and 3 are correct
   B. if 1 and 3 are correct
   C. if 2 and 4 are correct
   D. if 4 only is correct
   E. if all are correct

21. Abnormalities that have been reported to occur in the DES-exposed male include
   1. abnormalities in the semen analysis.
   2. cryptorchidism.
   3. epididymal cysts.
   4. carcinoma of the testis.

22. Genital tract smears for cytologic examination should be obtained from any DES-exposed woman. At a minimum, smears should be taken from the
   1. ectocervix.
   2. vaginal fornices.
   3. endocervix.
   4. endometrial cavity.

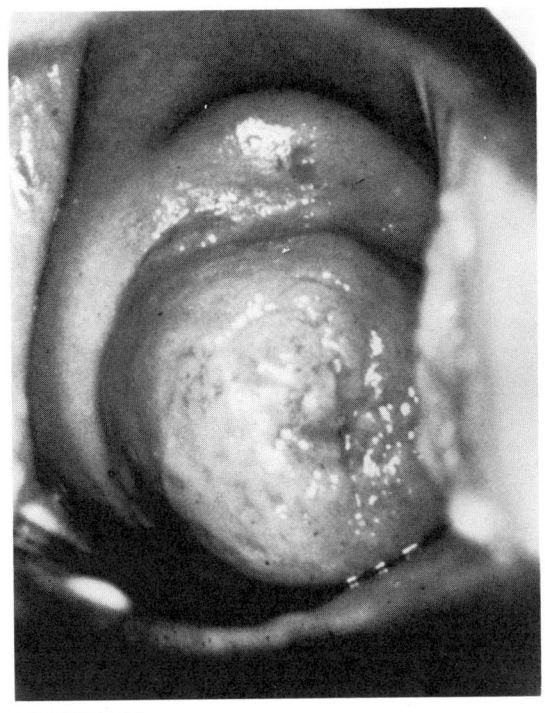

FIGURE 14-3.

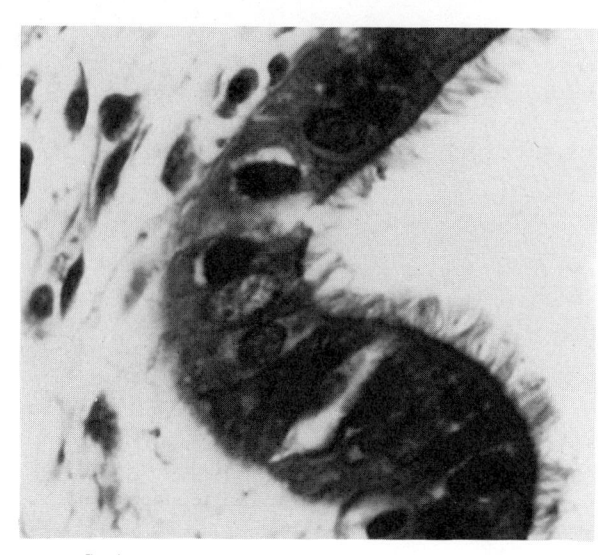

FIGURE 14-4.

23. Structural abnormalities of the cervix or vaginal fornices are not found in all women with an in utero exposure to Diethylstilbestrol. Factors that appear to increase the probability of a structural abnormality include a woman
    1. who has never been pregnant.
    2. who had her menarche at age 15.
    3. whose mother took more than 12,000 mg of Diethylstilbestrol during her pregnancy.
    4. whose mother started taking Diethylstilbestrol at 22 weeks of pregnancy.
24. A 27-year-old gravida 0, whom you have been following with a cervicovaginal ridge associated with an in utero DES exposure, is planning to get pregnant and seeks information. You would state that statistically she has a greater chance of
    1. aborting.
    2. having an ectopic pregnancy.
    3. delivering prematurely.
    4. not becoming pregnant.
25. Figure 14-4 is a photomicrograph of a biopsy specimen. It could have been taken from the
    1. fallopian tube.
    2. the vagina of a DES-exposed woman.
    3. endometrial cavity.
    4. the surface of a normal adult ovary.
26. A 20-year-old gravida 1, para 1, whom you have been following for vaginal adenosis due to in utero DES exposure, consults you for contraceptive advice. What would you recommend?
    1. A diaphragm.
    2. An intrauterine device.
    3. Condoms and foam.
    4. Oral contraceptives.
27. A 25-year-old gravida 0 is referred with a complaint of heavy vaginal discharge. The history includes known in utero exposure to DES.
    On examination the cervix appears as pictured in Figure 14-5 A. A sample of the vaginal discharge is placed on a slide and allowed to dry. It is then stained, as in Figure 14-5 B. What would you do next?
    1. Apply half-strength Lugol's solution.
    2. Prescribe appropriate antibiotic therapy.
    3. Perform colposcopy.
    4. Tell the patient she has a 50% chance of developing adenosis.
28. Which are synonyms for a cervicovaginal ridge?
    1. Collar
    2. Hood
    3. Pseudopolyp
    4. Cockscomb

ANSWERS

1. **B**, Page 363. The tuboendometrial cell of vaginal adenosis is believed capable of providing the origin of clear cell adenocarcinoma.

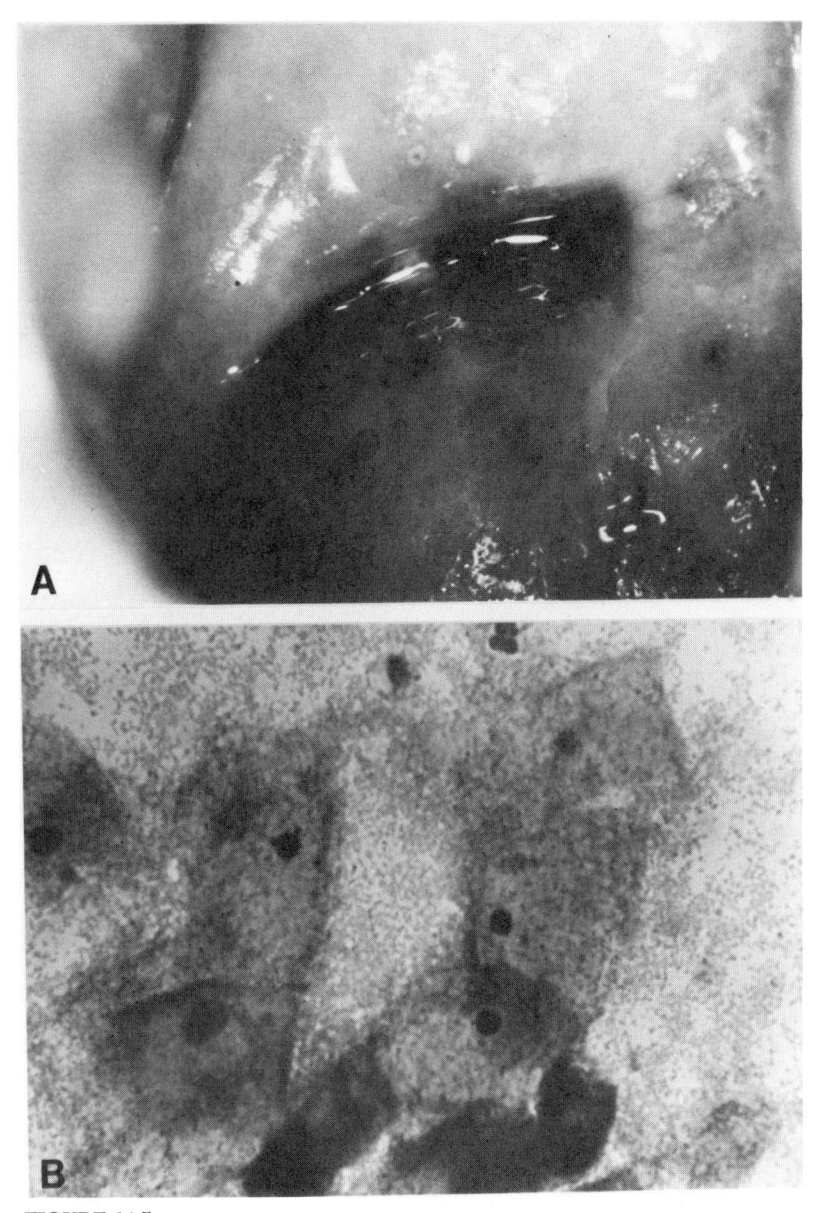

FIGURE 14-5.

2. E, Pages 369–371. Müllerian-derived columnar epithelium is replaced by a solid core of squamous epithelium that arises from the vaginal plate. The vaginal plate grows cephalad from the urogenital sinus, and the solid core of squamous epithelium ultimately canalizes to form the permanent lining of the vagina. In mice, when squamous transformation of columnar epithelium is arrested by estrogen treatment, persistence of müllerian-type columnar epithelium results in the upper vagina and cervix. In utero exposure to DES in humans may have a similar effect, that is, a DES-induced persistence of glandular epithelium in the vagina leading to adenosis.

3. B, Page 365. Tissues having a normal diploid (2N) distribution are "euploid" and normal. Polyploidy refers to the nuclear DNA measurement being increased by multiples of the diploid amount. Aneuploidy occurs when the DNA content reveals a wide distribution of intermediate modal values that differ from the diploid or polyploid ranges, and often a wide range of intermediate values are encountered. Metaplasia usually contains diploid values and occasionally some polyploid values. Tissues showing an aneuploid

distribution usually consist of CIN II, CIN III, or frank malignancy.
4. **E**, Page 363. The intervals for follow-up examinations depend on the findings as well as the completeness of the initial examination. Yearly intervals are adequate for most individuals.
5. **B**, Pages 363, 368. The initial examination of the DES-exposed woman is usually performed after menarche or by the age of 14 years unless abnormal bleeding or discharge necessitates a prior evaluation. Clear cell adenocarcinoma of the vagina is exceedingly rare before the age of 14.
6. **E**, Pages 363, 368, 372. Adenosis, ectropion, and cervicovaginal ridges heal spontaneously in many but not all DES-exposed females. The risk of developing clear cell adenocarcinoma in the DES-exposed female 24 years of age or younger is between 0.14 and 1.4 per 1000.
7. **D**, Page 369. Insofar as clear cell adenocarcinomas developed in the DES-exposed females through their 20s and early 30s, the cancers will continue to be diagnosed for a number of years, since DES usage in pregnancy is known to have continued, albeit on a limited basis, until 1971.
8. **E**, Pages 367–368. Cerclage is not indicated as an interval procedure. In fact, it only should be considered during pregnancy in patients who have undergone midtrimester losses. Indications for cerclage are no different than if the woman had not been exposed to DES. Although there may be an increased risk for an unfavorable outcome in DES-exposed females with an abnormal hysterosalpingogram, the results of the examination have not been correlated with any individual or specific adverse pregnancy outcome. Routine hysterographic evaluation of DES-exposed females is, therefore, not warranted. Ablation of the adenosis could destroy a large portion of the reproductive tract. Unless it is associated with dysplasia or malignancy, it is not indicated. In view of the higher rates of ectopic pregnancy among the exposed, some structural or functional alteration of the fallopian tubes appears likely. This is generally not recognized by laparoscopic examination.
9. **E**, Pages 364, 368, 369, 373. The risk of clear cell adenocarcinoma of the vagina and cervix is increased in DES-exposed women, but these tumors occur in less than 1 per 1000 exposed.
10. **E**, Page 363. This woman's age places her at low risk for DES-associated changes. In this case the figure is of a "mosaic" pattern in a hood surrounding the cervix of a DES-exposed woman. Figure 14-1 depicts a heavy mosaic pattern (histologically proven metaplasia) in a hood surrounding the cervix of a DES-exposed offspring (from DiSaia PJ, Creasman WT: Clinical gynecologic oncology, 2nd ed. St. Louis, the C.V. Mosby Company, 1984, p.58). Squamous metaplasia may give rise to an atypical-appearing transformation with areas of "mosaicism" and "punctation," findings that often suggest the presence of intraepithelial neoplasia in the *unexposed* female. However, in the DES-exposed offspring such changes often indicate the presence of active squamous metaplasia rather than a dysplastic process. Colposcopy does allow for the careful evaluation of the transformation zone in the DES-exposed woman and provides a guide for biopsy sites in individuals whose pap smears indicate atypia of the squamous cells. In this case, with known negative pap smears for 5 years, it would be reasonable to do nothing and see the patient in 1 year. The first time that a DES-exposed woman is examined, however, it is not unusual to want to biopsy areas with a colposcopic "mosaic" pattern. That is not the same as performing four quadrant biopsies.
11. **A**, Page 359. Both A (diethylstilbestrol) and B (dienestrol) are members of the stilbene group and differ only in the location of double bonds. Vallestril, C, is a napthalene. D is TACE, tri-p-anisylchloroethylene, and E is ethinyl estradiol.
12. **E**, page 366. Case control studies have had conflicting findings in regard to menstrual abnormalities and infertility. Some reports suggest a correlation between oligomenorrhea, hypomenorrhea, and infertility and DES exposure. Other studies have not.
13. **C**, Page 368. Clear cell adenocarcinomas are extraordinarily rare before age 14. Then there is a rapid rise in the age-incidence curve that plateaus at about age 19, followed by a drop to lower levels through the 20s.
14. **A**, Pages 360, 365. Figure 14-3 depicts a vaginal hood (from Robboy SJ, Scully RE, Herbst, AL: J. Reprod. Med. 15:13, 1975). Local destruction of the entire area of intraepithelial neoplasia is important. In the cervix, laser treatment can be utilized, and occasionally local surgical therapy in the form of conization is indicated. Although cryotherapy has been used extensively and successfully to treat intraepithelial neoplasia of the cervix in the unexposed woman, it has been reported to be followed by cervical stenosis in many DES-exposed women. For that reason, this modality of therapy should be avoided if possible. Trachelectomy, cervicectomy, is unwarranted in a young woman without any children. It represents undertreatment for a

malignant process and overtreatment for a benign one.

15–17. 15, **B**; 16, **B**; 17, **D**; Page 371. A constriction ring near the entrance of the fallopian tube and a cervical collar have been associated with DES exposure. Ingestion of steroidal estrogens during pregnancy has not been reported to be associated with such changes. Neither DES nor steroidal estrogen use has been reported to increase the incidence of a neural tube defect.

18–20. 18, **D**; 19, **B**; 20, **B**; Page 366. DES exposure does not appear to cause anatomic abnormalities of the urinary tract. Various types of abnormalities of the shape and size of the endometrial cavity have been identified on hysterosalpingograms performed on women who were exposed to DES in utero prior to 22 weeks.

21. **A** (1, 2, 3), Page 371. Cryptorchidism, hypoplasia of the testis, and more frequent epididymal cysts, as well as abnormalities in semen analyses, have been described in DES-exposed males. The testicular and semen changes have not been verified by some studies. An increased incidence of testicular cancer has not yet been reported. If cryptorchidism is verified, however, one would expect an increased incidence of carcinoma since cryptorchidism is a risk factor.

22. **A** (1, 2, 3), Page 363. When examining a DES-exposed woman, cytologic samples are obtained from the vagina, including the fornices, as well as from the ectocervix and the endocervical canal.

23. **A** (1, 2, 3), Page 361; see Jeffries JA, Robboy SJ, O'Brien PC, et al: "Structural anomalies of the cervix and vagina in women enrolled in the Diethylstilbestrol Adenosis (DESAD) Project." *Am J Obstet Gynecol* 148:59, 1984. Factors that appear to increase the frequency of structural changes of the cervix and vagina include nulligravidity and a late menarche. The dosage of DES and time started during pregnancy are important interrelated factors. A larger dosage of the drug or initiation of treatment early in pregnancy leads to a greater risk of adenosis.

24. **A** (1, 2, 3), Page 367. Unfavorable pregnancy outcomes, including premature live birth, ectopic pregnancy, and nonviable birth, have been reported more commonly among DES-exposed females. Although reproductive performance in DES progeny has been associated with an increased proportion of unfavorable outcomes, over 80% of DES women who desire pregnancy have delivered at least one live-born infant.

25. **A** (1, 2, 3), Pages 359, 360. Figure 14-4 is a photomicrograph of vaginal adenosis (from Herbst AL, ed: Intrauterine exposure to diethylstilbestrol in the human. Washington, DC, American College of Obstetricians and Gynecologists, 1978). The columnar epithelium of vaginal adenosis usually contains various cell types. One type resembles the epithelium of the endocervix, another contains cells that are similar to the epithelium of the endometrium and/or fallopian tube. The surface of the adult ovary does not contain ciliated cells.

26. **E** (All), Pages 365–366. No data indicate that any contraceptive method, including oral contraceptive steroids, is contraindicated in the DES-exposed female. There has been concern regarding the potential increased risk of endocrine-related tumors. In spite of these concerns, no current evidence indicates increased risk of these types of malignancies associated with the use of estrogen-containing compounds. Also, there has been concern about prescribing an intrauterine device because of the abnormal contours of the endometrial cavity that have been demonstrated on hysterosalpingogram. It has not yet been demonstrated, however, that the intrauterine device causes excessive risk for the DES-exposed female. The issue of an IUD might become academic since they are likely to become unavailable.

27. **A** (1, 2, 3), Pages 363, 372. Figure 14-5 depicts a normal cervix. Colposcopy and staining the vagina with half-strength Lugol's solution is part of the routine examination of a patient with known DES exposure. Vaginal adenosis occurs in about one third of DES-exposed females. The smear contains clue cells. Thus, the patient should be treated.

28. **E** (All), Page 358. A cervicovaginal ridge is a structural change in the cervix and/or upper vagina of DES-exposed females. It is also called a hood, cockscomb, pseudopolyp, or collar.

CHAPTER 15

Abortion

DIRECTIONS: Select the one best answer or completion.

1. A 23-year-old gravida 4, para 1, ab 3 registered for prenatal care. The patient's first pregnancy, 5 years ago, went to term. She delivered a 3000 g male. This was followed by spontaneous abortions at 8, 16, and 14 weeks. She did not remember the date of her last menstrual period and you obtained an ultrasound yesterday. Dates from this exam place the pregnancy at 14 weeks. Given this information at the time you are reviewing the ultrasound, depicted in Figure 15-1, the mostly likely explanation is
   A. in utero DES exposure.
   B. progestin ingestion during early pregnancy.
   C. a previous D&C which was traumatic.
   D. a previous cone biopsy.

2. A 40-year-old has a spontaneous abortion at 14 weeks of gestation. Previously, she had three normal pregnancies by a different husband. Her youngest child is 10 years of age. Given this information, it is most likely that
   A. the husband has an abnormal karyotype.
   B. the wife has an abnormal karyotype.
   C. the abortus is trisomic.
   D. the abortus is a mosaic.
   E. the abortus is euploidic.

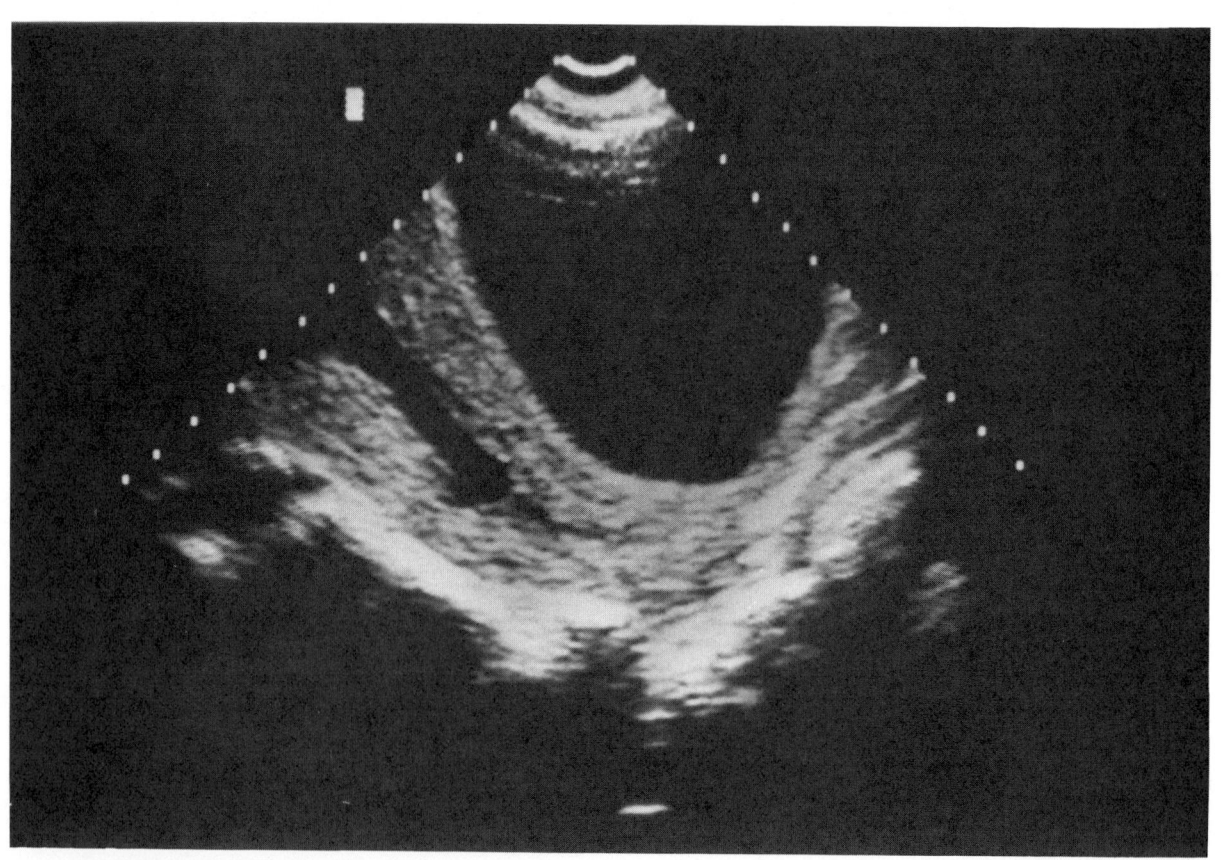

FIGURE 15-1.

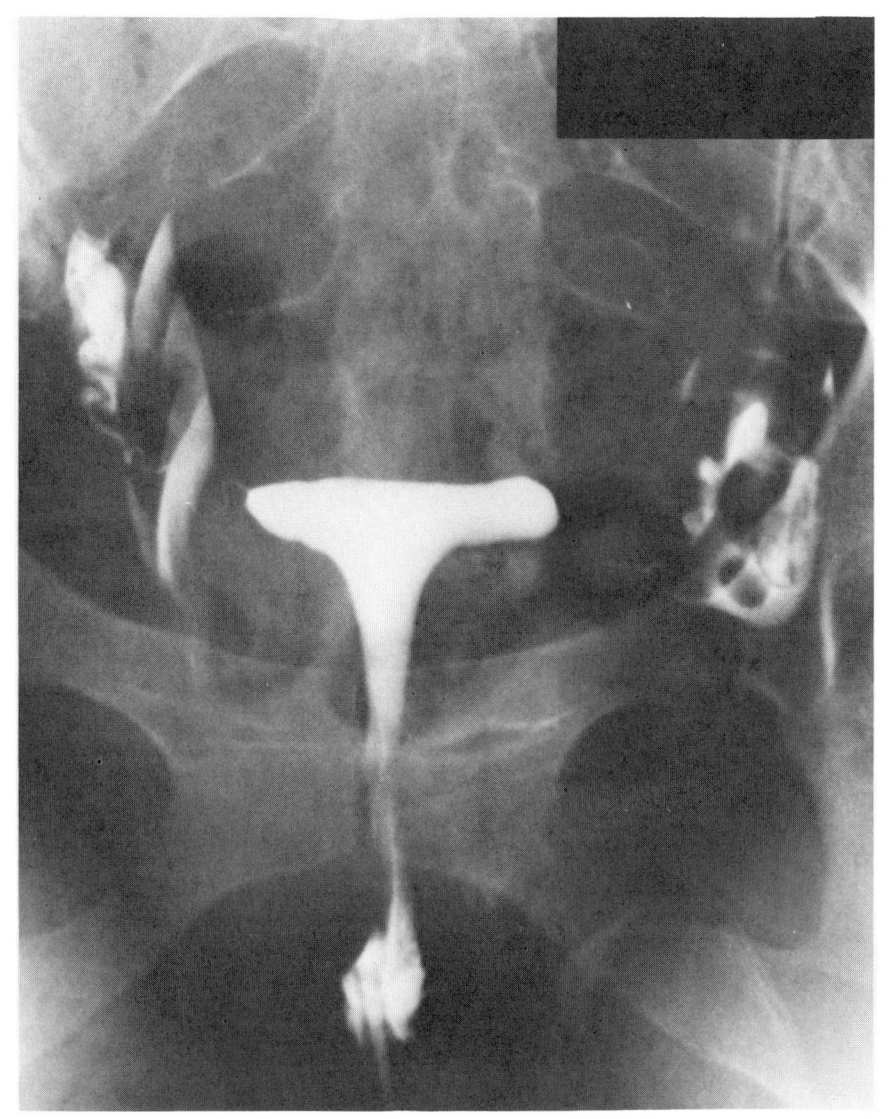

FIGURE 15-2.

3. An immunologic etiology for repetitive abortions is
   A. well established.
   B. suggested by the fact that couples with repetitive abortions have less sharing of more than one HLA at the A, B, and DR locus than a control population.
   C. suggested by the observation that this population has an increased amount of maternal blocking factor.
   D. highly unlikely because of the protective effect of progesterone.
   E. controversial. Some studies support such an etiology and others refute findings in the supporting study.
4. Lupus anticoagulant has been found in the circulation of women with
   A. lupus erythematosus.
   B. a variety of collagen vascular diseases.
   C. a history of recurrent thrombotic episodes.
   D. all of the above.
   E. none of the above.
5. A gravida 3, para 0, ab 3 has just had a hysterosalpingogram which is shown in Figure 15-2. While discussing this finding, you are told that the patient had an in utero DES exposure.
   Appropriate management should include
   A. Strassman metroplasty.
   B. Jones metroplasty.
   C. Tompkins metroplasty.
   D. uterine cerclage.
   E. none of the above.

6. A patient is 10 weeks pregnant by dates corroborated by sonography. Fetal heart activity is about 140 beats per minute. This woman had a serum HCG drawn 2 days ago because of significant vaginal bleeding, and this is reported back as 8800 mIU/ml. The patient denies any pain, and her bleeding has stopped. Given this information, you would tell the patient that
    A. all is well.
    B. if she carries beyond the 20th week, in all probability she will deliver at term.
    C. she is not at increased risk of having an anomalous child.
    D. in all probability she will abort.
    E. she is at greater risk for having an abruptio placentae in the third trimester.
7. The most common genetic cause of fetal loss is due to errors in
    A. maternal gametogenesis.
    B. paternal gametogenesis.
    C. fertilization.
    D. zygote division.
    E. implantation.

DIRECTIONS: For each numbered item, select the one heading most closely associated with it. Each lettered heading may be used once, more than once, or not at all.

Incidence of embryonic loss
    (A) 1% to 2%
    (B) 15% to 20%
    (C) 25%
    (D) 40%
    (E) 60%
8. Clinically recognized abortions
9. Total human embryonic loss before 12 weeks
10. Incidence of clinical abortions per week from weeks 5 to 12
    (A) Figure 15-3 A
    (B) Figure 15-3 B
    (C) Figure 15-3 C
    (D) Figure 15-3 D
11. Greatest incidence of spontaneous abortion
12. Metroplasty by the Strassman technique

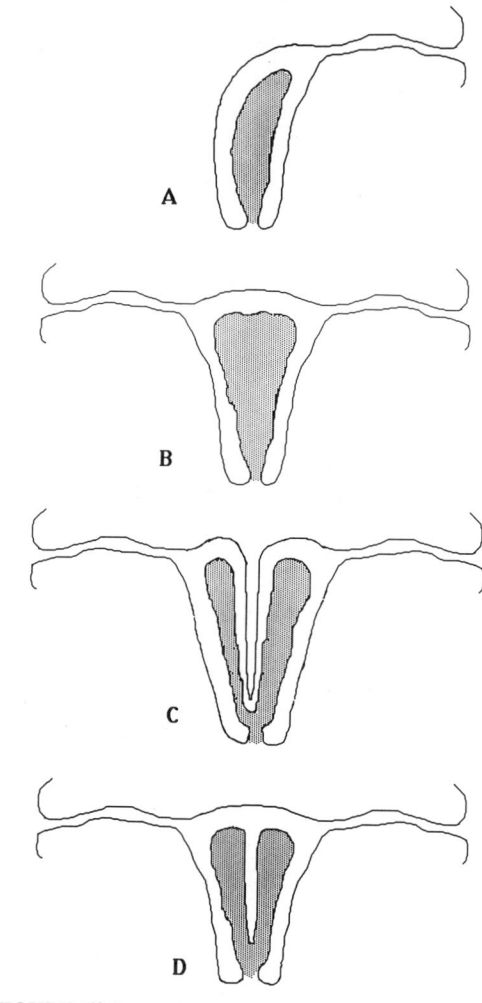

FIGURE 15-3.

DIRECTIONS: For each numbered item, indicate whether it is associated with
A. only (A)
B. only (B)
C. both (A) and (B)
D. neither (A) nor (B)

    A. Increased likelihood of abortion of chromosomally normal fetus.
    B. Increased likelihood of abortion of chromosomally abnormal fetus
    C. Both
    D. Neither
13. A woman who smokes 2 packs per day
14. A woman who has had GI series and IVP at about the time of implantation
15. A woman who imbibes an alcoholic beverage on an average of 3 times a week

DIRECTIONS: Each question contains four suggested answers of which one or more is correct. Choose the answer
A. if 1, 2, and 3 are correct
B. if 1 and 3 are correct
C. if 2 and 4 are correct
D. if 4 only is correct
E. if all are correct

16. Which modalities are acceptable in the treatment of a Rh negative patient with an inevitable or incomplete abortion?
    1. Oxytocin
    2. Curettage
    3. Iron sulfate
    4. Anti-D gamma globulin

17. An 18-year-old and her 20-year-old husband want an explanation for the fact that they have no live-born children. She has a history of two previous spontaneous abortions at 8 and 10 weeks. The last abortus was submitted for karyotype and was 45X. Which statements would be appropriate to share with this couple?
    1. The survival rate of 45X conceptions is about 1 in 300.
    2. This is the second most common **single chromosomal** abnormality found in abortus material.
    3. The karyotype of this abortus is associated with a younger maternal age.
    4. Another abortus with this karyotype is likely.

18. Worldwide, random, sporadic, spontaneous abortions associated with chromosomal abnormalities have been associated with
    1. conceptions occurring in the spring.
    2. advanced paternal age.
    3. abortions occurring before 6 weeks of gestational age (defined as from the LMP to the time of abortion).
    4. advanced maternal age.

19. Women who have repetitive abortions are more likely than individuals who have aborted once to
    1. abort after rather than before 12 weeks gestation.
    2. have a chromosomally normal abortus.
    3. have an uterine or cervical etiology.
    4. undergo emotional trauma after the abortion.

20. An 18-year-old gravida 1, para 0, on examination is noted to have blood coming through her closed cervix. Her LMP was 8 weeks ago, and the uterus is 6 weeks size. A β-HCG is positive. To her knowledge, she has not passed any tissue.
    Diagnostic considerations include
    1. ectopic pregnancy.
    2. inevitable abortion.
    3. threatened abortion.
    4. complete abortion.

21. A 30-year-old moved to the United States from India 5 years ago. She has never had a live-born infant, and she has tried to become pregnant for 8 years. She thinks she aborted on at least two occasions 6 years ago when she was 4 to 6 weeks late for her period. She showed her doctor the material she passed, and he assured her that she had aborted, but there was no histologic proof. For the last 5 years, her periods have been very scant and infrequent. She denies pelvic pain or dysmenorrhea. She does have premenstrual tension, but it is not severe enough to require medication.
    Her physical exam is completely normal. Her pelvic exam is also normal. The uterus is normal sized, anterior, and smooth. The ovaries are easily palpated. There is no pain.
    Which procedures do you anticipate will establish the most likely reason for her infertility?
    1. Hysterosalpingogram
    2. D&C
    3. Hysteroscopy
    4. Laparoscopy

22. A 23-year-old is 4 weeks late for her menstrual period. She did start spotting yesterday. You obtain a serum β-HCG that is 3770 mIU/ml. What should the differential diagnosis include **at this point**?
    1. An ectopic
    2. A normal pregnancy
    3. A threatened abortion
    4. A persistent corpus luteum

23. Which organisms are associated with septic abortion?
    1. *Escherichia coli*
    2. Group B beta-hemolytic streptococci
    3. *Bacteroides* species
    4. *Clostridium perfringens*

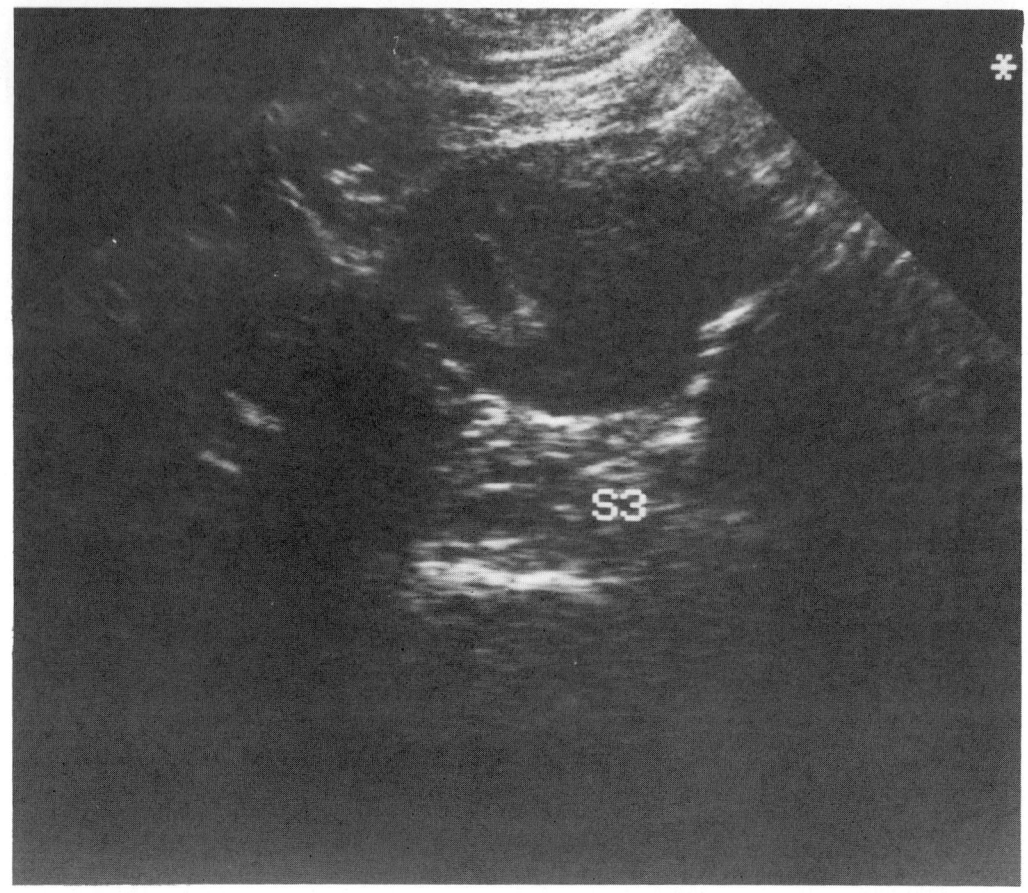

FIGURE 15-4.

24. Patients with systemic lupus erythematosus who have circulating lupus anticoagulant have an increased likelihood of aborting. It is postulated that this immunoglobulin is responsible for the abortion by
   1. promoting the activation of prothrombin by the prothrombin activator complex.
   2. decreasing platelet adhesiveness.
   3. causing complete fetal heart block.
   4. decreasing prostacyclin formation.
25. Luteal insufficiency is an entity that has been associated with repetitive pregnancy loss. Theoretically, this diagnosis can be associated with
   1. low levels of HCG.
   2. normal levels of serum progesterone.
   3. administration of a synthetic progestin.
   4. low levels of serum progesterone.
26. A 26-year-old gravida 2, para 1, is 14 weeks pregnant by dates. On pelvic examination the uterus felt smaller than you would have anticipated. A representative image of the ultrasound that you ordered is depicted in Figure 15-4. This patient should have
   1. an immediate determination of her serum fibrinogen level.
   2. her karyotype determined.
   3. a quantitative serum β-HCG level.
   4. an immediate D&C.
27. The management of a septic threatened abortion in 1987 should include
   1. single agent antibiotics.
   2. an intraarterial line.
   3. corticosteroids.
   4. uterine evacuation.

28. A 33-year-old gravida 4, para 0, ab 4 is now 8 weeks pregnant. On ultrasound a gestational sac containing a fetus of appropriate size is visualized. Cardiac activity is recorded at 140 beats/minute. Although the patient has bled for 3 days, a source is not seen on this scan. A serum β-HCG level is at the mean for 8 weeks. The patient states that she is currently staining 6 to 7 pads a day. She doesn't have any cramps.

    Your management would include
    1. thyroid replacement.
    2. absolute bed rest.
    3. progesterone suppositories.
    4. iron replacement.

29. A young couple with a history of repetitive abortions and a limited income is trying to decide how much of an investigation they can afford. You suggest parental chromosomes. The likelihood
    1. that either has an abnormal karyotype is greater than 10%.
    2. is greater that the maternal rather than the paternal karyotype is abnormal.
    3. is greater that an X chromosome mosaicism of the father, rather than the mother, is apt to be revealed.
    4. is that if an abnormality is uncovered, it is a translocation.

Questions 30–32

30. In counseling a woman about the possibility of a spontaneous abortion in a subsequent pregnancy, it would be important to know that she
    1. has had 3 previous abortions.
    2. is 35 years of age.
    3. has one living child.
    4. is Asian.

31. In order to determine the relative risk of another abortion and suggest management options, it also would be important to know that she
    1. is married to a 55-year-old.
    2. is a controlled insulin-dependent diabetic.
    3. aborted 1 month ago.
    4. spontaneously aborted her first pregnancy at age 16.

32. Assume all eight of the above statements were true. With this information, you should
    1. ask her to delay her attempt to get pregnant for 3 months.
    2. obtain serum thyroxine.
    3. request maternal chromosomes.
    4. obtain a serum progesterone 3 days before the expected period.

ANSWERS

1. **C, Page 385.** The ultrasound depicted in Figure 15-1 is a longitudinal view through the pelvis. One can see a well-filled bladder and the lower uterine segment and cervix. Since there is fluid in the cervical canal itself, the diagnosis is highly suggestive of an incompetent cervix. The woman is so young that DES exposure is not too likely. Furthermore, no mention of findings associated with DES is given in the short history. Progestin treatment has not been associated with an incompetent cervix. It is likely that with the first abortion a D&C was performed. Although conization can cause cervical incompetence, this operation is not described in the history.

2. **E, Page 381.** Based on medically verified abortions with tissue, the peak incidence of euploid abortions (chromosomally normal abortuses) is about 12 to 13 weeks of gestation; the peak incidence of aneuploid abortions is about 11 weeks. Even in cases of repetitive abortion, the incidence of an abnormal parental karyotype is less than 10%. In this case, it is even less likely. The incidence of chromosomally normal abortions increases markedly after a maternal age of 35 years, rising to more than 30% after age 40. The finding of a chromosomally normal abortus does not mean that there is not an abnormality at the gene level.

3. **E, Pages 381–382, 389.** An immunologic etiology for repetitive abortions is not well established but controversial in 1987. There are conflicting studies. Some studies suggest greater sharing of more than one HLA antigen at the A, B, and DR locus, while one study found no difference between couples with a history of repetitive abortion and normal controls. An immunologic etiology would be supported by a decreased rather than an increased maternal blocking factor. This factor, the circulating IgG antibody, coats the foreign fetal antigens and prevents the fetus from being rejected. Some protection of the fetus from an immunologic effect is provided by progesterone. This neither supports nor refutes the immunologic etiology.

4. **D, Page 389.** Lupus anticoagulant has been found in women with systemic lupus erythematosus as well as in those with other connective tissue diseases. It has been found in women with a history of recurrent thrombotic episodes as well as in women with no other disease process. About 50% of women with lupus anticoagulant have a false positive serologic test for syphilis. Lupus anticoagulant is found in a subset of women with recurrent abortions.

5. **E, Page 384.** No therapy has been shown to be beneficial in lowering the abortion rate in women exposed to DES who have abnormal-

ities of the uterine cavity (as illustrated in Figure 15-2) and recurrent abortion.

6. **D**, Pages 392, 402. There is no evidence that women with gestational bleeding who do not abort have an increased incidence of complications of pregnancy, but they may have a slightly increased incidence of fetal anomalies and preterm birth. A poor prognosis for pregnancy is associated with a serum HCG level less than 10,000 mIU/ml in a woman with a threatened abortion in the first trimester of pregnancy after the seventh week.

7. **A**, Page 379. Twenty-six percent of all fetal loss is due to errors of maternal gametogenesis, 5% to errors of paternal gametogenesis, 4% to errors of fertilization, and 4% to errors of zygote division.

8–10. 8, **B**; 9, **E**; 10, **A**; Pages 376, 400. The rate of human pregnancy loss is relatively high. Ova are not fertilized or fail to cleave or implant. Then, there are the recognized clinical abortions which equal 15% to 20% in most series. The total human embryonic loss before 12 weeks is estimated to be 60% to 70%. About 80% of abortions occur in the first trimester, with the incidence decreasing with increasing gestational age. The incidence of clinical abortion is relatively stable at 1% to 2% per week from weeks 5 to 12 and steadily declines thereafter.

11-12. 11, **A**; 12, **C**; Page 383. Figure 15-3 A is a unicornuate uterus, B is a normal uterus, C is bicornuate uterus, and D is a septate uterus. The unicornuate uterus is associated with the greatest incidence of spontaneous abortion, about 50%. This is higher than the 25% to 30% reported with either a septate or bicornuate uterus. A bicornuate uterus can be unified using the Strassman technique. Either a transfundal metroplasty, as described by Jones or Tompkins, or a transcervical hysteroscopic resection of the uterine septum are the methods used to correct a septate uterus. Surgical corrections should not be considered if the woman has never aborted and should not be performed until other causes of abortion have been ruled out.

13–15. 13, **A**; 14, **D**; 15, **A**; Pages 390–391. In one study, for women who smoked more than 14 cigarettes per day, the risk of having an abortion was 1.7 times greater than for women who did not smoke. There was no increased risk of an aneuploid abortion in smokers. There is little likelihood that irradiation of less than 5 rads (several times greater than the amount used in all diagnostic procedures listed) will cause an abortion in the human, even if it is administered during the time of implantation. The risk of abortion is threefold normal with daily ingestions of alcohol, and twofold greater in women who drink at least 2 days a week. Just as with smokers, the risk of abortion is confined to chromosomally normal embryos.

16. **E** (All), Page 396. A patient with an inevitable or incomplete abortion should receive intravenous oxytocin. The uterus should be emptied by gentle, complete sharp or suction curettage. This can often be done on an outpatient basis. It is important not to be too vigorous since intrauterine adhesions are a possible complication. The evacuation should be complete to minimize the chance of a septic abortion. Since there is always loss of a significant amount of blood, these patients should receive iron supplementation following the curettage. If the patient is Rh negative and the father Rh positive or Rh unknown, the woman should receive 50 micrograms of anti-D gamma globulin. Some physicians will place the patient on a 2 or 3 day regimen of ergonovine maleate after the D & C.

17. **B** (1, 3), Page 380. The survival rate of 45X conceptions is about 1 in 300. This is the **most common single** chromosomal abnormality found in abortus material. The most common **type** of chromosomal abnormality is an autosomal trisomy. There is evidence that monosomy 45X is associated with a younger maternal age than other aneuploid or euploid abortions. Karyotypes of abortuses of women who have had more than one abortion tend to be similar to the first if the first abortus was either normal or an autosomal trisomy.

18. **D** (4), Pages 379–381. Various surveys have revealed no seasonal variability in the incidence of any type of chromosomal abnormality in abortions. There is also no effect of paternal age. Some authorities, but not all, have suggested a slight increase in the number of live births with aneupoidy with a father whose age is 55 or greater. Single gene defects such as achondroplasia are more common with advanced paternal age. In one series the greatest prevalence of chromosomally abnormal abortions occurred at 9 weeks of gestation and gradually decreased thereafter. The failure to detect more chromosomal abnormalities earlier may be artifactual, as the success of karyotyping by culture is less likely if an embryo is not present, and the frequency of empty gestational sacs is greatest in abortions of 8 weeks or less. Maternal age is directly related to the incidence of trisomies, mainly in the D and G group. Advanced maternal age has no effect on the incidence of the other chromosomal anomalies in abortions.

19. **E** (All), Page 397. Women with recurrent abortions have a tendency to abort later in gestation, with two thirds of such abortions occurring beyond 12 weeks of gestation. The abortuses of women who have three or more abortions are more likely to be chromosomally normal (80% to 90%) than those of women with a single spontaneous abortion. If the cause of repetitive abortion is found, it is

likely to be associated with a uterine or cervical problem such as a müllerian fusion anomaly, leiomyomata, intrauterine adhesions, or cervical incompetence. With recurrent abortion the emotional trauma is magnified, and the physician needs to express sympathy and understanding as counseling is performed and a diagnostic regimen is outlined.

20. **B** (1, 3), Page 375, Chapter 16. With an ectopic pregnancy there is often vaginal bleeding. The β-HCG is usually positive and the uterus less than 8 weeks in size. An inevitable abortion is uterine bleeding from a gestation of less than 20 weeks accompanied by cervical dilation but without expulsion of any placental or fetal tissue through the cervix. A threatened abortion is the presence of any uterine bleeding from a gestation of less than 20 weeks without any cervical dilation or effacement. A complete abortion is the spontaneous expulsion of all fetal and placental tissue from the uterine cavity before 20 weeks of gestation.

21. **A** (1, 2, 3), Pages 386–387. This woman has a history that is compatible with intrauterine adhesions. The cause is not clear, but perhaps she contracted genital tuberculosis, which is still encountered in India. Adhesions in the uterine cavity can cause partial or complete obliteration of the endometrium, leading to menstrual abnormalities and amenorrhea as well as being a cause of abortion. The best means of diagnosis is hysteroscopy. The problem may be strongly suspected at the time of D&C and can be diagnosed by hysterosalpingogram.

22. **B** (1, 3), Pages 392–393. A β-HCG of 3770 mIU/ml is not compatible with a pregnancy of 8 weeks. The patient could have an unruptured tubal pregnancy. She should be evaluated by serial β-HCG, sonography, and/or laparoscopy. By definition this cannot be called normal, because the patient is bleeding; however, a significant number of these patients will go on to have a normal pregnancy. Patients with a persistent corpus luteum do not have detectable β-HCG.

23. **E** (All), Page 395. A septic abortion is usually polymicrobial, with *Escherichia coli* and aerobic gram-negative rods frequently involved. Group B beta-hemolytic streptococci, anaerobic streptococci, *Bacteroides* species, and on occasion *Clostridium perfringens* are other organisms that can cause this problem.

24. **D** (4), Page 389. It is thought that abortion occurs because of thrombosis in the placental blood supply. Abortions associated with this disease often occur during the second trimester. The antibody interferes with prostacyclin formation, leading to a relative excess of thromboxane A_2, thus causing a thrombotic tendency. There is interference with the activation of prothrombin by the prothrombin activator complex. Decreased platelet adhesiveness is a feature of von Willebrand's disease and is implicated in bleeding, not abortion. The fetus of a mother with systemic lupus erythematosus not infrequently has a complete heart block. It is unlikely that this is the cause of the increased rate of spontaneous abortion in patients with systemic lupus erythematosus.

25. **E** (All), Pages 387–388. Some investigators have reported luteal deficiency to occur in as many as one third of women with recurrent abortion, whereas others have reported it to be an infrequent cause of abortion. Maintenance of the endometrium for the first 7 weeks of gestation depends on progesterone produced by the corpus luteum. The function of the latter depends on HCG produced by the trophoblast. When progesterone secretion from the corpus luteum is lower than normal or the endometrium has an inadequate response to normal circulating levels of progesterone, endometrial development may be inadequate to support the implanted blastocyst and may lead to spontaneous abortion. Synthetic progestins are luteolytic. There is no evidence that their administration corrects luteal insufficiency. It has even been suggested that their use may contribute to the problem.

26. **D** (4), Pages 380, 395. The ultrasound is diagnostic of a blighted ovum or a missed abortion. One can see a large gestational sac but not a fetal pole. A quantitative β-HCG is unnecessary. Likewise, with only one pregnancy loss, a karyotype is not cost effective. The incidence of hypofibrinogenemia is uncommon in gestations of less than 14 weeks.

27. **D** (4), Pages 396, 397. Patients with a septic abortion should receive combination antibiotics, including an agent that will be effective against anaerobic bacteria. Newer antibiotics such as Imipenem may become an exception to this rule. The uterine cavity should be evacuated to provide drainage of the infected material. This may be accomplished surgically or medically. An intraarterial line may be preferred if the patient develops septic shock, but is unnecessary in the case of a septic abortion without shock. Likewise, corticosteroids are not indicated in this patient and their use in septic shock is controversial.

28. **D** (4), Pages 387–388, 395. Thyroid and progesterone have not proven effective in preventing an abortion. The presence of vaginal bleeding in some cases is the first sign of uterine evacuation of an already nonviable conceptus. The administration of a progestin may increase the probability of having a missed abortion. There is no evidence that bed rest is of value. Should she abort, the longer the patient is in bed, the greater the

emotional and possibly even the financial loss to the family. Iron replacement is indicated in women who are bleeding, especially when there is a good chance that there will be a significant blood loss.

29. **C** (2, 4), Page 380. A maternal and paternal karyotype is an accepted part of the workup of a couple with repetitive abortions. The yield is not large, however. More than 90% of couples in this category are chromosomally normal. The most common abnormal finding is a maternal abnormality, a balanced translocation. If the karyotype is abnormal, mosaicism in one of the parents (usually X chromosome mosaicism of the mother) is a frequent finding.

30. **A** (1, 2, 3), Pages 376, 378, 400. See answer 31.

31. **B** (1, 3), Pages 376–378, 388–389. When talking to a woman contemplating pregnancy, it is important to know facts about previous pregnancies. In this case the woman has a history of repeated pregnancy wastage. The risk of a pregnancy terminating in a spontaneous abortion increases with increasing maternal and paternal age. For women with no live births and a reproductive history of three prior pregnancies terminating in abortion, the chance of having an abortion in a subsequent pregnancy is about 50%, whereas women with at least one live birth and three spontaneous abortions only have a 30% chance that the next pregnancy will terminate in abortion. In the last 25 years, the incidence of a spontaneous abortion in a diabetic, when she is controlled either by diet or by insulin, is the same as the general population. If conception occurs within 3 months after a prior live birth, the incidence of abortion is increased compared to the relatively stable rate if conception occurs later than 3 months.

32. **B** (1, 3), Pages 376, 380, 387–388. If conception occurs within 3 months after a prior live birth, the incidence of abortion is increased compared to the relatively stable rate if conception occurs after 3 months. Although older studies indicate that hypothyroidism may be a cause of abortion, there is no definitive evidence that hypothyroidism is a cause of abortion in humans. Furthermore, a better screening test is a serum TSH. Some 90% of couples who have two or more spontaneous abortions are chromosomally normal. That means that obtaining both maternal and paternal chromosomes in cases of repetitive abortion will be fruitful in roughly 10% of cases. Several investigators have reported that in conception cycles the midluteal peak progesterone levels in the circulation are always greater than 9 ng/ml. Serum progesterone 3 days before menses will be close to the nadir for that cycle.

CHAPTER 16: Ectopic Pregnancy

DIRECTIONS: Select the one best answer or completion.

1. An 18-year-old is seen in the emergency room. She is 5 weeks late for her period. She is sexually active and has used foam irregularly for contraception. At the time you see her, her BP is 90/60 and her pulse 110. She is receiving Ringer's lactate. The intern has performed a culdocentesis and obtained 15 ml of nonclotting blood. A ELISA assay for HCG is negative.
   You would
   A. admit and observe.
   B. obtain a sonogram.
   C. repeat the culdocentesis.
   D. obtain a radioimmunoassay for HCG.
   E. perform a laparotomy.

2. What is the overall subsequent conception rate in women with an ectopic pregnancy?
   A. 30%
   B. 40%
   C. 50%
   D. 60%
   E. 70%

3. Of women with an ectopic pregnancy the number that have a subsequent live birth is about
   A. 1/4.
   B. 1/3.
   C. 1/2.
   D. 2/3.
   E. 3/4.

4. At the time of diagnosis, in patients with a ruptured tubal pregnancy
   A. less than half will have blood in the peritoneal cavity.
   B. the culdocentesis will be positive 40% to 50% of the time.
   C. blood obtained by culdocentesis has previously clotted and thus will not clot.
   D. blood obtained by culdocentesis will have a hematocrit of less than 15%.
   E. most of the blood found in the peritoneal cavity is of fetal origin.

5. The finding of nonclotting blood on culdocentesis is
   A. indicative of tubal rupture.
   B. present in more than 75% of patients with a ruptured ectopic pregnancy.
   C. only seen when signs of peritoneal irritation are present.
   D. incompatible with upper abdominal pathology.
   E. important in supporting the diagnosis of cervical ectopic pregnancy.

6. Women with ectopic pregnancies should receive Rh(D) immunoglobulin if they are
   A. Rh negative, antibody negative.
   B. Rh negative, antibody positive.
   C. Rh positive, antibody negative.
   D. Rh positive, antibody positive.
   E. Du positive, antibody negative.

7. In cases where a salpingectomy is the treatment of choice for a ruptured tubal pregnancy
   A. the ipsilateral ovary should also be removed.
   B. the contralateral ovary should also be removed.
   C. both ovaries should be removed.
   D. both ovaries should be preserved if at all possible.
   E. wedge excision of the ipsilateral ovary should be performed.

8. With currently available equipment for abdominal ultrasonography, the visualization of a "fetal" mass or embryonic sac in the oviduct can be accomplished in what percentage of patients with tubal pregnancies?
   A. $\geq 75\%$
   B. 66–75%
   C. 46–65%
   D. 26–45%
   E. $\leq 25\%$

98 *General Gynecology*

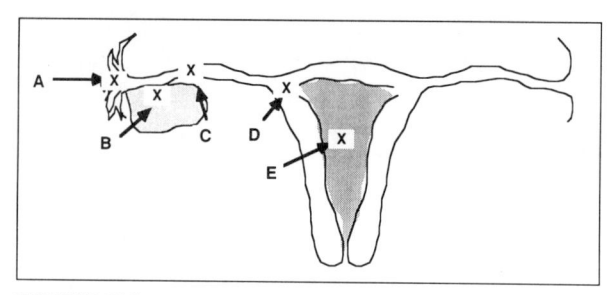

FIGURE 16-1.
Sites of implantation.

DIRECTIONS: For each numbered item, select the one heading most closely associated with it. Each lettered heading in Figure 16-1 may be used once, more than once, or not at all.

9. Associated with the highest morbidity
10. Most common location of ectopic gestations
11. Location of less than 1% of ectopic gestations
12. Most common location for implantation in women wearing IUDs
13. Most common location for implantation for a conception following an ectopic pregnancy
14. Associated with "tubal abortion"

DIRECTIONS: For each numbered item, indicate whether it is associated with
A. only (A)
B. only (B)
C. both (A) and (B)
D. neither (A) nor (B)

(A) β-HCG
(B) Progesterone
(C) Both
(D) Neither

15. Responsible for the decidual change in the endometrium
16. Generally reduced in ectopic as compared to intrauterine pregnancies at 8 weeks
17. Doubles about every 2 or 3 days in early intrauterine gestations
18. Responsible for the Arias-Stella reaction

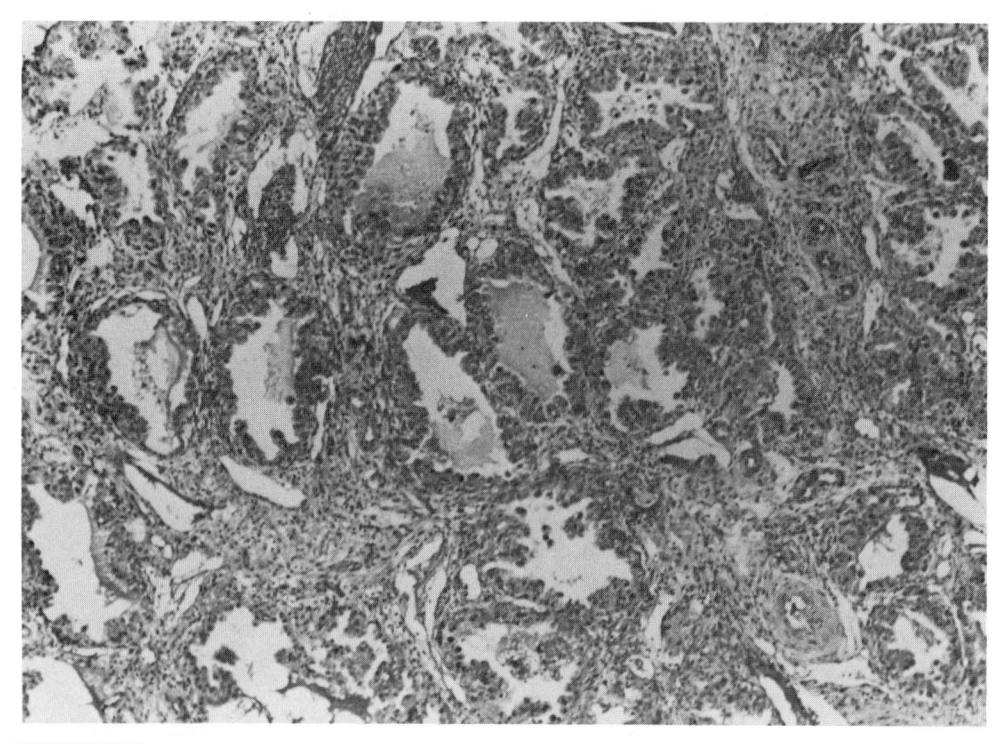

FIGURE 16-2.

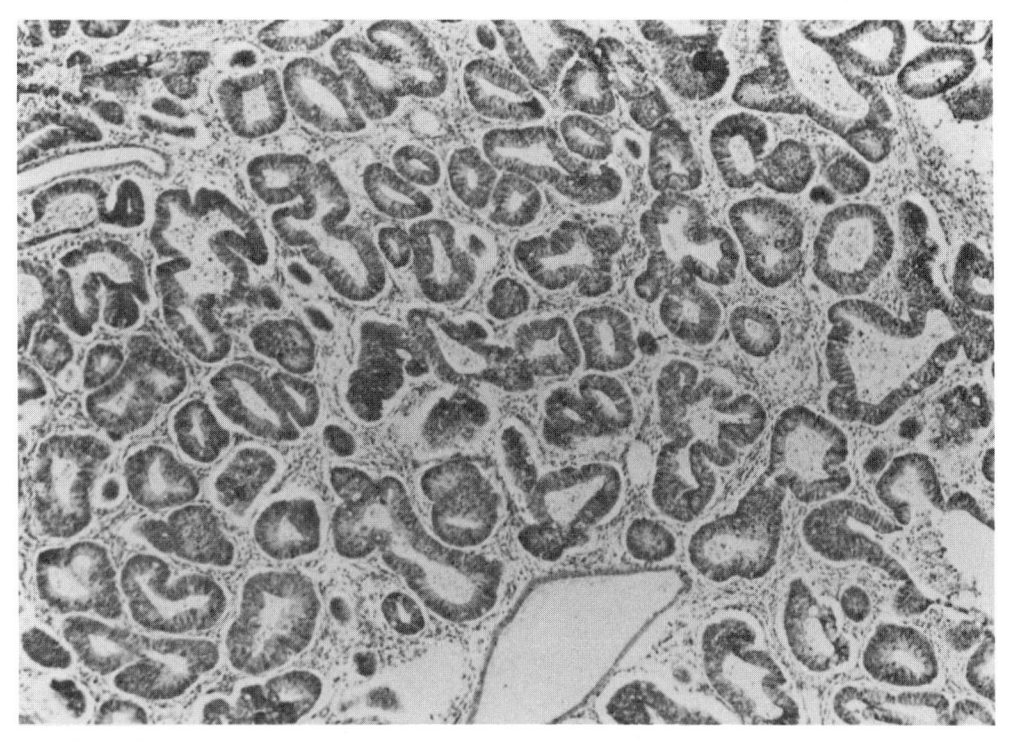

FIGURE 16-3.

19–21. Associated with
   A. An intrauterine pregnancy
   B. An extrauterine pregnancy
   C. Both
   D. Neither

19. See Figure 16-2.
20. See Figure 16-3.
21. See Figure 16-4.

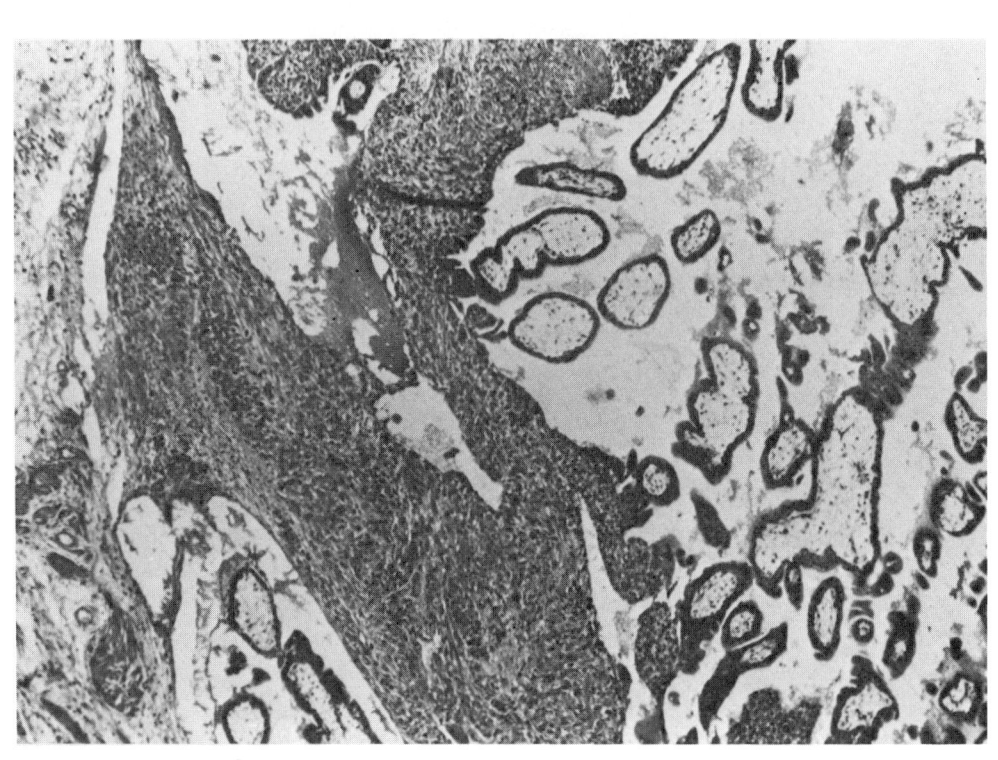

FIGURE 16-4

100   General Gynecology

DIRECTIONS: Each question contains four suggested answers of which one or more is correct. Choose the answer
- A. if 1, 2, and 3 are correct
- B. if 1 and 3 are correct
- C. if 2 and 4 are correct
- D. if 4 only is correct
- E. if all are correct

22. Which symptoms are found in more than half of the patients with diagnosed ectopic pregnancies?
    1. Abdominal pain
    2. Amenorrhea
    3. Vaginal bleeding
    4. Passage of decidual tissue

Questions 23 & 24

23. A 30-year-old has been on a progestin-only oral contraceptive agent. She is now 1 week late for her period, which usually is predictable at 28 days. A pregnancy test, UCG-Beta Slide, is weakly positive. The sonogram is pictured in Figure 16-5.

    Your differential diagnosis includes
    1. an ectopic pregnancy.
    2. an early intrauterine pregnancy.
    3. a blighted ovum.
    4. a delayed period.

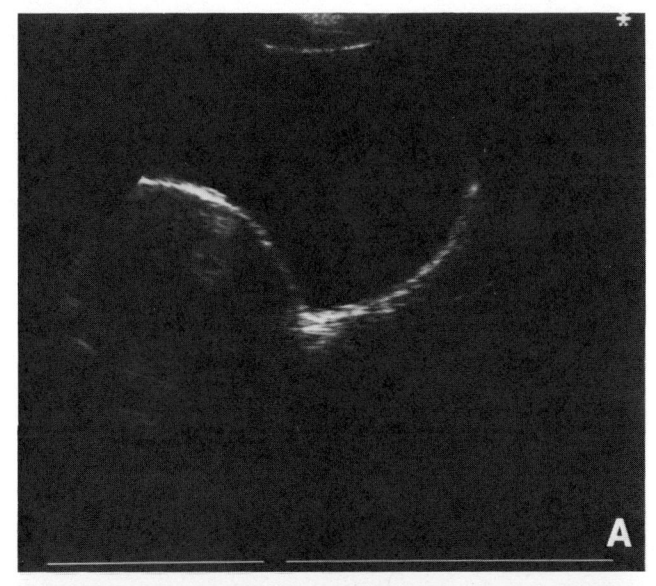

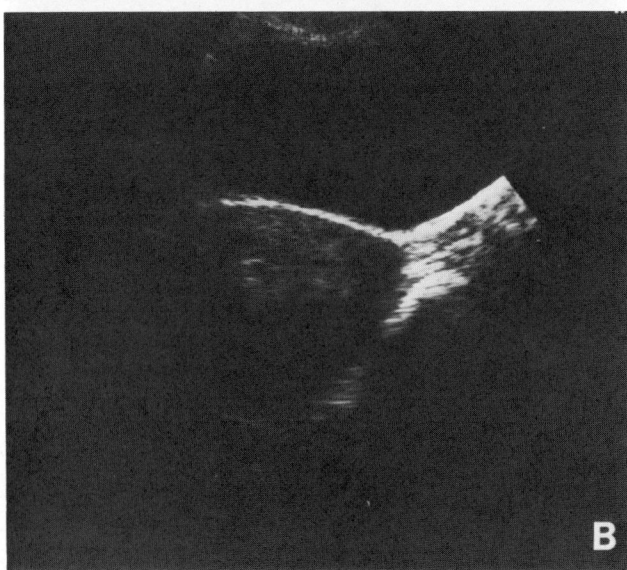

FIGURE 16-5.

24. A radioimmunoassay for HCG is obtained and reported to be 800 mIU/ml. A second test is performed 72 hours later. This time the value is 1200 mIU/ml. A sonogram is repeated. The picture is not changed. The patient sees you a day later, 96 hours after the first visit.
    Your updated differential diagnosis is
    1. an ectopic pregnancy.
    2. an early intrauterine pregnancy.
    3. a blighted ovum.
    4. a delayed period.
25. Factors that contribute to or cause death from ectopic pregnancy in more than half the cases include
    1. false positive culdocentesis.
    2. physician delay and misdiagnosis.
    3. anesthetic complications.
    4. blood loss.
26. You are an expert witness. The plaintiff, a 35-year-old woman, claims that she no longer can become pregnant as a result of the defendant's mismanagement. The plaintiff has been under the defendant's care for several years during which time he hospitalized her for acute pelvic inflammatory disease and the surgical removal of the organ depicted in Figure 16-6 (see page 102), a picture of which is the defendant's Exhibit A.
    On the witness stand you might emphasize that
    1. the physician did an inadequate surgical procedure.
    2. the patient's past history of pelvic inflammatory disease was a causative factor.
    3. the initial cervical cytology should have suggested the diagnosis.
    4. loss of fertility is usually a consequence of this clinical occurrence.
27. Conception rates following ectopic pregnancy are higher in women
    1. with parity greater than 3.
    2. under the age of 30.
    3. without a history of salpingitis.
    4. when rupture of the tube has not occurred.
28. Findings that do not rule out the diagnosis of an ectopic pregnancy include
    1. a rising β-HCG level.
    2. a negative culdocentesis.
    3. an ultrasound study showing an intrauterine sac.
    4. a history of tubal ligation.
29. In the United States, death from ectopic pregnancy
    1. is the most frequent cause of maternal death in black women.
    2. is more frequent in unmarried rather than married women.
    3. is 10 times more common than for childbirth.
    4. has risen at the same rate as the incidence of ectopic pregnancy.
30. Factors implicated in the etiology of ectopic pregnancies include
    1. previous salpingitis.
    2. delayed tubal ovum transport.
    3. abnormal embryonic development.
    4. genetic abnormalities of the blastocyst.
31. Women who are at an increased risk of ectopic pregnancy (expressed as incidence/1000 total pregnancies) include
    1. nonwhite women.
    2. nulliparous women.
    3. women with a history of salpingitis.
    4. women under the age of 24.
32. Spiegelberg's criteria for the diagnosis of ovarian pregnancy include
    1. the tube on the affected side must be intact.
    2. the gestational site must be in the normal position of the ovary.
    3. the gestational site must connect to the uterus by the ovarian ligament.
    4. histological evidence of ovarian tissue must be present in the sac wall.
33. Which signs are present in 50% or more of patients who present with ectopic pregnancies?
    1. Adnexal tenderness
    2. Uterine enlargement
    3. Adnexal mass
    4. Orthostatic hypotension

ANSWERS

1. **E**, Pages 423, 427. This patient appears to be in shock and should receive immediate attention. Both a sonogram and a radioimmunoassay would delay definitive treatment. A radioimmunoassay may be more sensitive, but the diagnosis is a hemoperitoneum. In this case, the most likely diagnosis is a ruptured corpus luteum. On occasion, an arteriole in the ovary is bleeding and requires suturing.
2. **D**, Page 430. The overall subsequent conception rate in women with an ectopic pregnancy is about 60%. Also see the comment for Answer 3.
3. **B**, Page 430. A little less than half of pregnancies subsequent to an ectopic pregnancy terminate in another ectopic gestation or a spontaneous abortion. Combined with the concep-

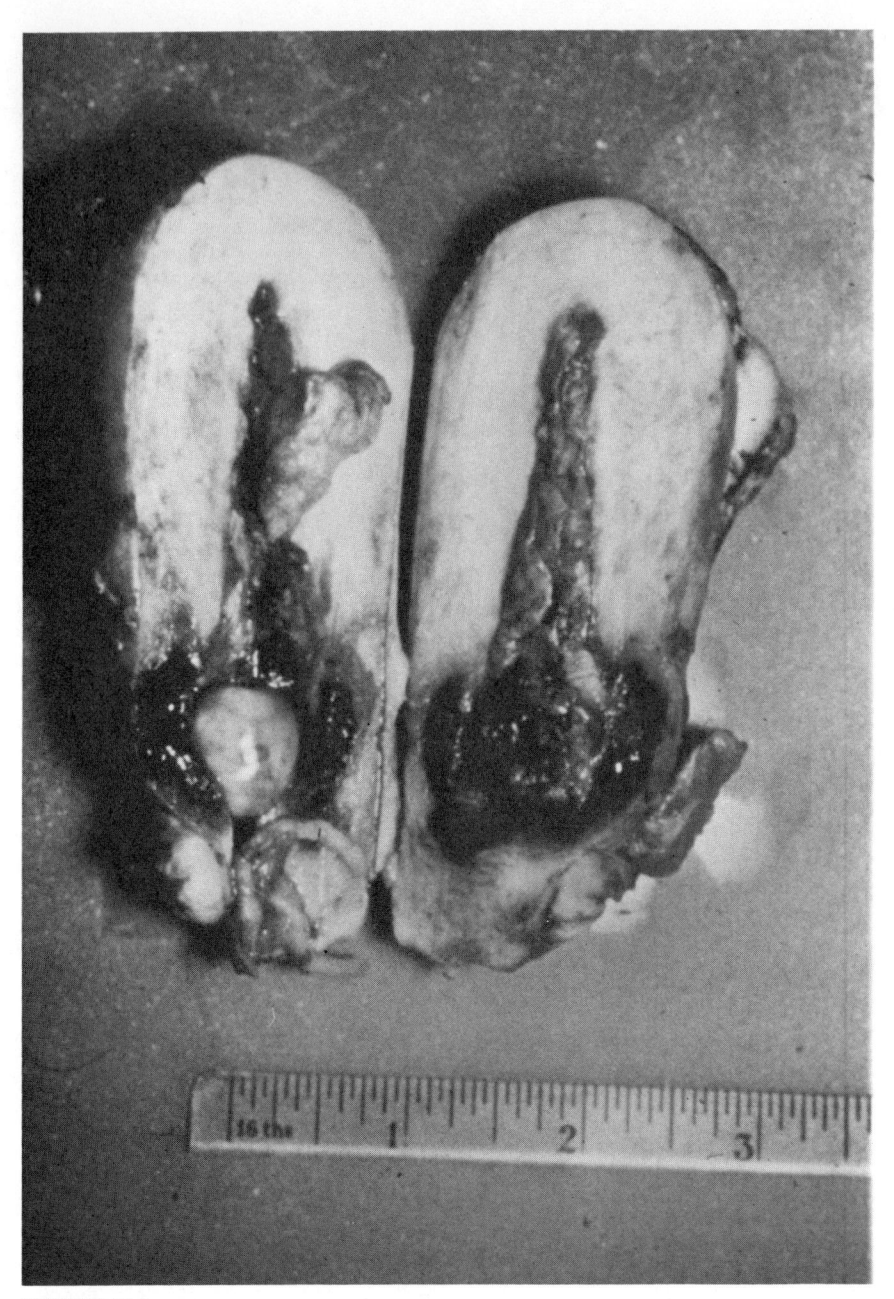

FIGURE 16-6.

tion rate of 60% found in women with a previous ectopic pregnancy, this means that only about one third of the women with ectopic pregnancies will have subsequent live births. However, these general figures are modified by several factors, particularly age, parity, evidence of contralateral tubal disease, and whether the tube was or was not ruptured.

4. **C**, Pages 419, 424. Blood is almost always found in the peritoneal cavity in patients with ruptured ectopic pregnancies of any location except cervical implantations. As we begin to make the diagnosis prior to rupture, the number with blood in the peritoneal cavity is likely to fall. The blood is from the mother. It is able to clot and does so in the same way that peripheral blood does. Following clotting, this blood undergoes lysis to yield the nonclotting blood found on culdocentesis. In patients with rapid catastrophic blood loss, the blood obtained by culdocentesis may clot on occasion because it has not had time to undergo lysis. Blood obtained by culdocentesis generally will have a hematocrit of greater

than 15%. In the presence of a ruptured tubal pregnancy, a culdocentesis is positive over 90% of the time.

5. **B**, Page 424. In 70% to 95% of patients with symptomatic ectopic pregnancies, nonclotting blood can be recovered by culdocentesis. Although other sources of bleeding (including the upper abdomen) may be responsible, 85% of patients with hemoperitoneum who are suspected of having an ectopic do have one. No matter what the anticipated cause of the intraabdominal bleeding, the case must be handled as a ruptured ectopic pregnancy until proven otherwise. Hemoperitoneum can be found prior to the onset of peritoneal irritation or rupture of the ectopic implantation. Bleeding into the peritoneal cavity generally does not occur with cervical ectopic pregnancies.

6. **A**, Page 430. While the risk of Rh sensitization of an Rh negative mother by an ectopic pregnancy is low, all Rh negative patients who are not already sensitized should receive Rh(D) immunoglobulin. A person who is classified as RhDu positive rarely develops antibodies when challenged by Rho(D) antigen.

7. **D**, Pages 428–429. While data concerning the removal of the ipsilateral ovary is conflicting, most authors agree that there should be as little as possible done to or around the ovary in order to preserve future fertility options.

8. **E**, Page 426. In 1987, using abdominal scanning techniques, the visualization of an ectopic gestation occurs in only about 25% or less of patients. Transvaginal scanning techniques eventually may raise this rate to 50%. Improvements in imaging are occurring at such a rapid rate that it is difficult to predict their efficacy in the future. Visualization of an intrauterine gestational sac containing a fetal pole is possible at 5 to 7 weeks of gestational age (menstrual dates).

9–14. 9, **D**; 10, **C**; 11, **B**; 12, **E**; 13, **E**; 14, **A**; Pages 409, 413–415. While most ectopic gestations implant in the mid to distal portion of the tube, the area of implantation associated with the greatest morbidity and mortality is the interstitial portion due to the catastrophic consequences of a rupture in that area. Implantations at or near the fimbrial end of the tube may abort without causing tubal rupture. Less than 1% of ectopic pregnancies are found implanted in the ovary. About 2% of all ectopic pregnancies are interstitial. Most pregnancies after previous ectopic pregnancy or while wearing an IUD are intrauterine.

15–18. 15, **B**; 16, **C**; 17, **A**; 18, **B**; Pages 411, 419, 421, 424. Both progesterone and HCG are generally lower in ectopic pregnancies in comparison to normal intrauterine pregnancies. The rate of increase in HCG is much slower in ectopic pregnancies. Normally it doubles in 48 to 72 hours. The progesterone produced by the corpus luteum is responsible for both the decidual and the Arias-Stella reaction.

19. **C**, Pages 421–422. Sometimes the secretory cells of the endometrial glands become hypertrophied with hyperchromatism, pleomorphism, and increased mitotic activity (Figure 16-2). This is known as the Arias-Stella reaction, and it can be confused with neoplasia (Question 20). It is not unique for an ectopic pregnancy; it can occur with an intrauterine pregnancy as well as following stimulation with clomiphene.

20. **D**, Page 810. Figure 16-3 is a microscopic section of a grade I endometrial adenocarcinoma. There is glandular atypia. The glands are closely packed. They are not uniform in size or shape. In some areas the glands are stratified with beginning tufting and papillae. The cells are irregular in size and shape.

21. **B**, Page 411. Figure 16-4 is a photomicrograph of a tubal pregnancy. Chorionic villi can be identified on the right. A well-developed myometrium is not seen. Instead, adipose tissue (on the left) is seen in close proximity to the villi.

22. **A** (1, 2, 3), Page 422; Table 16-7 (from Droegemueller). Abdominal pain is present in 90% to 100% of patients with ectopic pregnancies, while 75% to 95% of patients report amenorrhea. Vaginal bleeding is found in one half to more than three quarters of patients. Only 5% to 10% of patients with ectopic pregnancies report the passage of any tissue.

23. **A** (1, 2, 3), Pages 423, 426. The possibility of a pregnancy, either intrauterine or ectopic,

should be considered whenever a woman is late for a period. In this case the patient was on a progestin-only contraceptive. This is a risk factor for an ectopic pregnancy. On sonogram one sees a gestational sac or perhaps a pseudosac. Since a fetal pole is not identified, the picture is compatible with a very early but normal intrauterine pregnancy, a blighted ovum, or even an ectopic pregnancy. The latter is less likely, because this probably is not a pseudosac. If the patient merely was having a missed period, the pregnancy test would be negative and the endometrial cavity empty.

24. **B** (1, 3), Page 425. See comment for Answer 23. The HCG has increased 40% in 72 hours. This indicates an abnormal pregnancy, either a blighted ovum or an ectopic. In a normal pregnancy the HCG level should be at least 66% higher than the initial value in 48 hours.

25. **C** (2,4), Pages 206, 409. Over half of all deaths from ectopic pregnancy occur as a result of blood loss and physician delays or misdiagnosis. Anesthetic complications account for less than 2% of all ectopic pregnancy deaths. The incidence of a false positive culdocentesis is less than 2%.

26. **D** (4), Page 418. This is a hysterectomy specimen from a cervical pregnancy. Most cervical pregnancies occur after sharp uterine curettage. More than half the patients with cervical pregnancy require hysterectomy for treatment. Even if hysterectomy is not performed, the prognosis for future fertility is poor.

27. **E** (All), Pages 430–431. Conception rates following an ectopic pregnancy are much higher if tubal rupture has not occurred. Conception rates are also higher in women under the age of 30 or those who have had three or more children. Conception rates will be much lower when a history of salpingitis is present.

28. **E** (All), Pages 427–428. A patient with an ectopic pregnancy may not have blood on culdocentesis, either because there may have been no leakage or because adhesions prevent the culdocentesis needle from reaching the blood. Ectopic pregnancies occur in the presence of an intrauterine gestation or after a failed tubal ligation, but these are rare events. Levels of β-HCG will rise in patients with ectopic pregnancies, but the rate of increase is slower than for intrauterine gestations.

29. **A** (1, 2, 3), Pages 407–409. Death from ectopic pregnancy is three times greater for blacks than whites and is the most frequent cause of maternal mortality for blacks. Unmarried women are 1.7 times more likely to die from ectopic pregnancy than married women. The risk of death from ectopic pregnancy is about 10 times greater than with childbirth and more than 50 times greater than with legal abortions. The risk of death-per-case of ectopic pregnancy has dropped by a factor of 4 from 1970 to 1980.

30. **A** (1, 2, 3), Pages 410–411. Although the greatest single cause of ectopic pregnancies is the sequela of salpingitis, in almost 40% of ectopic pregnancies no direct cause can be found. One cause is presumed to be a physiologic disorder that results in delay of passage of the embryo into the uterine cavity so the embryo remains in the oviduct at the gestational age of 7 days when implantation occurs. While migration of a fertilized egg to the opposite tube does occur, it is considered neither common nor causative. Studies indicate that there is no difference in the chromosomal complement of ectopic compared with intrauterine pregnancies. Gross structural abnormalities occur in only about one half of those embryos studied. These types of abnormalities could interfere with normal tubal transport.

31. **B** (1, 3), Pages 407–408. The incidence of ectopic pregnancy is approximately twice as high for nonwhite women as it is for whites. More than half of all ectopic pregnancies occur in women with three or more pregnancies. Salpingitis is a major risk factor for ectopic pregnancy and there has been a parallel rise in the rates of salpingitis and ectopic pregnancies over the past few years. Fifty-three percent of all ectopic pregnancies occur in women aged 25 to 34.

32. **E** (All), Page 406. To make the diagnosis of ovarian ectopic pregnancy, these four criteria must be met:
    (1) The tube on the affected side must be intact.
    (2) The gestational site (ovary) must be in the normal position of the ovary.
    (3) The gestational site must connect to the uterus by the ovarian ligament.
    (4) Histological evidence of ovarian tissue must be present in the sac wall.

33. **B** (1, 3), Page 422; Table 16.8 (from Droegemueller). Abdominal and adnexal tenderness are the most common presenting signs in patients with ectopic pregnancies. An adnexal mass may be found in half the patients. On bimanual examination the uterus is enlarged in only one third of the patients, and it is nearly always less than 8 weeks size. Orthostatic changes in blood pressure indicate significant loss of blood volume, but these changes are found in only 10% to 15% of patients.

CHAPTER 17

Benign Gynecologic Lesions

DIRECTIONS: Select the one best answer or completion.

1. A 25-year-old gravida 1, para 0 at 24 weeks of gestation with a known history of leiomyomata presents with severe uterine pain. Fetal status is normal. On palpation a 6 cm tender area is found on the uterus. The examination is otherwise unremarkable. What is the most likely diagnosis?
   A. Ruptured uterus
   B. Placental abruption
   C. Hyaline degeneration of a myoma
   D. Red degeneration of a myoma
   E. Premature labor

2. An asymptomatic 25-year-old patient who is sexually active presents for a routine gynecological examination. A 3 cm sausage-shaped cystic mass is found protruding from the anterolateral wall of the upper vagina. What is the treatment of choice?
   A. Expectant management
   B. Oral antibiotics
   C. Laparoscopy and cystoscopy
   D. Marsupialization of cyst
   E. Excision of cyst

3. Which of the following dermatologic diseases of the vulva should *not* be treated with topical steroids?
   A. Contact dermatitis
   B. Psoriasis
   C. Lichen planus
   D. Hidradenitis suppurativa
   E. Seborrheic dermatitis

4. Given an asymptomatic 30-year-old gravida 5, para 5 patient with a 16-week irregular pelvic mass which you suspect is uterine myomas, what should your next step be?
   A. Abdominal x-ray
   B. Ultrasound
   C. CT scan
   D. Hysteroscopy
   E. Hysterectomy

5. A 27-year-old gravida 1, para 1, who is 6 weeks postpartum and breastfeeding, comes to the emergency department with heavy vaginal bleeding since having intercourse 2 hours ago. This was the first time in several months she has attempted coitus. Although the examination is difficult, a 1 cm transverse bleeding laceration of the posterior fornix is identified. What is the proper management?
   A. Vaginal estrogen cream
   B. Vaginal packing
   C. Suturing of the laceration
   D. Hospitalization for observation
   E. Discharge to be followed by the office in the morning

6. A 30-year-old patient has a 6 month history of dyspareunia, dysuria, and dribbling of urine. A palpable, tender mass is apparent in the anterior vagina. What is the most likely diagnosis?
   A. Skene's glands cysts
   B. Chronic cystitis
   C. Vaginal inclusion cyst
   D. Urethral diverticulum
   E. Gartner's duct cyst

7. A 40-year-old patient complains of intermenstrual and postcoital spotting (see figure 17-1). What is the appropriate therapy for this patient's condition?
   A. Hysterectomy
   B. Fractional D&C
   C. Removal of mass in the office
   D. Laser conization
   E. Vaginal estrogen cream

8. A 28-year-old gravida 0 whose LMP was 6 weeks ago presents with a 1 week history of left lower quadrant pain. She uses a diaphragm for contraception. Her previous menstrual history was normal. She denies any history of PID. Abdominal examination is normal. On pelvic examination, there is a tender 3 cm left adnexal mass that is confirmed by ultrasound. The Hct is 38%, WBC is 6000, and serum pregnancy test is negative. What is the most likely diagnosis?
   A. Ectopic pregnancy
   B. Tubo-ovarian abscess
   C. Salpingitis
   D. Endometriosis
   E. Corpus luteum cyst

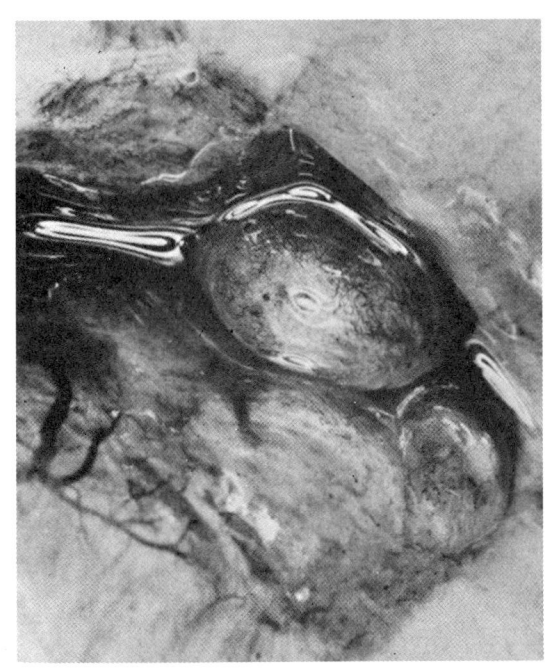

FIGURE 17-1.
(From Kolstad P, Stafl A, eds: Atlas of colposcopy, 2nd ed. Baltimore, University Park Press, 1977, p. 66.)

9. A 48-year-old asymptomatic patient is found to have an 8-week sized irregular myomatous uterus. What should be proper management at this point?
   A. Return in 6 to 12 months for re-evaluation
   B. Administration of GnRH analogues
   C. Fractional D&C
   D. Myomectomy
   E. Hysterectomy
10. After the delivery of twins at term by cesarean section, bilateral ovarian masses similar to those in Figure 17-2 are found. You should proceed to
    A. total abdominal hysterectomy with bilateral salpingo-oophorectomy.
    B. bilateral oophorectomy.
    C. bilateral wedge resection.
    D. needle aspirate cysts.
    E. close the abdomen.
11. A 22-year-old college student is found to have an asymptomatic 5 cm ovarian cyst. Her menstrual periods are regular. She is not sexually active and does not use oral contraceptives. The cyst is freely mobile and not tender to palpation. What is the treatment of choice?
    A. Reexamination in 6 months
    B. Oral contraceptives
    C. Needle aspiration under ultrasound
    D. Laparoscopy
    E. Laparotomy
12. A 25-year-old on birth control pills whose LMP was 1 week ago complains that she was awakened by a sudden onset of severe left lower quadrant pain. She had several milder episodes over the last week for which she did not seek medical care. She is nauseated and has vomited three times.

    On physical examination, her temperature is 100 degrees, there is tenderness of the left lower quadrant and there is an exquisitely tender 5 cm left adnexal mass. Pregnancy test is negative. What is the most appropriate action?
    A. Administer parenteral broad-spectrum antibiotics
    B. Perform IVP
    C. Perform a barium enema
    D. Perform laparoscopy or laparotomy
    E. Perform culdocentesis

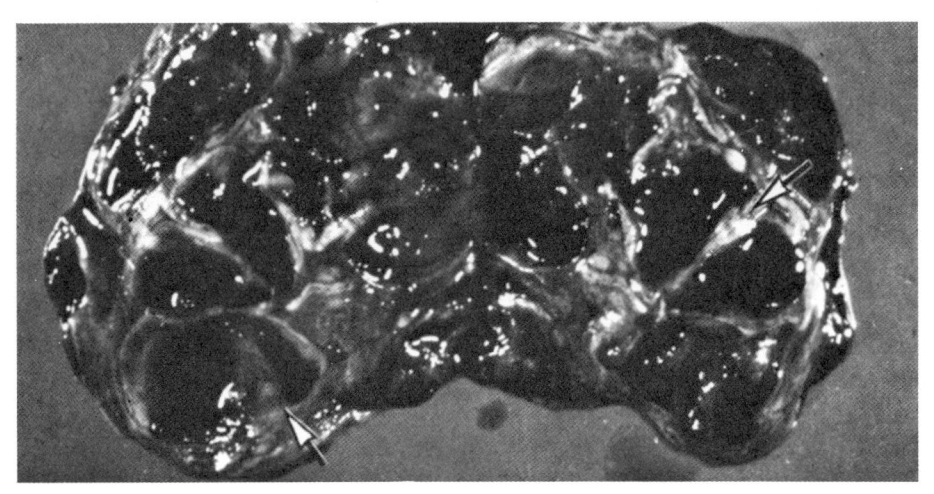

FIGURE 17-2.
(From Blaustein A: In Blaustein A, ed. Pathology of the female genital tract. New York, Springer-Verlag, 1977, p. 397.)

13. What is the most common complication of a cystic teratoma?
    A. Infection
    B. Torsion
    C. Rupture
    D. Hemorrhage
    E. Malignant degeneration

DIRECTIONS: For each numbered item, select the one heading most closely associated with it. Each lettered heading may be used once, more than once, or not at all.

Match the description with the most closely associated vulvar lesion.
   (A) Fibroma
   (B) Lipoma
   (C) Hidradenoma
   (D) Granular cell myoblastoma
   (E) Bowen's disease
14. Most common benign, solid vulvar tumor
15. Arise from neural sheath cells
16. Histologically similar to adenocarcinoma
   (A) Cystic teratoma
   (B) Fibroma
   (C) Serous cystadenoma
   (D) Dysgerminoma
   (E) Endometrioma
17. Tubercle of Rokitansky
18. Meig's syndrome
19. Brenner tumor

DIRECTIONS: For each numbered item, indicate whether it is associated with
   A. only (A)
   B. only (B)
   C. both (A) and (B)
   D. neither (A) nor (B)

   (A) Leiomyoma of oviduct
   (B) Paratubal cyst
   (C) Both
   (D) Neither
20. May undergo torsion
21. Mesonephric duct origin
22. Simulate ovarian mass
23. Salpingectomy indicated
   (A) Hematometra
   (B) Pyometra
   (C) Both
   (D) Neither
24. May be the result of cervical stenosis
25. Associated with amenorrhea
26. Associated with endometriosis
   (A) Follicular cyst
   (B) Corpus luteum cyst
   (C) Both
   (D) Neither
27. Arise from mature graafian follicle
28. Intraperitoneal hemorrhage extremely rare
29. Surgical excision

DIRECTIONS: Each question contains four suggested answers of which one or more is correct. Choose the answer
   A if 1, 2, and 3 are correct
   B if 1 and 3 are correct
   C if 2 and 4 are correct
   D if 4 only is correct
   E if all are correct

30. Which medical conditions have been associated with the ovarian tumor pictured in Figure 17-3?
    1. Autoimmune hemolytic anemia
    2. Thyrotoxicosis
    3. Carcinoid syndrome
    4. Diabetes mellitus
31. True statements concerning benign cystic teratomas of the ovary include:
    1. There is a preponderance of ectodermal tissue.
    2. Malignant transformation occurs in 1–2%.
    3. Bilateral tumors occur in 15% of cases.
    4. The chromosomal makeup is 46, XY.
32. Indications for surgery in the management of an adnexal mass include
    1. a solid tumor.
    2. a prepubertal patient.
    3. a cystic mass greater than 8 cm.
    4. a postmenopausal patient.
33. Indications for hysterectomy include uterine myomas that
    1. are the size of a 14-week gestation.
    2. grow after menopause.
    3. prevent adequate evaluation of adnexa.
    4. are associated with partial ureteral obstruction.
34. Topical estrogen is appropriate initial therapy for which of the following lesions?
    1. Vulvar granular cell myoblastoma
    2. Vulvar fibroma
    3. Vulvar hemangioma
    4. Urethral caruncle
35. Which are clinical features of early malignant melanoma?
    1. Asymmetry
    2. Variation of the color
    3. Irregularity of the border
    4. Larger than 6 mm
36. Which are symptoms associated with cervical myomas?
    1. Urgency
    2. Dysmenorrhea
    3. Dyspareunia
    4. Abnormal bleeding

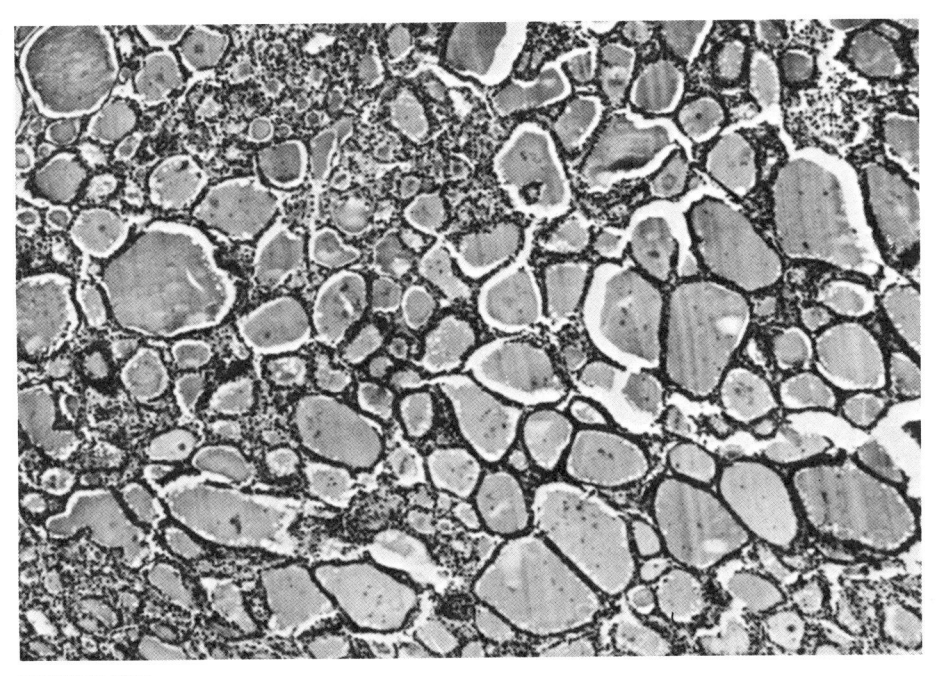

FIGURE 17-3.
(From Talerman A: In Blaustein A, ed. Pathology of the female genital tract. New York, Springer-Verlag, 1977, p. 563.)

37. A 65-year-old patient is undergoing office endometrial sampling because of vaginal spotting. With difficulty, a 1 mm dilator is passed into the endometrial cavity resulting in a purulent discharge from the cervical os. Proper management includes:
    1. intravenous broad-spectrum antibiotics.
    2. pelvic ultrasound.
    3. laparoscopy.
    4. fractional D&C at a later time.
38. Which are symptoms attributable to uterine myomas?
    1. Infertility
    2. Dysmenorrhea
    3. Urinary frequency
    4. Menorrhagia

ANSWERS

1. **D,** Page 463. The blood supply to myomas is less than to a similar-sized area of normal myometrium. Therefore, as the myoma grows, it outgrows its blood supply, resulting in degeneration. The most acute form of degeneration is red or carneous degeneration typified by the rapidly growing myoma during the midtrimester of pregnancy. The sudden muscular infarction causes pain and localized peritonitis. Treatment should be medical since surgical intervention in a pregnant patient results in profuse blood loss. Placental abruption at 24 weeks is unusual and the uterus would be expected to be diffusely tender.

2. **A,** Page 452. Gartner's duct cysts are dysontogenetic cysts of mesonephric origin, usually found in the upper half of the vagina. They occur in approximately 1 out of 200 women and are usually asymptomatic. Unless symptoms such as vaginal pain, dyspareunia, difficulty with urination, or a large palpable mass occur, they may be followed conservatively.

3. **D,** Pages 449–450. Hidradenitis suppurativa is a chronic, refractory infection of the skin and subcutaneous tissue. It may progress from subcutaneous nodules to draining abscesses and sinuses. The treatment of choice is early, aggressive, wide excision. Dermatologic conditions such as contact dermatitis, psoriasis, lichen planus, and seborrheic dermatitis can all be treated with a topical steroid.

    It should be emphasized that pruritis and vulvodynia are only symptoms. Treatment should be based upon establishing a specific diagnosis from a differential list that includes skin infections, sexually transmitted diseases, dermatoses, vulvar dystrophies, malignancies, neurodermatitis, and psychologic causes.

4. **E,** Pages 464–465. The diagnosis of uterine myomas is usually confirmed by palpating an enlarged, firm irregular uterus during pelvic examination. In experienced hands further verification is unnecessary. On occasion, concentric calcifications on abdominal x-ray or characteristic findings on ultrasound and CT scan may aid in the diagnosis.

Submucous myomas may be observed during hysteroscopy. They also appear as filling defects on hysterosalpingogram. If the patient does not desire surgery, frequent follow-up is mandatory.

5. **C, Page 453.** Coitus is the most frequent cause of trauma to the lower genital tract of adult women. Predisposing factors include virginity, pregnancy, postpartum and postmenopausal vaginal epithelium, prolonged abstinence, hysterectomy, and inebriation. Intercourse may be painful with 25% of patients complaining of persistent pain after coitus. Often the history of coital injury cannot be obtained. Management includes suturing the laceration under adequate anesthesia. It should be noted that patients such as the one described have vaginas that show little estrogen effect and are thereby at greater risk for trauma if not exogenously lubricated prior to coitus.

6. **D, Page 451.** The most common symptoms associated with a urethral diverticulum are urinary urgency, frequency, and dysuria. Dyspareunia and postvoid dribbling have also been reported by the 80% of patients with urethral diverticulum who are symptomatic.

    The diagnosis may be confirmed by several techniques including voiding cystourethrography, cystourethroscopy, and positive pressure urethrography using a Davis catheter.

7. **C, Pages 453–456.** The patient with intermenstrual and postcoital spotting has symptoms suggestive of a cervical polyp. The differential diagnosis of this pictured lesion includes endometrial polyp, prolapsed myoma, and cervical malignancy. In most instances, an endocervical polyp may be removed by twisting it off its base using a surgical clamp. If the intermenstrual and postcoital spotting continue after removal of the polyp, endometrial sampling is indicated to identify endometrial lesions whose symptoms mimicked those of a polyp.

8. **E, Page 472.** Halban's syndrome describes a persistently functioning corpus luteum cyst that clinically mimics an ectopic pregnancy. This triad includes a delay in normal menses with subsequent spotting, unilateral pelvic pain, and a small, tender adnexal mass. With the advent of rapid, sensitive pregnancy tests that measure β-HCG, the distinction between ectopic pregnancy and persistent corpus luteum cyst is made more easily because the pregnancy test is almost always positive in the presence of an ectopic pregnancy.

9. **A, Page 465.** Most women with uterine myomas do not require surgery. This is particularly true for asymptomatic perimenopausal patients since the condition tends to improve with declining levels of circulating estrogen. Reexamination allows determination of the rate of growth. Symptomatic patients must be evaluated appropriately with therapy ultimately depending on severity and persistence of symptoms, age, parity, and reproductive plans. D&C would be warranted in cases of abnormal bleeding. Myomectomy, both transabdominal and hysteroscopic, is reserved for symptomatic women who have not completed childbearing A few small series of cases using danazol, GnRH analogues or medroxyprogesterone have reported reduction in tumor size. Myomas tend to return after the medication is discontinued.

10. **E, Pages 473–474.** Pregnancies producing large placentas such as twins, diabetes, and Rh sensitization are more likely to be associated with theca lutein cysts. The ovaries should be handled delicately to avoid cyst rupture and hemorrhage. No further surgery is warranted since the cysts will regress as gonadotrophin stimulation is removed.

11. **B, Pages 469–470.** The initial management of a suspected functional ovarian cyst is observation. Since most follicular cysts resorb spontaneously or silently rupture within 4 to 8 weeks, reevaluation should not be unnecessarily delayed. A 6 month delay would be excessive, whereas reevaluation in 6 weeks would be an acceptable alternative. A 6-week rather than a 4-week interval is preferable so that the patient may be examined at a different point in her cycle. Oral contraceptives remove any influence by pituitary gonadotrophins and may be prescribed for a short-term trial. Surgical intervention is not warranted initially in the asymptomatic patient.

12. **D, Page 486.** Most patients with adnexal torsion, like the one described, are ill enough to warrant operative intervention. When the diagnosis is in doubt, laparoscopy may be needed to rule out conditions such as abscess and ruptured corpus luteum. In selected cases of partial torsion, it is acceptable to untwist the pedicle, perform a cystectomy, then stabilize the ovary. This does carry the risk of releasing venous thrombi. In cases of vascular compromise, unilateral salpingo-oophorectomy is the operation of choice.

13. **B, Page 477.** The most frequent complication of a cystic teratoma is torsion, which occurs in approximately 11% of patients. The overall incidence of rupture is less than 5%, occurring more commonly in pregnancy and the puerperium with resultant leakage and incitement of a chemical peritonitis. Infection, hemorrhage, and malignant degeneration are all unusual complications, occurring in less than 1% of patients.

14. **A, Pages 445–446.** Fibromas are the most common solid tumor of the vulva; lipomas are

the other common benign tumor of mesenchymal origin. Both grow slowly, have a low-grade malignant potential, and are typically excised to establish the diagnosis.

15. **D**, Page 447. Granular cell myoblastomas arise from neural sheath (Schwann) cells and are sometimes called *schwannomas*. These rare, slow-growing, solid tumors are painless and benign, but they infiltrate surrounding tissue. If the initial excision is not wide enough, these tumors tend to recur.
16. **C**, Pages 446–447. A hidradenoma may be mistaken histologically for adenocarcinoma because of its hyperplastic, adenomatous pattern.
17. **A**, Page 477. Most of the solid elements in a cystic teratoma are contained in a nipple of the cyst wall termed the protuberance or tubercle of Rokitansky.
18. **B**, Page 480. Meig's syndrome is the association of an ovarian fibroma with ascites and hydrothorax. Both ascites and hydrothorax resolve when the tumor is removed. Although classically described with ovarian fibroma, these clinical features are also found with other ovarian tumors.
19. **C**, Pages 482–485. Thirty percent of Brenner tumors are found in association with serous or mucinous cystademonas of the ipsilateral ovary. There is, however, a lack of mitotic figures and nuclear pleomorphism. The tumor arises from apocrine sweat glands and may be solid or cystic. It typically occurs in Caucasian women between the ages of 30 and 70. The treatment of choice is excisional biopsy.
20. **C**, Pages 466–467. Both tubal myomas and paratubal cysts may undergo acute torsion resulting in acute lower abdominal and pelvic pain. Most cases of paratubal cyst torsion are associated with pregnancy or the puerperium.
21. **B**, Page 466. Tubal myomas arise from smooth muscle cells as do the commonly coexistent uterine myomas. Paratubal cysts may be of mesonephric, paramesonephric, or mesothelial origin.
22. **C**, Pages 466–467. Both tubal myomas and paratubal cysts may mimic an ovarian tumor. The former simulates a solid tumor while the latter is often indistinguishable from a cystic ovarian mass.
23. **D**, Pages 466–467. The treatment of a tubal myoma is excision of the myoma in cases where it is symptomatic. Similarly, cases of paratubal cysts do not require salpingectomy unless tubal torsion has occurred.
24–26. 24, **C**; 25, **C**; 26, **A**; Pages 457–459. Both pyometra and hematometra may be the result of cervical stenosis. Hematometra is the consequence of complete genital tract obstruction in a reproductive age woman who has an intact hypothalamic-pituitary axis. Postmenopausal women develop pyometra and are usually asymptomatic. Retrograde menstruation in a patient with hematometra is commonly associated with endometriosis.
27. **B**, Pages 468–471. Follicular cysts are by far the most common cystic structures in normal ovaries and result from either the dominant mature follicle's failure to rupture or an immature follicle's failure to undergo normal atresia. A corpus luteum cyst develops from a mature graafian follicle.
28. **A**, Pages 468–473. Corpus luteum cysts may produce dull, unilateral pelvic pain. It is not uncommon for rupture to be associated with significant intraperitoneal hemorrhage. Rupture of a corpus luteum cyst must be considered in the differential diagnosis of ectopic pregnancy. Significant bleeding associated with a follicular cyst is rare.
29. **D**, Pages 468–473. In both follicular and corpus luteum cysts, management of the unruptured cyst should be conservative observation. In cases of cyst rupture resulting in significant intraperitoneal hemorrhage, the ovary should be preserved if at all possible.
30. **A** (1, 2, 3), Page 478. Adult thyroid tissue is identified in 12% of cystic teratomas. If thyroid is the predominant tissue, the term *struma ovarii* is applied. Thyrotoxicosis develops in less than 5% of patients with struma ovarii. On rare occasions, carcinoid syndrome and autoimmune hemolytic anemia have also been described in association with cystic teratomas.
31. **A** (1, 2, 3), Page 475. Benign cystic teratomas contain elements from all three germ cell layers, ectodermal tissue being predominant. Malignant transformation of a benign cystic teratoma occurs in no more than 1% or 2% of cases, usually in patients over 40. The malignant component is usually a squamous carcinoma. Benign teratomas are bilateral 10% to 15% of the time. The chromosomal makeup is 46XX and is different from the host.
32. **E** (All), Page 470. Any adnexal mass present prior to puberty or after the menopause requires surgical intervention. It should be noted that approximately 50% of ovarian cysts in prepubertal girls are follicle cysts. Similarly, a solid adnexal mass of any size or a cystic mass larger than 8 cm warrants surgery. A 5 to 8 cm cystic mass that persists despite either oral contraceptive suppression or normal menstruation should also be evaluated surgically.
33. **E** (All), Pages 462, 464–465. In addition to symptomatic myomas, there are situations in which asymptomatic uterine myomas may be removed. Myomas larger than 12- to 14-week size are expected to eventually produce symptoms and may obscure the palpation of the adnexa. Growth of myomas after menopause is the classic finding in cases of

leiomyosarcoma. Myomas that expand into the broad ligament may compress the ureter, resulting in hydroureter and possibly even renal compromise.

34. **D** (4), Pages 441–447. Urethral caruncles are fleshy outgrowths from the edge of the urethra. They are most commonly found in postmenopausal women and may respond to initial therapy of topical or oral estrogen. If it does not regress or is symptomatic, therapeutic modalities include operative excision, laser ablation, fulguration, or cryosurgery.

    Excision is the definitive treatment for the other vulval tumors listed: granular cell myoblastoma, fibroma, and hemangioma. Topical estrogen has very little therapeutic value on the vulva.

35. **E** (All), Page 444. Although vulvar nevi are usually asymptomatic, it should be recalled that approximately 30% of malignant melanomas arise from a preexisting nevus. Since a disproportionate number of malignant melanomas (5% to 10%) arise in the vulvar area, all vulvar nevi should be excised and examined histologically. Characteristic clinical features of an early malignant melanoma may be remembered by thinking of ABCD as described by Friedman: asymmetry, border irregularity, color variegation, and a diameter greater than 6 mm.

36. **E** (All), Pages 456–457. Cervical myomas constitute up to 8% of all myomas. Symptoms depend upon the direction in which the myoma expands; urinary difficulty, pain with intercourse, and painful menses are all possible symptoms. Prolapsed cervical myomas also may become ulcerated and infected, resulting in abnormal bleeding.

37. **D** (4), Page 457. Cervical stenosis resulting in pyometra in a postmenopausal patient may be caused by a previous operation, radiation, infection, neoplasia, or atrophic changes. Pyometra in postmenopausal patients usually does not require antibiotics since the primary goal of therapy is achieved with transcervical drainage. Ultrasound and laparoscopy would have no diagnostic or therapeutic value at this time. After the acute infection has subsided, however, a fractional D&C should be performed to rule out carcinoma of the endometrium.

38. **E** (All), Page 464. Most women with uterine myomas are asymptomatic. When symptomatic, severity is often related to number, location, and size of the myomas. One third of women with myomas have pelvic pain with dysmenorrhea the most common symptom. Large myomas may press on the bladder and/or rectum, resulting in difficulty with voiding or bowel movements. Menorrhagia is the most common type of abnormal bleeding caused by myomas although intermenstrual spotting also occurs. Myomas infrequently contribute to infertility, either as the sole factor or as one of several identifiable abnormalities. Successful term pregnancy rates are reported to be as high as 50% after myomectomy.

CHAPTER 18

Endometriosis and Adenomyosis

DIRECTIONS: Select the one best answer or completion.

1. Which of the following is **not** a widely accepted theory regarding the etiology of endometriosis?
   A. Endometriosis is due to implantation of endometrial cells shed as a result of retrograde menstruation.
   B. Cells of müllerian duct, derived from coelomic epithelium, undergo metaplasia to form endometrial tissue.
   C. Endometrial tissue can be transplanted via both lymphatic and vascular systems.
   D. The presence of endometriosis is dependent upon a generalized immunologic defect.
   E. There is a genetic predisposition transmitted by polygenic or multifactorial inheritance patterns.

2. Which is the most common site for endometriosis?
   A. Rectosigmoid
   B. Ovary
   C. Appendix
   D. Uterosacral ligament
   E. Fallopian tube

3. Most cases of suspected endometriosis are confirmed by
   A. initial history.
   B. repeat pelvic exam on first day of menstrual flow.
   C. laparoscopic visualization.
   D. speculum visualization.
   E. hysterosalpingogram.

4. A 22-year-old gravida 0 undergoes laparoscopy for progressive dysmenorrhea and chronic pelvic pain. She is found to have minimal endometriosis. She is not sexually active but does plan to marry in 6 months. She and her fiance look forward to having children someday. What is optimal therapy for her?
   A. Laparotomy and resection of endometriotic lesions
   B. Danazol therapy
   C. Conception
   D. Oral contraceptives
   E. Total abdominal hysterectomy with bilateral salpingo-oophorectomy

5. A 42-year-old gravida 3, para 3 is found to have endometriosis with extensive ovarian involvement at laparoscopy performed for progressive dysmenorrhea and dyspareunia. What is optimal therapy for her?
   A. Laparotomy and resection of endometriotic lesions
   B. Danazol therapy
   C. Oral contraceptives
   D. Hysterectomy
   E. Hysterectomy with bilateral salpingo-oophorectomy

6. Which figure shows the chemical structure of danazol?
   A. Figure 18-1, A
   B. Figure 18-1, B
   C. Figure 18-1, C
   D. Figure 18-1, D
   E. Figure 18-1, E

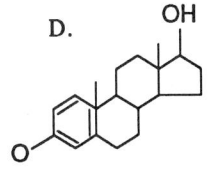

FIGURE 18-1.

7. All of the following are true statements concerning the natural history of endometriosis **except**:
   A. Serial pelvic exams may not reflect disease progression.
   B. The optimal preventive therapy is unknown.
   C. Approximately 10% of teenagers who develop endometriosis have associated congenital outflow obstruction.
   D. Pregnancy invariably improves endometriosis.
   E. Postmenopausal endometriosis is often related to the use of exogenous estrogens.
8. Of the 5 photomicrographs shown on pp. 114 to 116, the one diagnostic of endometriosis is:
   A. Figure 18-2
   B. Figure 18-3
   C. Figure 18-4
   D. Figure 18-5
   E. Figure 18-6
9. Of the 5 photomicrographs shown, the one diagnostic of adenomyosis is:
   A. Figure 18-2
   B. Figure 18-3
   C. Figure 18-4
   D. Figure 18-5
   E. Figure 18-6
10. A 42-year-old gravida 4, para 4 complains of secondary progressive dysmenorrhea and menorrhagia. On pelvic examination the uterus is globular, tender, boggy, and approximately twice normal size. What is the most likely diagnosis?
    A. Endometriosis
    B. Adenomyosis
    C. Leiomyomata uteri
    D. Endometrial carcinoma
    E. Leiomyosarcoma
11. Which is the least common symptom associated with endometriosis involving the GI tract?
    A. Cramping
    B. Lower abdominal pain
    C. Pain with defecation
    D. Constipation
    E. Rectal bleeding

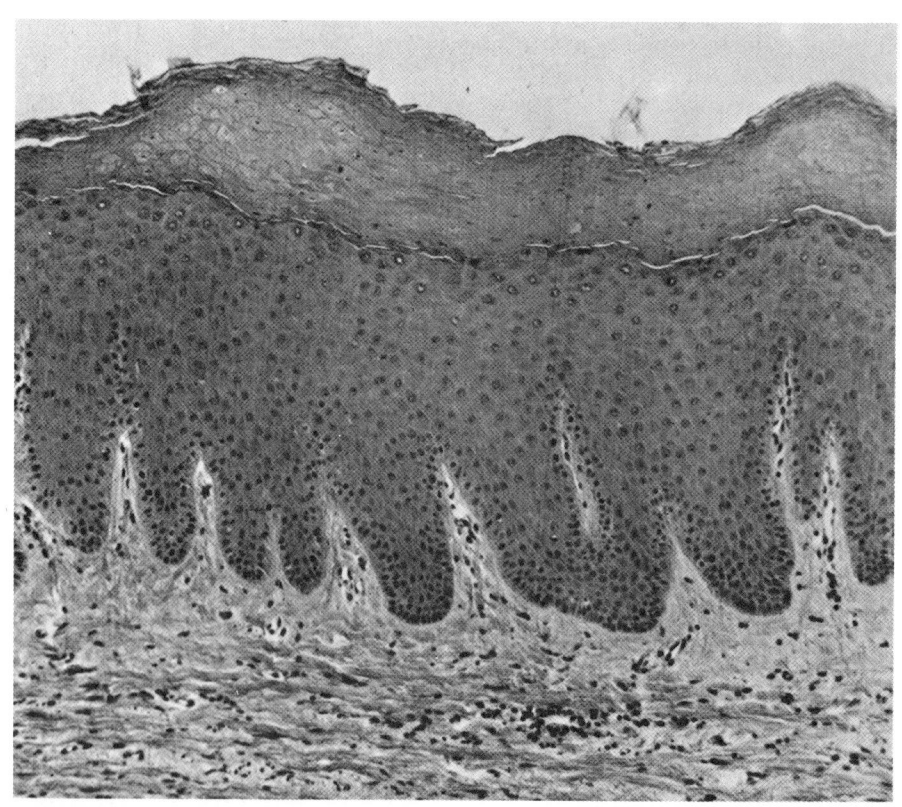

FIGURE 18-2.
(From Friedrich EG, Wilkinson EJ: The vulva. In Blaustein A, ed: Pathology of the female genital tract, 2nd ed. New York, Springer-Verlag, 1982.)

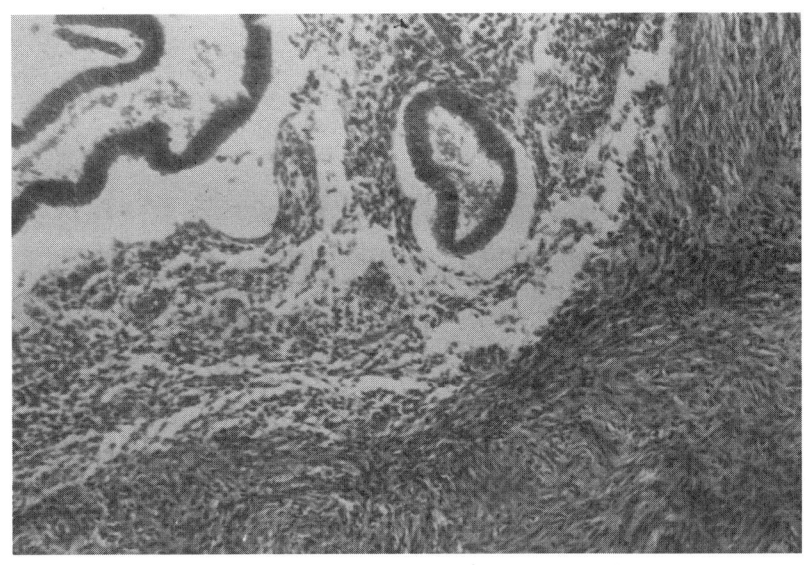

FIGURE 18-3.
(From Droegemueller W, Herbst AL, Mishell DR, Stenchever MA: Comprehensive Gynecology. St. Louis, The C. V. Mosby Co., 1987.)

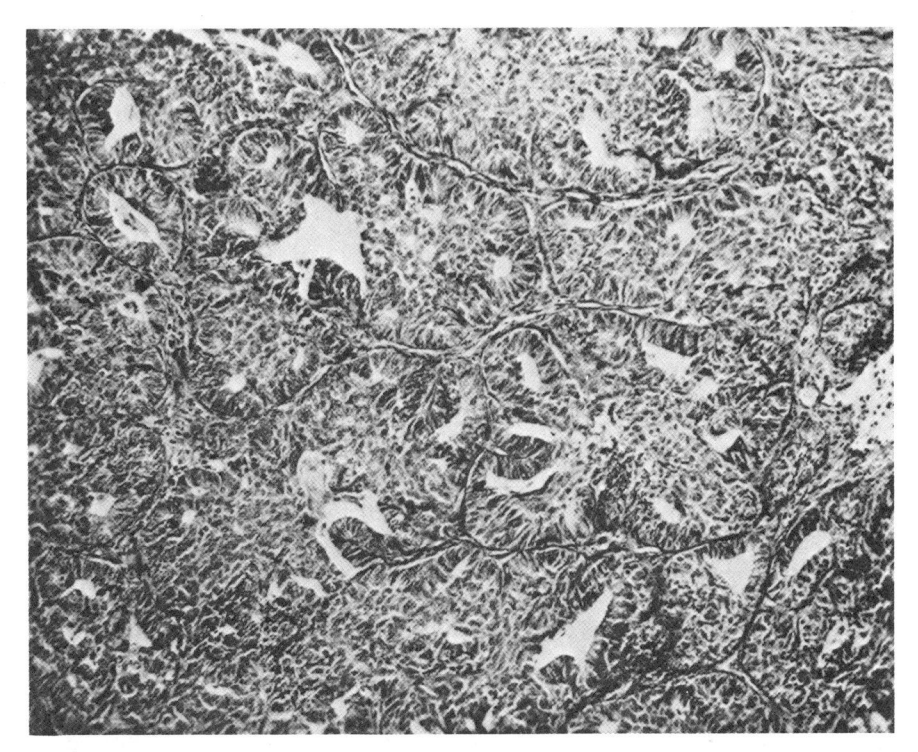

FIGURE 18-4.
(From Kurman RJ, Norris HJ: In Blaustein A, ed: Pathology of the female genital tract, 2nd ed. New York, Springer-Verlag, 1982.)

116 General Gynecology

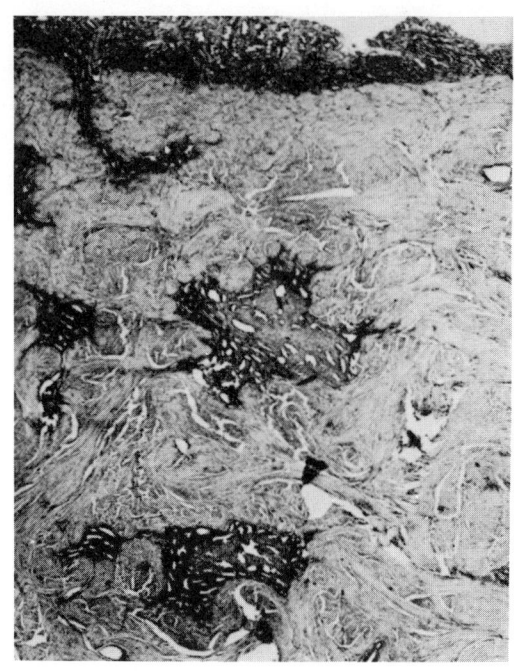

FIGURE 18-5.
(From Janovski NA, Dubranszky V: Atlas of gynecologic and obstetric diagnostic histopathology. New York, McGraw-Hill, 1967, p. 217.)

12. A 30-year-old patient has completed her childbearing and has confirmed mild endometriosis. She complains of dyspareunia and dysmenorrhea. Which is the most reasonable operative procedure?

A. D&C
B. Uterine suspension
C. Total abdominal hysterectomy
D. Presacral neurectomy
E. Resection of uterosacral ligaments

DIRECTIONS: For each numbered item, indicate whether it is associated with
  A. only (A)
  B. only (B)
  C. both (A) and (B)
  D. neither (A) nor (B)

13–16. In the treatment of endometriosis
(A) LH-RH agonist
(B) Intramuscular progestin
(C) Both
(D) Neither

13. Prompt resumption of ovulation expected
14. Amenorrhea
15. Breakthrough bleeding
16. Therapeutic success rate similar to oral contraception

DIRECTIONS: Each question contains four suggested answers of which one or more is correct. Choose the answer
  A if 1, 2, and 3 are correct
  B if 1 and 3 are correct
  C if 2 and 4 are correct
  D if 4 only is correct
  E if all are correct

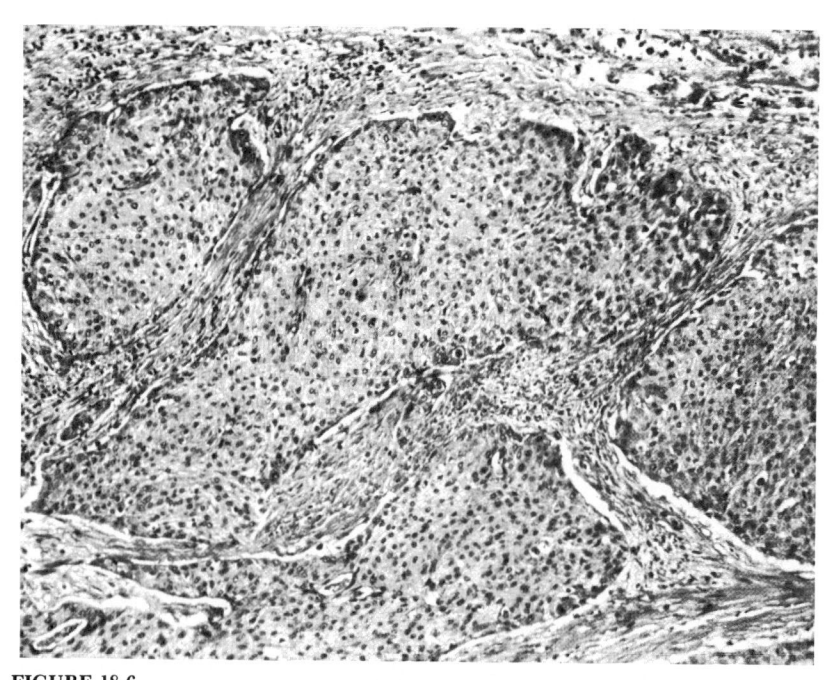

FIGURE 18-6.
(From Clement PB, Scully RE: Semin Oncol 9:251, 1982.)

17. True statements about endometriosis include:
    1. It is a benign but progressive and recurrent disease limited to the pelvic organs.
    2. The incidence of endometriosis is higher among infertile women.
    3. It should be considered an advanced stage of adenomyosis.
    4. Approximately 5% of cases are diagnosed following the menopause.
18. Which are uncommon sites of endometriosis?
    1. Surgical incisions
    2. Nasal mucosa
    3. Lung
    4. Spinal column
19. Which are classic signs of endometriosis?
    1. Tender nodularity of uterosacral ligaments.
    2. Scarring and tenderness in the posterior vaginal fornix.
    3. Fixed retroverted uterus.
    4. Bilateral symmetric adnexal enlargement.
20. Which of the following descriptions are consistent with the diagnosis of endometriosis?
    1. 0.5 cm blood-filled cyst
    2. Chocolate cyst
    3. Raspberry spot
    4. Powder burn
21. Which are indications for steroid hormone therapy after definitive surgical treatment for endometriosis?
    1. Menopausal symptoms
    2. Residual macroscopic endometriosis
    3. Suspected microscopic endometriosis
    4. In order to improve postoperative healing
22. Which are indications for danazol?
    1. Menorrhagia
    2. Benign cystic mastitis
    3. Hereditary angioneurotic edema
    4. Endometriosis
23. True statements regarding the histologic features of endometriosis include:
    1. Endometrial glands and stroma must be identified in order to make a presumptive diagnosis of endometriosis.
    2. The aberrant endometrial stroma usually undergoes decidual changes when exposed to physiologic levels of progesterone.
    3. The inflammatory response seen in endometriosis is primarily polymorphonuclear.
    4. The aberrant endometrial glands usually respond to estrogen and progesterone in cyclic fashion.
24. A 29-year-old female presents with a chief complaint of progressive dysmenorrhea for 2 years. She has had dyspareunia for 12 months, the duration of her marriage. She has never used contraception. The differential diagnosis should include
    1. adenomyosis.
    2. chronic pelvic inflammatory disease.
    3. primary dysmenorrhea.
    4. endometriosis.
25. A 24-year-old female reports that several of her friends have been found to have endometriosis. She is concerned that she also might have endometriosis. Clinical histories compatible with the diagnosis include
    1. secondary dysmenorrhea, infertility, intermittent constipation.
    2. dyspareunia, pelvic heaviness, hematuria.
    3. Premenstrual spotting.
    4. No symptoms.
26. True statements about danazol include:
    1. Some side effects are related to its anabolic properties.
    2. "Pseudomenopause" is a descriptive term because of a similarity in gonadotrophin levels in the menopausal woman and danazol treated patient.
    3. Danazol is less androgenic than testosterone.
    4. Free testosterone levels are decreased with danazol treatment.
27. According to the staging of endometriosis (Puleo and Hammond) used to follow patients with pain, criteria for mild disease include
    1. no significant adhesions.
    2. tubal obstruction.
    3. superficial ovarian implants.
    4. scattered, scarred implants on other abdominal structures.
28. In discussing danazol therapy with a patient, she should be told that side effects
    1. are uncommon.
    2. include muscle cramps, acne, and flushes.
    3. cause 1% to 2% of patients to discontinue the drug.
    4. occasionally include irreversible deepening of the voice.
29. Danazol
    1. binds to androgen receptors.
    2. inhibits steroidogenesis in ovary.
    3. binds to progesterone receptors.
    4. inhibits steroidogenesis in adrenal gland.
30. Surgery is mandatory in the treatment of endometriosis for cases in which there is
    1. ureteral obstruction.
    2. compromise of large bowel function.
    3. presence of an 8 cm ovarian endometrioma.
    4. progressive dysmenorrhea.

31. A 26-year-old patient is started on danazol for the treatment of moderate endometriosis. She should be told that the drug
    1. is most effective using 200 mg twice a day.
    2. costs approximately $60 per month.
    3. should be given on an empty stomach.
    4. should be started on the first day of the menstrual cycle.
32. True statements about the clinical outcome of patients with endometriosis treated with danazol include:
    1. 75% of patients report significant symptomatic improvement.
    2. 90% have objective improvement based on second look laparoscopy.
    3. Uncorrected fertility rate is approximately 40% after danazol.
    4. Between 5% and 10% have recurrent symptoms within 2 years of discontinuing therapy.
33. Which are regimens used today in treating endometriosis?
    1. Oral progestin
    2. LH-RH agonist
    3. Intramuscular progestin
    4. Methyltestosterone
34. The glands and stroma of adenomyosis are
    1. derived from aberrant glands of the basalis layer of the endometrium.
    2. relatively deficient in estrogen receptors in comparison with glands and stroma of the endometrium.
    3. most commonly diffusely involved throughout the myometrium.
    4. relatively deficient in progesterone receptors in comparison with glands and stroma of the endometrium.

ANSWERS

1. **D**, Pages 493–495. Most authorities feel that several factors are probably involved in the etiology of endometriosis. These include retrograde menstruation, metaplasia of coelomic epithelium, transport of endometrial cells via blood and/or lymphatics, a genetic predisposition, and a local rather than a generalized immunologic defect.
2. **B**, Pages 495–496. The ovaries are the most common site for endometriosis in two out of three patients.
3. **C**, Page 500. In most cases, the diagnosis of endometriosis is confirmed by direct laparoscopic visualization. In many cases this is discovered during an infertility work-up. Some people feel that pelvic exam on the first day of the cycle allows evaluation at the time of maximal swelling and tenderness. As with the history, the pelvic examination does not confirm the diagnosis. Because vaginal implants are rare, confirmation via speculum exam is unlikely. Abnormalities found on hysterosalpingogram are not specific for the diagnosis of endometriosis.
4. **D**, Page 502. For a symptomatic young patient with minimal endometriosis, medical suppression is a logical first step in therapy. Laparoscopic laser ablation is a surgical modality often used at the time of diagnosis and could have been done in this patient. Danazol is an appropriate drug for patients whose symptoms persist or whose disease progresses despite oral contraceptives. Laparotomy with resection of endometriotic lesions or hysterectomy are procedures reserved for more advanced or debilitating endometriosis. Recommending conception must be individualized to the patient's personal needs and circumstances and carries with it an inherent paradox since infertility is more common in patients with endometriosis.
5. **E**, Pages 506–507. In a 42-year-old multigravid patient, the most logical therapy to recommend is hysterectomy with bilateral salpingo-oophorectomy. The extirpative procedure removes not only macroscopic disease, but removes the potential stimulus for future endometriosis, that is, the ovaries. Although this is optimal treatment, the patient must share in the decision regarding oophorectomy. Any medical regimen would be considered less acceptable because of the patient's age and extent of disease.
6. **B** (Figure 18-1, B), Page 502. Danazol is an attenuated, orally active androgen. Chemically it is a synthetic steroid, the isoxasole derivative of ethisterone (17-α-ethinyltestosterone). (B is testosterone, C is progesterone, D is estradiol, and E is estrone.)
7. **D**, Pages 501-502. Endometriosis is dependent upon ovarian hormones to stimulate growth, but there is extreme variability in the rate of progression of the disease from one patient to another. There is no chemical marker or test available to follow its growth except laparoscopy. The natural history is largely speculation as is the optimal preventive therapy. There are cases of endometriosis that have increased in size during the first few weeks of pregnancy. Teenagers with endometriosis should be examined for the rare possibility of outflow obstruction. With a natural menopause, a gradual relief of symptoms is typically seen. It should be noted, however, that 5% of symptomatic cases present after the menopause.
8. **B**, Page 498. The three cardinal histologic features of endometriosis are ectopic endometrial glands, ectopic endometrial stroma, and hemorrhage into adjacent tissue. In addition, previous hemorrhage can be discovered by identifying large macrophages filled with hemosiderin near the periphery of the lesion. It has been estimated that no specific pathologic diagnosis can be made in about one third of typical endometriosis cases. (Figure 18-2 is hyperplastic dystrophy of the vulva; Figure 18-4 is adenocarcinoma of the endometrium; Figure 18-5 is adenomyosis;

Figure 18-6 is squamous cell carcinoma of the cervix.)

9. **D,** Page 510. The standard criterion of adenomyosis is the finding of endometrial glands and stromas that are more than one low-powered field (2.5 mm) from the basalis layer. Glands are typically inactive or proliferative. Cystic hyperplasia is seen occasionally, but secretory patterns are rare. The myometrium reacts to the ectopic endometrium by undergoing both hypertrophy and hyperplasia, thus producing the globular enlargement of the uterus.

10. **B,** Pages 510, 512. Patients with adenomyosis are usually asymptomatic. Symptomatic adenomyosis usually presents in women between 35 and 50 years of age, often in a parous woman with the classic symptoms of menorrhagia, dysmenorrhea, and occasional dyspareunia. The tender, boggy, and enlarged uterus described in this patient is typical. The degree of tenderness and consistency of the uterus may vary, depending on the time of the patient's menstrual cycle.

11. **E,** Pages 507–508. GI involvement occurs in one third of the cases of endometriosis. Involvement of small bowel is rare. Most cases of GI endometriosis are asymptomatic. If they are symptomatic, however, rectal bleeding is less likely than cramping, lower abdominal pain, pain on defecation, or constipation.

12. **C,** Page 507. No control studies have documented the benefit of D&C or uterine suspension in endometriosis. Occasionally, presacral neurectomy or uterosacral resection is performed for midline pain. In women who have completed childbearing and are in their late 20s or early 30s, hysterectomy with ovarian preservation can be optimal. In 10% of women the disease is subsequently found to be progressive and a second operation for oophorectomy is needed.

13. **A,** Pages 505–506. It may take as long as a year for ovulation to resume after the last injection of intramuscular progestin. With LH-RH, ovulation is expected to resume within 45 days of stopping the drug.

14. **C,** Pages 505–506. Amenorrhea is expected with both progestin and LH-RH therapy. Breakthrough bleeding is a common side effect of IM progestin therapy, which can be managed with low doses of estrogen.

15. **B,** Page 506. Breakthrough spotting or bleeding is the most persistent side effect of taking progestin. This symptom can be managed by the addition of small doses of oral estrogen.

16. **B,** Page 506. Therapeutic success rates for LH-RH exceed those of oral contraceptives and progestins.

17. **C (2, 4),** Pages 493–494. Endometriosis is a benign, progressive, recurrent disease that can both invade locally and disseminate to distant sites in the body. It is present in 5% to 15% of laparotomies performed on reproductive-age females. Its incidence in infertile women is 30% to 45%. It is a clinically different disease from adenomyosis. About 5% of cases are diagnosed following the menopause, usually stimulated by exogenous estrogen.

18. **E (All),** Page 496; Figure 18-1 (from Droegemueller). Rare sites of endometriosis include surgical incisions, nasal mucosa, lung, the spinal column, the umbilicus, bladder, arms, legs, kidney, and the male urinary tract.

19. **A (1, 2, 3),** Page 500. The most prominent pelvic finding associated with endometriosis is a fixed retroverted uterus with scarring and tenderness posterior to the uterus. The characteristic nodularity of the uterosacral ligaments and cul-de-sac of Douglas may be palpated on the rectovaginal exam. Ovaries may be enlarged, tender, and often fixed. The adnexal enlargement is rarely symmetric.

20. **E (All),** Page 498. New lesions are small, usually blood-filled cysts less than 1 cm in diameter. Clinically, they are often described as "raspberry" or "blueberry" spots. Initially, they are raised above the surrounding tissue and are either red or bluish-black. With time they become larger and assume a light or dark brown color with more intense scarring. These may appear more like a blood-filled cyst or "chocolate cyst." These are usually puckered or retracted from the surrounding tissue.

21. **A (1, 2, 3),** Page 507. Postoperative hormones can be given for a variety of indications. If not all the endometriosis has been removed, medroxyprogesterone is recommended for one year. To treat menopausal symptoms, cyclic estrogen and progestin can be used. Postoperative danazol or oral contraceptives may help eradicate microscopic endometriosis.

Steroidal hormones, including glucocorticoids, have not been proven efficacious in improving postoperative healing.

22. **E (All),** Page 502. Danazol has been an important medication in the treatment of endometriosis since its FDA approval in 1975. It may also be useful in cases of menorrhagia, benign cystic mastitis, and hereditary angioneurotic edema. In cases of menorrhagia, the use of danazol should not be considered an initial therapy.

23. **C (2, 4),** Page 498. In approximately 25% of cases, glands and stroma cannot be identified. In the majority of cases, the aberrant glands and stroma respond appropriately to estrogen and progesterone. Depending on the local blood supply, these changes may or may not be in synchrony with the uterine lining. Repetitive episodes of hemorrhage may lead to severe inflammatory changes and result in necrobiosis due to pressure atrophy or lack of blood supply. If so, a presumptive diagnosis is made by visualizing the intense chronic (**not** polymorphonuclear) inflammatory reaction and large macrophages filled with blood pigment.

24. **C (2, 4),** Page 500. The patient described is most likely to have endometriosis. There is no history of prior infection to warrant a diagnosis of

chronic PID, but this must still be included in the differential. Adenomyosis is most likely in a multiparous patient. Since the dysmenorrhea is of recent onset, it is, by definition, not primary dysmenorrhea.

25. **E** (All), Page 499. The classical symptoms are cyclic pelvic pain and infertility; however, approximately one third of patients are asymptomatic, the disease being discovered incidentally during an abdominal operation or visualized at laparoscopy for an unrelated problem.

26. **B** (1, 3), Pages 502–503. Danazol is mildly androgenic and anabolic, but the androgenic effects are approximately 1/200 that of testosterone. The drug also binds to sex hormone binding globulin, resulting in an increased level of free testosterone. FSH and LH are normally elevated in patients with ovarian failure (e.g., menopause). Danazol decreases FSH and LH more in menopausal patients than in the reproductive-age group. The term *pseudomenopause* is a misnomer and refers to side effects of the drug such as hot flashes and the histologic appearance of the endometrium.

27. **B** (1, 3), Page 500; The staging in Table 18-3 allows for systematic follow-up of patients who have been treated for endometriosis. A separate classification by the American Fertility Society is useful for patients with infertility (see Fig. 39-19 from Droegemueller). Tubal obstruction is associated with severe disease, and scattered, scarred implants on other structures are associated with moderate disease.

28. **C** (2, 4), Page 504; Table 18-4 (from Droegemueller). Side effects of danazol are seen in 80% of patients causing 10% to 20% to discontinue this medication. Reported side effects include acne, edema, weight gain, hirsutism, deepening of the voice, atrophic vaginitis, flushes, sweats, decreased breast size, uterine spotting, change in libido, GI disturbances, weakness, dizziness, cramps, and rashes. Except for occasional reports of deepening of the voice, all side effects usually resolve upon stopping the drug.

29. **E** (All), Page 503. Danazol binds to androgen and progesterone receptors and also binds to sex hormone binding globulin. It directly inhibits several steroidogenic enzymes in both the ovary and the adrenal gland.

30. **A** (1, 2, 3), Page 506. Although the choice between medical and surgical management for endometriosis depends on many considerations, certain findings warrant surgical management. Ureteral obstruction can ultimately lead to renal failure. Large bowel involvement by endometriosis must be managed surgically to avoid extensive compromise of bowel function. A large endometrioma poses risks of acute accident such as torsion, rupture, and hemorrhage. Furthermore, it should be remembered that an ovarian malignancy and an endometrioma can present the same clinical picture. In cases of progressive dysmenorrhea, medical therapy such as nonsteroidal anti-inflammatory agents should be used before surgery is considered.

31. **D** (4), Pages 503–504. The standard danazol regimen is 400–800 mg daily for 6 to 9 months. The half-life is between 4 and 5 hours, so that a single 200 mg tablet 4 times a day is preferable to 2 tablets twice daily. Because of the high monthly cost of $120 to $180, lower doses of drug have been tried. Symptomatic relief has been directly related to incidence of amenorrhea, but lower doses have been less successful in producing amenorrhea. Since food does not interfere with absorption, danazol can be taken with meals. If one is certain that the patient is not pregnant, it is better to start danazol on the first day of menstrual bleeding. By starting the hormone on the first day of the cycle rather than the fifth day as is commonly recommended, the patient will experience less breakthrough bleeding during the first 4 to 6 weeks.

32. **A** (1, 2, 3), Page 504. Standard danazol therapy for 6 to 9 months results in both symptomatic and objective improvement in a large portion of patients. The uncorrected fertility rate is 40%, but 15% to 30% of patients have recurrent symptoms within 2 years.

33. **A** (1, 2, 3), Pages 502–506. Both oral and injectable progestin have been shown to be effective, particularly useful in patients who cannot tolerate high dose estrogen or in whom estrogen is contraindicated. Progestin success rates are similar to oral contraceptives.

   LH-RH agonists cause a downward regulation of LH-RH receptors through prolonged receptor occupation, thus causing a medical castration without side effects in end organs. Continuous therapy for 6 months has resulted in regression of 85% of endometriosis.

   Methyltestosterone is no longer in common usage for endometriosis. Side effects range from acne and hirsutism to liver toxicity. The possibility of pregnancy and masculinizing effects on a female fetus were of constant concern.

34. **E** (All), Page 510. Adenomyosis and endometriosis are different clinical entities. The glands in adenomyosis are not as responsive to hormones as those in the endometrium. This may, in part, be due to the relative lack of estrogen and progesterone receptors in the glands and stroma of adenomyosis. In most cases, adenomyosis is diffusely distributed in the myometrium.

CHAPTER 19

Disorders of Abdominal Wall and Pelvic Support

DIRECTIONS: Select the one best answer or completion.

1. A 72-year-old para 3 presents with a history of recently noticed "bulge" protruding through the vaginal introitus. Fifteen months prior to this visit, a vaginal hysterectomy was performed on this patient for uterine decensus. What is her "bulge" most likely to be?
   A. Cystocele
   B. Rectocele
   C. Enterocele
   D. Prolapsed ovaries
   E. Sigmoid diverticulum

2. In performing a lower abdominal midline incision, the major anatomic landmark encountered in the abdominal wall involves a change in the fascial investiture of the rectus muscle. This change occurs at which anatomic landmark?
   A. Hesselback's triangle
   B. Linea semilunaris
   C. Linea alba
   D. Linea nigra
   E. Umbilicus

3. A 52-year-old para 4 woman complains of a bulging vaginal mass, constipation, and incomplete stool evacuation. Which anatomic defect is most likely to contribute to these symptoms?
   A. Cystourethrocele
   B. Uterine prolapse
   C. Poor anal sphincter tone
   D. Rectocele
   E. Enterocele

4. An 82-year-old woman with total vaginal vault prolapse is referred to you with a 2 month history of noticing a "bulge" between her labia. She is being treated for congestive heart failure. She had a total abdominal hysterectomy and bilateral oophorectomy 25 years prior and has been sexually inactive for more than 15 years. Which would be the best choice for surgical correction of this patient?
   A. Abdominal suspension from the rectus fascia.
   B. Abdominal sacral colpopexy.
   C. Abdominal enterocele reduction.
   D. Vaginal colpocleisis.
   E. Vaginal sacrospinous ligament suspension.

5. Which of the following defects in pelvic anatomy can be termed a true hernia?
   A. Cystocele
   B. Enterocele
   C. Rectocele
   D. Urethrocele
   E. Ureterocele

6. What is the goal for anatomic restoration of anterior colporrhaphy when done to correct stress urinary incontinence associated with a cystourethrocele?
   A. To foreshorten the pubovesical fascia.
   B. To lengthen the urethra.
   C. To make the bladder smaller.
   D. To correct the urethrovesical angle.
   E. To replace the bladder neck behind the pubic symphysis.

7. Which structures in Figure 19-1 lend the most support in the repair of a rectocele?
   A. Levator ani muscle group.
   B. Perirectal connective tissue.
   C. Proximal fibers of the superficial transverse perinei muscle.
   D. The trimmed posterior vaginal mucosa.
   E. The anal sphincter.

8. At the time of preoperative evaluation of a patient upon whom you anticipate performing a postpartum tubal sterilization, you notice a 5 cm umbilical hernia. What should you do at this point?
   A. Proceed with the operation as planned and repair the hernia upon completion of the sterilization.
   B. Proceed with the tubal sterilization and plan repair of the hernia at a later date.
   C. Abort the entire operation.
   D. Proceed with the sterilization only and make a lower midline vertical incision.
   E. Proceed with the operation using the laparoscope.

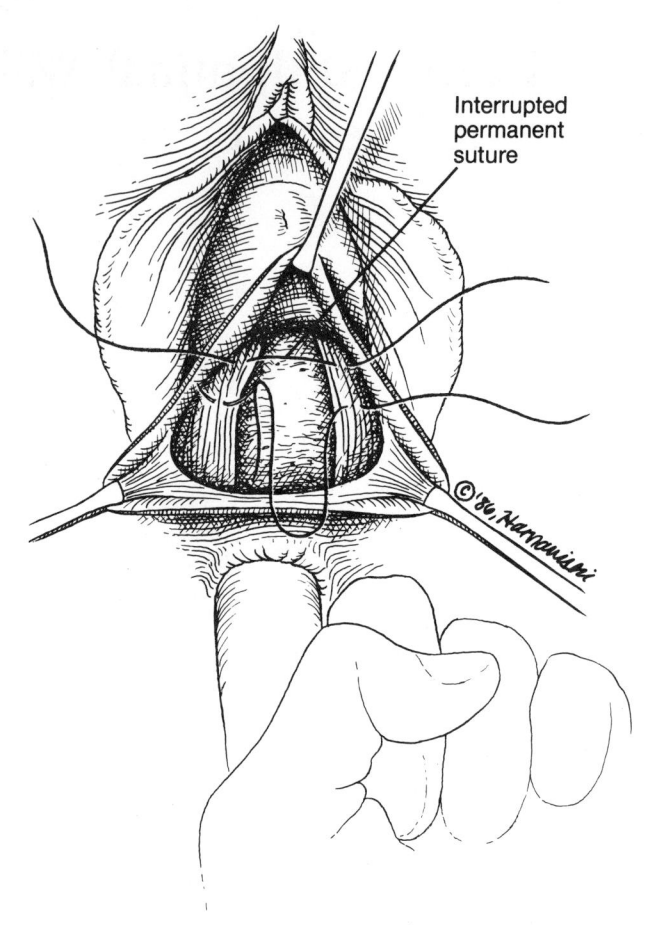

FIGURE 19-1.
(From Droegemueller W, Herbst AL, Mishell DR, Stenchever, MA: Comprehensive gynecology. St. Louis, The C.V. Mosby Co., 1987.)

9. A 48-year-old patient with these anatomic findings (Fig. 19-2) presents with symptoms of pelvic pressure, urethral irritation, and consistent stress urinary incontinence with mild valsalva. Assuming the completion of an appropriate urologic workup that documents stress urinary incontinence, which of the following surgical procedures is indicated?
   A. Marshall-Marchetti-Krantz procedure.
   B. Vaginal hysterectomy with anterior colporrhaphy.
   C. Anterior wall colporrhaphy.
   D. Burch procedure.
   E. Pereyra operation.

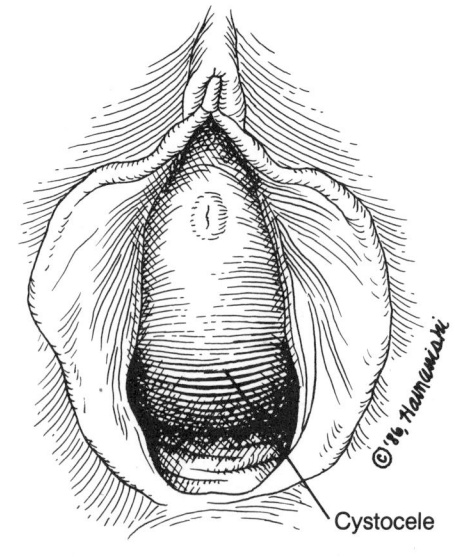

FIGURE 19-2.
(From Droegemueller W, Herbst AL, Mishell DR, Stenchever MA: Comprehensive gynecology. St. Louis, The C.V. Mosby Co., 1987.)

DIRECTIONS: For each numbered item, select the one heading most closely associated with it. Each lettered heading may be used once, more than once, or not at all.

(A) Vaginal hysterectomy and anterior-posterior colporrhaphy
(B) Manchester-Fothergill + anterior colporrhaphy
(C) Le Fort (modified)
(D) Goodal-Power
(E) Watkins interposition

10. Total procidentia; 85 years old; widowed; congestive heart failure
11. Elongated cervix; well-supported uterus; cystourethrocele with stress urinary incontinence
12. Second degree cystocele and rectocele; 78 years old; sexually inactive
13. 45 years old; second degree cystourethrocele with stress urinary incontinence

DIRECTIONS: For each numbered item, indicate whether it is associated with
A. only (A)
B. only (B)
C. both (A) and (B)
D. neither (A) nor (B)

(A) Vaginal colpopexy
(B) Abdominal colpopexy
(C) Both
(D) Neither

14. Correction of attendant enterocele.
15. Sexual function preserved.
16. Sacrospinous ligaments used for support.

(A) Cystocele
(B) Urethrocele
(C) Both
(C) Neither

17. Considered a true hernia.
18. Attenuation of pubovesical cervical fascia.
19. Contributes to urinary incontinence.

(A) Femoral canal
(B) Inguinal canal
(C) Both
(D) Neither

20. Aperture resulting from embryonic descent of testes from original retroperitoneal site to the scrotum.
21. Herniated peritoneum into this space may occur in both sexes.
22. In the woman, the round ligament courses through this aperture.
23. A hernia sac into this space may contain a portion of bowel.

DIRECTIONS: Each question contains four suggested answers of which one or more is correct. Choose the answer

A. if 1, 2, and 3 are correct
B. if 1 and 3 are correct
C. if 2 and 4 are correct
D. if 4 only is correct
E. if all are correct

24. During the performance of a vaginal hysterectomy, a postoperative enterocele is prevented by appropriate surgical disposition of which of the following structures?
    1. Uterosacral ligaments
    2. Cardinal ligaments
    3. Cul-de-sac peritoneum
    4. Round ligaments

25. Appropriate surgical correction in cases of vaginal vault (stump) prolapse include a recognition of the
    1. normal axis of the vagina in a standing position.
    2. perineal body anatomy.
    3. specific vaginal wall defects.
    4. urodynamic function by cystometrogram.

26. A cystourethrocele is more likely to develop if a woman has
    1. recurrent urinary tract infections.
    2. wide pubic arch.
    3. prominent ischial spines.
    4. delivered several children.

27. Which specific anatomic defects are identified in cases of total vaginal vault (stump) prolapse?
    1. Cystocele
    2. Rectocele
    3. Enterocele
    4. Attenuated perineal body

28. The differential diagnosis of a bulging anterior vaginal wall includes
    1. urethral diverticulum.
    2. Skene's gland enlargement.
    3. bladder diverticula.
    4. cystourethrocele.

29. Which are characteristics of an umbilical hernia?
    1. It is a vestige of extra embryonic coelomic cavity.
    2. When repaired, remnants of umbilical cord can be found.
    3. Fascial defect usually closes in first 3 years of life.
    4. A fascial defect in its severe form presents as gastroschisis.

30. Anatomic characteristics of abdominal hernias
    1. contain visceral organ structures (e.g., bowel).
    2. contain a reflection of peritoneum (sac).
    3. are congenital.
    4. are a fascial defect.

ANSWERS

1. **C,** Pages 526, 528. Enteroceles frequently occur after hysterectomy and generally are due to weakened support of the pouch of Douglas. Lack of attention to surgical repair of supporting structures at the time of original surgery may contribute to the formation of postoperative enterocele, especially one that presents this soon after the antecedent hysterectomy. A small preexisting herniation of peritoneum may have been overlooked during the vaginal hysterectomy. Lack of obliteration of this hernia sac and improper attention to the plication of uterosacral or cardinal ligaments may contribute to the development of an immediate postop enterocele. In this situation, there is often a degree of total vault prolapse perceived by the patient as a "bulge" passing through the vaginal introitus.

   Although cystocele and rectocele may be associated with this postoperative herniation, they are usually secondary rather than primary offenders. Prolapsed adnexal structures are rare and usually are not involved in cases of vaginal vault prolapse. Likewise, prolapse of the sigmoid colon or parts of the sigmoid colon do not present in this fashion.

2. **B,** Pages 517–518; Figure 19-2 (from Droegemueller). The investing fasciae of the external oblique, internal oblique, and transversus abdominis muscles completely encase the rectus abdominis muscles cephalic to the linea semilunaris. Caudally from the semiunar line, the muscle is completely posterior to the aponeurosis of the fasciae of these muscles and lies directly on the peritoneum. In making a midline incision, this change is apparent after mobilizing the rectus muscle laterally and just prior to entry into the peritoneal cavity. In the repair of this incision, it is important to remember that this area of relative weakness contributes to a higher incidence of postoperative abdominal incisional hernias.

   Hesselback's triangle defines that anatomic area in which a defect in the transversalis fasciae may result in a femoral type of groin hernia. The linea alba is the midline fusion of the rectus fasciae and is not used as a superficial anatomic landmark. The linea nigra is a vertical discoloration of the skin occurring between the umbilicus and the top of the pubic symphysis.

3. **D,** Pages 525–526. In a patient with these complaints referable primarily to lower bowel dysfunction, the most likely contributing anatomic defect is a rectocele. The other anatomic defects may be associated with the presence of a rectocele but do not contribute to these symptoms. Patients may often need to "splint" the posterior vaginal wall in order to ameliorate those symptoms associated with difficulty in having bowel movements. Chronic constipation in these patients with retention of firm stool in the lower colon can be associated with degrees of discomfort during sexual intercourse.

   It should be pointed out that a symptomatic rectocele, illustrated by this patient, is the only disorder of pelvic support that can be corrected by vaginal repair. Poor anal sphincter tone may be secondary to incompletely healed perineal lacerations incurred during childbirth. Symptoms related to this defect, such as incontinence of stool or flatus, are not manifest in this patient and, when present, are not necessarily associated with other disorders of pelvic support.

   Operative management of a rectocele is generally performed at the time of other vaginal surgery. Likewise, perineal body reconstruction (perineorrhaphy) is also indicated in those patients where there is a marked defect in perineal support. However, this does not routinely imply reconstruction of the anal sphincter.

4. **D,** Pages 534–535. Although there are a variety of procedures to manage vaginal vault (stump) prolapse, selection of the appropriate procedure is guided by a number of factors. This includes the age of the patient, sexual activity, the specific anatomic defects involved, and general health of the patient.

   In this geriatric patient who is sexually inactive with congestive heart failure, an extensive abdominal operation involving either suspension of the wall to the rectus fascia or any of a variety of sacral suspensions using inert gauze material is not needed. Abdominal reduction of an enterocele in this patient also would not be indicated, as this would not correct the anatomic defect presenting. Because this patient is sexually inactive, a more extensive procedure such as vaginal sacrospinous ligament suspension is not necessary. The most logical choice for this situation would be some form of vaginal closure by colpocleisis. This could be vaginectomy or vaginal colpocleisis modified after the LeFort procedure. When doing this procedure, it is important to identify enterocele if it is present so that appropriate dissection, ligation, and excision of redundant peritoneum can be performed to prevent an enterocele forming posterior to the colpocleisis.

5. **B,** Page 528. An enterocele is a true hernia of the peritoneal cavity emanating from the pouch of Douglas between the uterosacral ligaments and into the rectovaginal septum. It may be noticed as a separate bulge above the rectocele and at times it may be large enough to prolapse through the vagina. A hernia by definition must contain a serosal sac, although it may also contain bowel or omentum. The other defects noted above are not true hernias

in that they do not contain herniated peritoneum through a fascial defect. They are prolapsed distal bowel (rectocele), bladder (cystocele), or urethra (urethrocele). The latter is usually a detachment of the urethra rather than a ballooning out of this structure. The ureterocele is the most unusual of those listed above and represents saculation of the distal ureter into the bladder as a result of stenosis of the *ureteral* meatus.

6. **E,** Pages 524–525. The overall goal of anterior colporrhaphy to correct urinary incontinence is to replace the bladder neck behind the symphysis pubis in order to increase the amount of pressure transmitted to the proximal urethra during valsalva. The anatomic abnormality associated with urinary incontinence is discussed further in Chapter 20.

The other corrections noted in this question may all occur in the process of performing an adequate anterior colporrhaphy. That is, the pubovesical fascia may be drawn more closely towards the midline by appropriately placed Kelly plication sutures. Depending on the degree of urethrocele, the urethra may be somewhat lengthened, although this is not thought to lend appreciably to urinary continence. Bladder capacity may be reduced by cystocele repair, which results in the urge to void sooner than when there is marked laxity in the vaginal wall. Finally, the urethrovesical angle may be increased in the process of anterior colporrhaphy because of appropriate elevation of the bladder neck behind the symphysis. However, the angle in and of itself is probably not important in correcting incontinence.

7. **A,** Page 526. The major contribution in restoration of pelvic floor anatomy when performing posterior colporrhaphy is made by reducing the aperture of the levator hiatus. Although the levator plate is made up of a number of muscles, restoration of the anatomy of the pubococcygeus and puborectalis are probably most important. Plication of the lower margins of the bulbocavernosis and transverse perinei muscles also strengthens the support of the urogenital diaphragm. During dissection in the operating room, separation and identification of these muscles is very difficult. The superficial transverse perinei do not lend appreciably to pelvic muscle support, nor does the relatively attenuated perirectal connective tissue. The trimmed vaginal mucosa likewise does not lend much in the way of strengthening. The anal sphincter is usually not involved in this repair procedure. Knowledge of the anatomy of the levator plate is important in planning the appropriate operation for patients with marked posterior vaginal wall defects.

8. **A,** Page 520. In this unexpected situation, the presence of a small umbilical hernia need not deter the surgeon in performing the original operation. A Pomeroy Tubal sterilization can be carried out with appropriate repair of the umbilical hernia after completion of the sterilization. Care should be taken in this situation to completely dissect the peritoneal sac away from the point of intraperitoneal entry. Likewise, care should be taken to find the lateral extent of the fascial defect and repair this by either direct approximation from superior to inferior using nonabsorbable sutures (close the fascia in a "vest over pants" manner.) There is no point in delaying the repair of this hernia for a later date if it can be repaired at the time of this operation. There is no need to abort the operation or change the incision, nor is there any need to use the laparoscope.

Knowledge of this anatomic defect at the time of surgery should alert the surgeon to the possibility of adherent bowel just under the peritoneal sac or the presence of a Meckel's diverticulum just beneath the peritoneal surface.

Another consideration in this question has to do with the issue of informed consent. With potential alteration of the umbilicus, the surgeon should be aware that surgical alteration of this structure may carry with it the risk of patient dissatisfaction. Ideally, if this defect is appreciated prior to the actual surgery, appropriate informed consent should be obtained.

9. **B,** Pages 523, 553–557. Although a number of options exist for surgical repair of patients with stress urinary incontinence, certain principles can be used to guide surgical decisions.

The point of this question is to consider a general approach based on specific anatomic findings. Accordingly, this patient with marked anterior wall relaxation (cystourethrocele) with related pelvic pressure and irritation should have a vaginal procedure. This will best treat the anatomic defect (cystourethrocele) while at the same time offering a high degree of success in curing the incontinence. Most surgeons would agree that in a patient of this age, concomitant vaginal hysterectomy would also be indicated. Although it could be argued that a combined operation might be beneficial, it should be appreciated that the performance of a retropubic operation such as in Marshall-Marchetti-Krantz or Burch procedure is not indicated as the sole operation. Likewise, the Pereyra operation will not correct the vaginal wall defect.

10–13. 10, **C;** 11, **B;** 12, **D;** 13, **A;** Pages 531–534. This series of questions deals with the choice of surgical treatment for symptomatic pelvic relaxation under different circumstances. It must be realized that there is no consensus among surgeons about the appropriate surgical treatment in every case; however, the situations described above do delineate the types of operations to be considered in certain instances. In general, eponyms should be avoided, but certain surgical procedures are named for the surgeon or surgeons who first described and popularized them. It is realized that some of these operations are rarely indicated. This series of operations underscores the need for the consultant to know a wide range of surgical options and thus assist the occasional individual patient.

The Le Fort operation is usually considered the procedure of choice in elderly patients with total prolapse. This is in contrast to the Goodall-Power modification, which is used with lesser degrees of prolapse in the geriatric age group. This operation involves removing smaller triangular portions of anterior and posterior vaginal wall mucosa instead of the traditional rectangular portions removed in the Le Fort operation. Thus, when sutured together after reduction of the uterus, effective colpocleisis has been accomplished. Both operations will obliterate the vagina and should be reserved for sexually inactive women. Both operations usually are done in conjunction with perineorrhaphy as an additional measure to assure a better long-term result.

The Manchester-Fothergill operation is rarely indicated today. It is reserved for the occasional patient who has appreciable stress urinary incontinence, elongated cervix, and excellent uterine support either by previous operation or by intercurrent inflammatory or adhesion disease. An adequate anterior colporrhaphy and plication of the vesical neck can be accomplished with this operation, which involves amputating the elongated cervix and using the uterosacral ligaments to improve support of the residual cervix and cul-de-sac.

The Watkins interposition or transposition operation was used extensively for uterine prolapse in patients with a large cystocele. The operation consisting of amputating the elongated cervix and suturing the fundus of the uterus beneath the large cystocele. The fundus therefore was used as an obturator to fill the defect in the anterior segment of the pelvic diaphragm. This operation is rarely used today in lieu of more popular forms of vaginal plastic procedures.

Most instances of symptomatic vaginal relaxation associated with uterine prolapse can be surgically treated by vaginal hysterectomy and anterior posterior colporrhaphy. This will maintain a degree of vaginal depth and caliber suitable for sexual function while at the same time correcting anatomic defects that may be associated with urinary incontinence or problems with bowel evacuation. The gynecologic surgeon should realize that although vaginal hysterectomy with colporrhaphy usually can be done, other operations are available when indicated by special circumstances to ensure the overall health of the patient.

14–16. 14, C; 15, C; 16,A; Page 535. There are a variety of vaginal or abdominal procedures to reconstruct vaginal stump prolapse. Within each category there are specialized surgical nuances that may be applied to individual cases. In choosing a vaginal procedure, the best results occur in those patients where adequate vaginal length is maintained and the vagina is positioned against the rectum nearly parallel to the horizontal. Similarly, when choosing an abdominal colpopexy of some variety, there should be attention to restoration of anatomy that is as nearly normal as possible. Both vaginal and abdominal colpopexy correct attendant enteroceles if they are identified. In the case of vaginal reconstructive surgery, recognition of a dissecting enterocele sac should result in surgical attention and removal. In the abdominal operation, the deep cul-de-sac or beginning enterocele should be closed prior to the attachment of the vaginal vault to a fixed structure. Otherwise, continued enterocele sac dissection may take place despite adequate support of the vaginal vault.

Both abdominal or vaginal procedures may preserve sexual function. This is especially important to consider in vaginal repair. Adequate caliber and depth can be maintained with careful attention to anatomic principles.

The sacrospinous ligaments may be used for additional vaginal vault support in selected cases. This operation is technically more difficult and potentially riskier than routine vaginal colporrhaphy, but occasionally should be chosen as a means for ensuring vaginal vault support.

17–19. 17, D; 18, C; 19,B; Page 523. Neither the cystocele nor urethrocele is considered a true hernia since neither condition includes the protrusion of a peritoneal reflection or sac through a true fascial defect. Attenuation or rupture of the pubovesical cervical fascia for any reason may allow the descent of the urethra (urethrocele), bladder neck, or bladder (cystocele) into the vaginal canal. Often a cystocele is present, and in this situation the patient is generally continent of urine. When a urethrocele also is present, the woman usually suffers from stress urinary incontinence, because the urethra has rotated posteriorly. The urethra and bladder neck now lie in a position where intraabdominal pressure is not transmitted to the periurethral tissues. In other words, there is little compensatory pressure around the bladder neck and proximal urethra during times of valsalva. In this situation, relatively more pressure is exerted on the bladder and relatively less pressure on the urethra, thereby creating urinary incontinence. Even in the presence of the cystocele, with maintenance of normal intraurethral pressures, patients generally will remain continent of urine. This observation is useful when considering surgical techniques to correct anatomically related stress urinary incontinence.

20–23. 20, **B**; 21, **C**; 22, **B**; 23, **C**; Pages 517–518; Figure 18-2 (from Droegemueller). Because of embryonic descent of the testis from its original retroperitoneal site to the scrotum, the internal inguinal ring is formed at the level of the transversalis fascia. The inguinal canal runs from the internal inguinal ring obliquely medial and caudal, emerging through the external inguinal ring, opening in the external oblique aponeurosis just above the pubic tubercle, and continuing into the scrotum. In the female, the round ligament courses similarly and ends just short of the labium majus. (The femoral canal represents a potential space under the inguinal ligament medial to the femoral vessels and lateral to the lacunar ligament.) Because there is no embryonic movement of the testicle in women, their inguinal canal is less likely to be associated with herniated peritoneum. Femoral hernias are more common in women than in men. Either potential space (canal) may be involved with a hernia that includes a portion of the bowel.

24. **A** (1, 2, 3), Page 528. Enteroceles may occur after abdominal or vaginal hysterectomy and generally are due to a weakened support system around the cul-de-sac or pouch of Douglas. Inasmuch as an enterocele may form by herniation of the cul-de-sac past the uterosacral ligaments into the rectovaginal septum, appropriate surgical disposition of the uterosacral ligaments, cardinal ligaments, and peritoneum overlying the cul-de-sac are imperative. Generally, if there is redundant peritoneum beginning to herniate into the rectovaginal septum, this space should be closed after the removal of the uterus to prevent further extension. Likewise, the uterosacral and cardinal ligaments should be plicated in the midline or into the vaginal cuff. Each of these procedures has a number of variations, but all are termed as types of culdoplasty.

The round ligaments do not lend significantly to posthysterectomy vault support and generally are not considered important to incorporate into the vaginal cuff in an effort to prevent postoperative enterocele or other vaginal wall relaxation.

25. **A** (1, 2, 3), Page 534. There is some controversy with respect to the choice of procedure for vaginal vault (stump) prolapse. Nevertheless, certain principles and facts are important. The first is that the normal position of the vagina in the standing position is against the rectum and no more than 30 degrees from the horizontal. This is important for the occasional patient in whom abdominal colpopexy is anticipated. The second principle is that pelvic relaxation is part of the problem and dictates that an existing cystocele, rectocele, or enterocele must be repaired as part of this procedure to ensure long-term success. Defects are likely to recur when appropriate recognition and repair has not taken place during the initial surgery for vaginal prolapse. The third principle acknowledges that the perineal body is almost always severely weakened in women with total vaginal vault prolapse and must therefore be reconstructed.

It is not necessary to perform routine urodynamic function tests on these patients if incontinence is not a major component of their presenting complaint.

26. **C** (2, 4), Page 523. The factors associated with the development of a cystourethrocele are numerous and difficult to state in very specific terms, but some general associations can be noted. These include parity and a wide pelvic arch typical of the gynecoid type pelvis. Although a cystourethrocele may develop in nulliparous women, this is unusual. In such cases, the patients will often have concomitant neurologic or metabolic disease contributing to loss of pelvic support, or they may be overweight or have chronic obstructive pulmonary disease. The presence of a wide pubic arch in a gynecoid type of pelvis allows the full force of the fetal head to compress against this area during descent in the second stage of labor. Narrower arches, such as those associated with the android or anthropoid pelvis, seem to protect this region from descent of the fetal head. This may account in part for the observation that a cystourethrocele is much less common in the black race, in whom the android or anthropoid pelves are common. Similarly, prominent ischial spines are more consistent with these latter two types of pelves than with the gynecoid type and therefore makes this choice incorrect.

Rather than a cause for developing a cystourethrocele, recurrent urinary tract infections may be a result of significant defects in the anterior vagina and/or bladder resulting in excessive amounts of residual urine in the bladder even after micturition.

Although it can be argued that obesity may increase chronic intraabdominal pressure on the pelvic supporting structures, obesity in and of itself has not been documented to be associated with a higher incidence of cystourethrocele.

27. **E** (All), Page 534. All of the above anatomic defects can be noted in cases of total vaginal vault (stump) prolapse. Usually some combination of defects is seen. Only occasionally will the prolapse involve one of these entities and not the entire vaginal barrel. This includes 6% that are cystocele only, 5% rectocele only, 9% primarily enterocele, and 72% of mixed type.

It is important to recognize the specific anatomic defects involved in these cases so that appropriate surgical repair can be planned. For example, repairing a cystocele and rectocele without recognizing an enterocele may result in progressive enterocele formation behind the previously repaired cystocele and rectocele. This is a special problem in a patient on whom colpocleisis has been performed.

28. **E** (All), Page 523. On physical examination, defective anterior vaginal wall support usually is apparent and will consist of varying degrees of a cystourethrocele. However, other entities should be considered depending on the visual and palpable characteristics of these defects. A urethrocele must be differentiated from inflamed and enlarged Skene's glands and urethral diverticula. With a urethral diverticulum, a palpable mass usually is present. Inflamed Skene's glands are tender. With both a urethral diverticulum and inflamed Skene's glands, it may be possible to express pus from the urethra when they are palpated. Cystoceles must be differentiated from bladder tumors and bladder diverticula, both of which are rare. A cystocele is generally soft, pliable, and nontender, as are bladder diverticula.

Correct anatomic diagnosis and documentation of unusual findings are important in determining therapy, especially if surgical intervention is indicated. This is discussed further in Chapter 20.

29. **B** (1, 3), Page 519. The umbilical hernia is an example of a congenital malformation. Before 10 weeks of gestation, the abdominal contents are partially herniated through the umbilicus into the extra embryonic coelomic cavity. Shortly thereafter, the visceral contents return to the abdominal cavity and the defect in the abdominal wall closes during subsequent fetal growth. Generally, at birth this space contains only the umbilical cord. Following the cutting of the cord the area heals so that the skin in the area of the umbilicus fuses over the closed fascial layer. Small umbilical hernias at birth usually close in the first 3 years of life.

In rare cases, with less complete closure of the abdominal wall, an omphalocele forms, which is a hernia sac at the umbilicus covered only by peritoneum and including bowel and other abdominal contents. This is in contrast to gastroschisis, which is a failure of midline fusion of the abdominal wall not solely related to absence of fusion around the umbilical cord.

In the repair of the umbilical hernia, usually all that is encountered is an empty hernia sac protruding through the small fascial defect.

30. **E** (All), Pages 517–519. Characteristics of abdominal hernias by definition include a reflection of peritoneum through a fascial defect. When intraperitoneal organ structures are part of the hernia, they are called sliding hernias.

Although most hernias occur at anatomic weak sports, they generally are not considered congenital anomalies. The only exception is the persistence of an umbilical hernia resulting from failure of the fascia of the abdominal wall to close over the site of the umbilical cord insertion. When considering surgical repair of abdominal hernias, it is important to remember that there is almost always a peritoneal reflection to dissect and close, in addition to closing the original fascial defect.

CHAPTER 20: Gynecologic Urology

DIRECTIONS: Select the one best answer or completion.

1. A 24-year-old, healthy appearing woman complains of a recent onset of urgency with loss of urine. She has never had such symptoms before. Which is the best single test in this case?
   A. Residual urine
   B. Cystometrics
   C. Urine analysis
   D. Bonney test
   E. Urethroscopy

2. What is the major action of urethral support operations?
   A. Decrease bladder activity
   B. Increase urethral sphincter tone
   C. Decrease the parasympathetic nerve supply to the urethra
   D. Decrease the caliber of the urethral lumen
   E. Increase the transmission of abdominal pressure to the urethra

3. Which is a major concern with the Bonney test when evaluating incontinence?
   A. It damages the vaginal mucosa.
   B. It causes osteitis pubis in 1% to 3% of patients.
   C. It is only of use if the functional length of the urethra is over 2 cm.
   D. It cannot be used when the patient is standing.
   E. It may be falsely positive if too much pressure is used.

4. What is the major risk for a patient who has had a Mersilene sling procedure for urethral suspension?
   A. Intraoperative hemorrhage
   B. Infection
   C. Transection of the urethra by the Mersilene
   D. Reabsorption of the sling
   E. Loss of bladder innervation

5. A 72-year-old diabetic female has been sent to you from a nursing home for evaluation because she is always incontinent. She has no complaints other than the wetness. How can the most likely etiology be tested?
   A. Urinalysis
   B. Urethroscopy
   C. Residual urine test
   D. Bonney stress test
   E. Transurethral injection of methylene blue.

6. A woman complains that a large volume of urine is lost shortly after coughing or jumping. She occasionally has a loss of urine while in bed at night if she happens to cough vigorously. She is unable to stop the urinary stream once it has begun. With this history, what is she most likely to have?
   A. Stress incontinence
   B. Fistula
   C. Detrusor dyssynergia (bladder instability)
   D. Urinary tract infection
   E. Ectopic ureter

7. A 24-year-old woman complains of frequency, urgency, and dysuria of 2 days duration. What is the most common etiologic agent causing these symptoms?
   A. *Enterobacter aerogenes*
   B. *Streptococcus faecalis*
   C. *Chlamydia trachomatis*
   D. *Klebsiella aerogenes*
   E. *Escherichia coli*

8. Four weeks after a MMK (Marshall-Marchetti-Krantz) repair for stress incontinence, a patient complains of increased pain in the suprapubic area that is aggravated by walking. She is continent, afebrile, and has a white blood count of 11,000. Her urinalysis is clear. On examination, she has pain over the mons pubis. On bimanual, the pubic symphysis is exquisitely tender with no other findings. What is the mostly likely diagnosis?
   A. Urinary tract infection
   B. Retropubic abscess
   C. Osteitis pubis
   D. Osteomyelitis
   E. Unresolved hematoma in the space of Retzius

9. A 44-year-old woman complains of copious (approximately one-half cup) urine loss that she is unable to stop once it begins to flow. She states that the loss begins shortly after a cough or sneeze and that she frequently feels she has to void. If she doesn't void within a few minutes after this sensation, she will also lose urine. What is the most likely etiology?
   A. Urge incontinence
   B. Stress incontinence
   C. Urethrovaginal fistula
   D. Urethral diverticula
   E. Overflow incontinence

10. A premenopausal woman who has completed her family and has mild genuine stress incontinence without infection asks you to describe the methods available for treatment in her case. Which is most appropriate as an initial step?
    A. Estrogen replacement
    B. Kegel exercises
    C. Alpha adrenergic agents
    D. Kelly plication
    E. Marshall-Marchetti-Krantz procedure

11. A 50-year-old woman has a history of recurrent dysuria and frequency as well as dyspareunia and postvoid dribbling. On examination she has a tender nodule palpable through the anterior vaginal wall. What is the most likely diagnosis?
    A. Ectopic ureter
    B. Bartholin duct abscess
    C. Urethral diverticulum
    D. Urethrocele
    E. Gartner's duct cyst

12. A cystourethrocele is a ballooning out of
    A. the bladder.
    B. the urethra.
    C. both the urethra and the bladder.
    D. the bladder and a detachment of the urethra.
    E. the bladder and a diverticulum of the urethra.

13. What is a patient with genuine stress incontinence most apt to have?
    A. A short urethra.
    B. An abnormal bead chain cystourethrogram.
    C. Loss of the pubourethral vesical angle.
    D. A positive Q-tip test.
    E. Lack of transmission of intraabdominal pressure to the urethra.

14. When counseling a patient on how to use Kegel exercises, you should tell her to contract the pelvic floor muscles
    A. whenever she thinks of it.
    B. five times every 4 hours during the day.
    C. five times every half hour during the day.
    D. five times whenever she urinates.
    E. ten times every 4 hours during the day.

DIRECTIONS: For each numbered item, select the one heading most closely associated with it. Each lettered heading may be used once, more than once, or not at all.

(A) Passing a needle with a suture from the rectus fascia through the space of Retzius to the paravaginal tissue.
(B) Suturing lateral paravaginal fascia together beneath the urethra to support the bladder neck.
(C) Suturing the paravaginal fascia to the symphysis pubis.
(D) Suturing the rectus fascia beneath the urethra.
(E) Suturing the paravaginal fascia to Cooper's ligament.

15. Burch
16. Kelly
17. Marshall-Marchetti-Krantz
18. Pereyra

DIRECTIONS: For each numbered item, indicate whether it is associated with
A. only (A)
B. only (B)
C. both (A) and (B)
D. neither (A) nor (B)

(A) Urge incontinence
(B) Genuine stress incontinence
(C) Both
(D) Neither

19. An objectively demonstrated involuntary loss of urine that is a social or hygienic problem.
20. Involuntary loss of urine associated with bladder pressure greater than urethral pressure in the absence of detrusor contractions.
21. Involuntary loss of urine associated with uninhibited detrusor contractions.
22. Involuntary loss of urine due to a bladder pressure greater than the urethral pressure because of bladder distension without detrusor activity.

(A) Inhibits bladder contraction
(B) Stimulates urethral contraction
(C) Both
(D) Neither

23. The micturition feedback nerve circuit from the cortex to the brain stem (loop I).
24. Parasympathetic stimulation.
25. Stimulation of adrenergic receptors.

DIRECTIONS: Each question contains four suggested answers of which one or more is correct. Choose the answer
A. if 1, 2, and 3 are correct
B. if 1 and 3 are correct
C. if 2 and 4 are correct
D. if 4 only is correct
E. if all are correct

26. To diagnose detrusor dyssynergia (bladder instability), which of the following must be present?
    1. Incontinence.
    2. Response to bladder retraining drills.
    3. Failure to respond to surgical suspension of the urethra.
    4. Uninhibited bladder contractions.

27. A woman has genuine stress incontinence and symptoms and signs of anterior vaginal wall excoriation from a fourth degree cystourethrocele. Her stress incontinence has improved minimally with adequately performed Kegel exercises. She wishes to remain fertile, but she wants to have a surgical procedure to relieve her symptoms. Which is the appropriate surgical procedure(s)?
    1. Vaginal hysterectomy and anterior and posterior repair.
    2. MMK (Marshall-Marchetti-Krantz) procedure.
    3. Burch procedure.
    4. Anterior colporrhaphy with Kelly plication.

28. Before a surgical correction procedure, you are counseling a patient in whom the diagnosis of genuine stress incontinence has been made. Factors to discuss include the risk of
    1. damage to other organs and structures.
    2. increased incontinence.
    3. failure to achieve correction.
    4. difficulty in urinating after the procedure.

29. Urinary continence is achieved by maintaining urethral pressures greater than the intravesical pressures. Factors that contribute to the maintenance of intraurethral pressure include
    1. smooth and striated muscle in the urethral wall.
    2. vascularity of the urethral submucosa.
    3. transmission of intraabdominal pressure to the urethra.
    4. the distal 1 cm of the urethra.

ANSWERS

1. **C, Pages 543–544.** In an otherwise healthy woman who has had recent onset of urinary urgency and loss of urine, the differential diagnosis should include urethritis, trigonitis, or cystitis. If the clean void urinalysis has WBCs and bacteria, cystitis is likely. If only WBCs are found, urethritis with an organism such as chlamydia is likely. In such a case, treatment of the infection is the first priority and other tests (with the exception of urine culture to determine the type of organism) are not indicated unless symptoms persist later in the absence of an infection.

2. **E, Page 557.** The basic defect in genuine stress incontinence is lack of transmission of abdominal pressure to the urethra. The urethral support procedures all attempt to accomplish the same goal. This goal is to ensure adequate intraabdominal pressure transmission so that it, together with the sphincter muscles of the urethra and the epithelium of the urethra, combine to make the intraurethral pressure greater than the intravesical pressure, thereby insuring continence.

3. **E, Page 545.** The Bonney test is the use of pressure to elevate the urethra, thereby preventing urine loss with stress. Too much pressure may occlude the urethra, giving a false positive test and this is a significant drawback for this maneuver. The Bonney test does not damage the vagina or cause osteitis pubis or urinary infections, and it may be used with patients supine or standing, regardless of urethral length.

4. **B, Page 557.** A foreign body left in place always creates a risk of infection. This is a major complication of a urethral sling, which utilizes synthetic materials. The Mersilene will not absorb, but it has been known to work its way into, or through, the urethra with resulting fistula. The patient is at no greater risk of hemorrhage or loss of bladder innervation than with any other suspension procedure.

5. **C, Pages 544–545.** This patient is quite likely to have overflow incontinence secondary to a neurogenic bladder with incomplete emptying. Her age, history of diabetes, and the history of constant wetting are significant clues to this etiology. If this is the case, large amounts of urine will remain in the bladder after voiding and may easily be detected by simple catheterization after an attempt to void. If the diagnosis of a neurogenic bladder is established, treatment of the underlying disease may be helpful to decrease incontinence, but usually it is not. Voiding frequently at specific times or using intermittent catheterization may be the best management.

6. **C, Page 558.** Detrusor dyssynergia (bladder instability) is associated with uninhibited bladder contractions. These are often triggered by an intraabdominal stress, such as coughing. Therefore it is easily confused with genuine stress incontinence. However, careful history usually will reveal that a few seconds of time elapse between the stress

and the onset of the urine flow. The bladder hyperactivity should be demonstrated by a cystometrogram. Treatment with bladder drills, such as voiding at specific time intervals, and anticholinergic or beta-adrenergic drugs are often helpful.

7. **E, Page 547.** *Escherichia coli* is the most frequently found bacterium in uncomplicated urinary tract infections. The causative bacteria are usually present in accumulations of more than 100,000 organisms per ml, but in symptomatic women with a single organism, even 100 organisms per ml are highly predictive of a true bladder infection. At least 20% of all women will have urinary tract infections.

8. **C, Page 556.** It is possible that this patient, who has suprapubic pain 4 weeks after an MMK, could have a urinary tract infection, an abscess, or a hematoma. However, the lack of WBCs in the urine, a low white count, absence of fever, and no mass on exam make these all unlikely. Osteitis pubis is rare, but with this presentation of pain over the symphysis without fever or mass, it is the most likely diagnosis. Osteomyelitis is another possibility, and clinical differentiation between osteomyelitis and osteitis pubis may be difficult. Diagnosing osteomyelitis requires X-ray changes of cortical bone, marrow biopsy demonstrating infection, and recovery of microorganisms. Osteomyelitis pubis may be the severe end of a continuum of an inflammatory process of the pubic bone, whereas osteitis pubis represents the early and less severe manifestation.

9. **A, Page 558.** With a history of short delay after the cough, the copious uncontrollable urine loss, and the urgency she often feels, urge incontinence is likely. Stress incontinence is usually described as loss of a small amount of urine and occurs immediately after or during the cough or valsalva. A urethro vaginal fistula causes an unpredictable urinary stream and/or loss of urine from the vagina, whereas overflow incontinence causes constant leakage when the bladder is full. Urethral diverticula tend to leak after voiding. In any event, the patient should be evaluated for infection and detrusor contractility prior to any surgery.

10. **B, Page 553.** As this woman is premenopausal, estrogen is probably not indicated, although it is helpful in treating postmenopausal women. Kegel pubococcygeal muscle exercises often yield good results if done correctly and frequently, especially in younger women. Alpha adrenergic drugs are mildy effective in increasing urethral pressure, but usually are not the best choice for the initial treatment of patients with mild symptoms of stress incontinence. Surgical treatment, whether by vaginal or abdominal route, should be reserved until the effect of Kegel exercises can be evaluated.

11. **C, Page 549.** With a history of dysuria, frequency, urinary dribbling, and dyspareunia, coupled with a palpable tender nodule, urethral diverticulum is highly suspect. Ectopic ureter causes constant incontinence. The anatomic location is wrong for both Bartholin and Gartner's duct pathology. A urethrocele is not detected as a tender nodule, whereas a urethral diverticulum often presents with a tender suburethral mass. Urethral diverticula are relatively uncommon, but are seen frequently enough to be considered when these signs and symptoms occur.

12. **D, Page 553.** A urethrocele is somewhat of a misnomer, as the urethra most often does not balloon out. The urethra instead becomes detached. Then both the urethra and bladder rotate caudally out of the space beneath the symphysis pubis so that pressure from the intraabdominal cavity can no longer be transmitted to the urethra. Loss of this pressure transmission often results in genuine stress incontinence as the pressure transmission to the bladder continues increasing the intravesical pressure above that of the urethra.

13. **E, Pages 551–552.** Genuine stress incontinence is due mainly to a lack of transmission of intraabdominal pressure to the urethra. The length of the urethra or its angle, as measured by the Q-tip test, or the amount of funneling of the bladder neck, as determined by the bead chain cystourethrogram, do not correlate well with the presence or absence of genuine stress incontinence. However, in all cases the pressure differential between the bladder and urethra will be present.

14. **C, Page 553.** Patients are frequently told to do Kegel exercises, but they are not told how often to perform them. If they are not done frequently, they are ineffective. Kegel reported excellent results (84%) when the pelvic floor muscles were intermittently contracted and relaxed for 20 minutes three times per day. An alternate method is to contract the same muscles five times every half hour throughout the day. Adequate pelvic floor musculature must remain in order for the exercises to cause hypertrophy and yield a beneficial result. If the pelvic floor muscles have been attenuated or are in any way obliterated, the exercise regime is less helpful as muscles cannot be developed if they are not present.

15–18. **15, E; 16, B; 17, C; 18, A; Pages 553–556.** In the Marshall-Marchetti-Krantz procedure, the paravaginal fascia is sutured to the symphysis pubis in the space of Retzius. The Burch procedure is a modification of the MMK and requires suturing the paravaginal fascia to Cooper's ligament. The Kelly plication sutures lateral paravaginal fascia in the midline beneath the urethra. The Pereyra procedure involves passing a needle with a suture attached through the space of Retzius from the rectus fascia to the paravaginal fascia on either side of the urethra. Each procedure is designed to place the proximal third of the urethra in an area where the intraabdominal pressure can be transmitted to it, while maintaining support of the urethra that will not allow it to move out of that pressure zone. This results in an increase in intraurethral pressure which, together with the urethral sphincters and mucous membrane, creates an intraurethral pressure greater than the intravesical pressure resulting in urinary continence.

19–22. 19, **C**; 20, **B**; 21, **A**; 22, **D**; Page 538. All incontinence with an intact urinary system (that is, without a fistula) results from a greater pressure in the bladder than in the urethra. Urine then flows from a high pressure area to a low pressure area in accordance with physical laws. The various types of incontinence are defined according to the cause of the pressure gradient. Successful treatment is based on correcting the specific reason for the higher bladder pressure, the lower urethral pressure, or both. Therefore, diagnostically it is important to determine the reason for the pressure differential as the treatment differs depending on the underlying cause.

23–25. 23, **A**; 24, **D**; 25, **C**; Pages 539–541, Figure 20-1 (from Droegemueller). Loop I of the micturition feedback nervous system circuit runs from the cortex to the brain stem to inhibit urination by modifying sensory stimuli from loop II, thereby inhibiting the bladder. Loop I mediates the learned suppression of autonomic voiding and can be modified by bladder drills. The parasympathetic system generally initiates voiding with detrusor muscle stimulation and relaxation of urethral sphincters. Activating the beta adrenergic receptors of the sympathetic system inhibits the detrusor muscle while activation of the alpha adrenergic receptors cause urethral muscle constriction. Knowing these facts allows one to plan rational therapy for

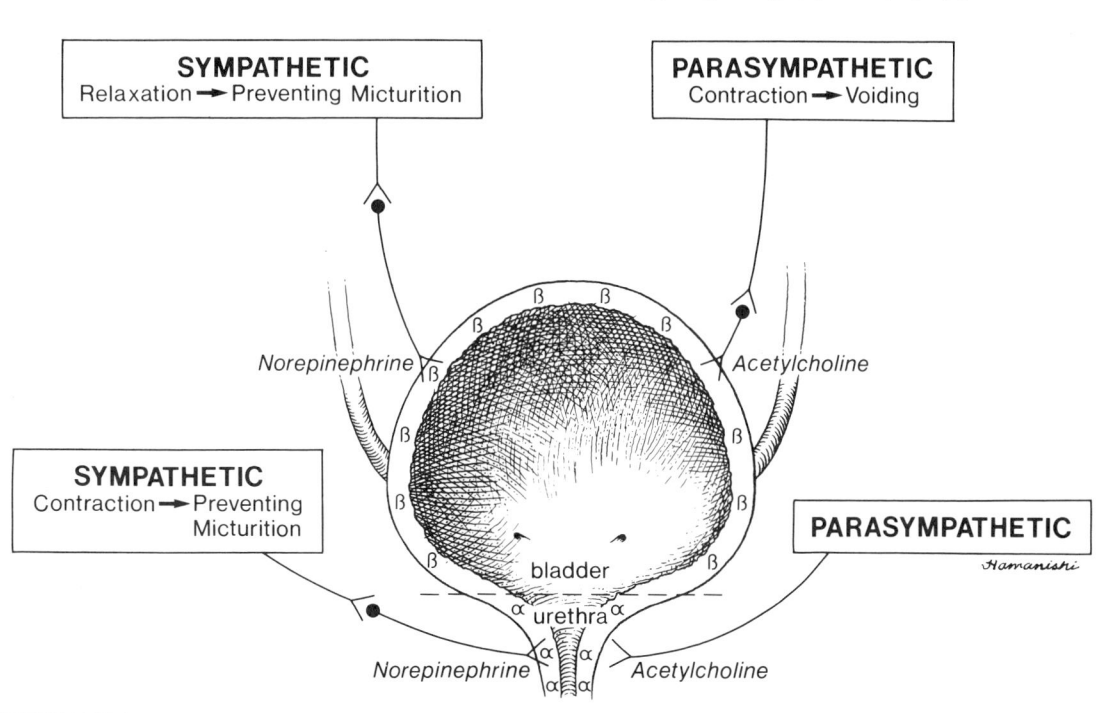

FIGURE 20-1.
The innovation of the bladder and urethra. Parasympathetic fibers arising in S2 through S4 have long preganglionic fibers and pelvic ganglia close to the bladder and urethra. These parasympathetic fibers excrete acetylcholine. Sympathetic fibers that have long postganglionic fibers discharge norepinephrine to beta receptors, primarily in the bladder, and alpha receptors, primarily in the urethra.
(Redrawn and modified from Raz S: Urol Clin North Am 5:323, 1978).

urge incontinence, which is due to uninhibited bladder muscle spasms.

26. **D** (4), Page 558. The requirement for the diagnosis of detrusor dyssynergia (bladder instability) is uninhibited bladder contraction. This may or may not lead to incontinence, depending upon whether the intraurethral pressure is exceeded by the intravesical pressure. While it is true that detrusor dyssynergia does not often respond to surgical repair, such failure is not necessary for diagnosis. In fact, the diagnosis should be made before surgery is attempted. Detrusor dyssynergia frequently but not always responds to bladder retraining drills. Therefore, response to such drills is not required for the diagnosis.

27. **D** (4), Pages 554–555. In this patient, who wishes to remain fertile, removal of the uterus is contraindicated. Anterior repair with a Kelly plication will support the bladder and urethra, thereby relieving her symptoms. There is no need for posterior repair if there are no symptoms of posterior relaxation. A Marshall-Marchetti-Krantz procedure will relieve her stress incontinence, but it will not replace the cystocele; therefore, her anterior vaginal wall will still be excoriated from extrusion. Modifications of the MMK, such as the Burch procedure, also would be of little benefit in this case.

28. **E** (All), Page 557. Any surgical candidate should be informed of several basic surgical risks—infection, hemorrhage, damage to other structures, failure to achieve cure, and risks of anesthesia. These general risks should all be documented on the patient's record. Specific procedures carry specific complications and these should also be outlined. In the case of urethral suspension, failure to spontaneously void may be a major factor. The patient should recognize the possible need for long-term urinary catheterization. Eventually nearly all patients with these repairs will void spontaneously. Some patients—particularly those who have minimal stress incontinence or have urge incontinence rather than stress incontinence, will actually have more incontinence postoperatively.

29. **A** (1, 2, 3), Page 541. The muscles, the vascularity, and the transmission of increased intraabdominal pressure are all important factors in maintaining a high urethral pressure with resultant continence. The vascularity and mucosal thickness of the urethra increase in response to estrogen. This may be the reason that estrogen helps in the treatment of incontinence in some estrogen-deficient women. The ability to transmit intraabdominal pressure to the urethra is a major factor in preventing stress urinary incontinence. The achievement of anatomic relationships that allow this pressure transmission is the aim of surgical corrective procedures for stress urinary incontinence. The distal urethra is usually not important in maintaining continence as it is beyond the sphincter action of the striated muscle and beyond the area of intraabdominal pressure transmission.

Chapter 21: Infections of the Lower Genital Tract

DIRECTIONS: Select the one best answer or completion.

1. A 22-year-old woman complains of urgency, frequency, and dysuria. Urinalysis reveals more than 20 WBCs per hpf, and culture reveals 10 colonies per ml. The most likely diagnosis is
   A. pyelonephritis.
   B. vulvovaginitis.
   C. cystitis.
   D. cervicitis.
   E. acute urethral syndrome.

2. A 19-year-old woman complains of headache, myalgia, dizziness, and low grade fever with each menstrual period for the past 6 months. She feels well at other times and denies depression or dysmenorrhea. She takes birth control pills and uses tampons. Of the following the most likely diagnosis is
   A. Weil's disease.
   B. premenstrual syndrome.
   C. flu.
   D. measles.
   E. forme fruste of toxic shock syndrome.

3. A 22-year-old woman complains of severe itching of her perineum, wrists, and breasts. The symptoms are worse at night. Exam reveals excoriation in all of the above areas. No hives are seen. The most likely diagnosis is
   A. allergy.
   B. scabies.
   C. molluscum contagiosum.
   D. lice.
   E. Pityriasis rosea.

4. A 26-year-old woman from the British Virgin Islands is found to have several painless, beefy red ulcers on the vulva. Biopsy reveals the following histology (Figure 21-1). The diagnosis is
   A. syphilis.
   B. chancroid.
   C. herpes simplex.

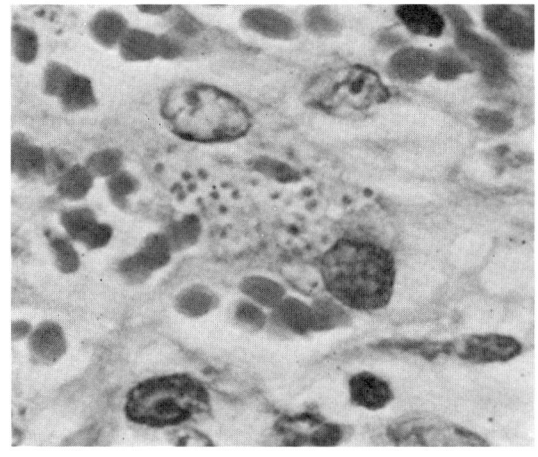

FIGURE 21-1.
(From Hart G. In Holmes KK, Mårdh PA, Sparling PF, et al, eds: Sexually transmitted diseases. New York, McGraw-Hill, 1984, p. 394.)

   D. lymphogranuloma venereum.
   E. granuloma inguinale.

5. You suspect a patient has gonococcal cervicitis and obtain a single gonorrhea culture from her endocervix. What percentage of identifiable gonococcal cervicitis infections would be diagnosed by this technique?
   A. 100%
   B. 95%
   C. 85%
   D. 70%
   E. 50%

6. A patient with severe toxic shock syndrome is most likely to have
   A. total lymphocytes greater than 1000 per cc.
   B. polymorphonuclear cells less than 80%.
   C. SGOT less than 30 units per liter.
   D. BUN greater than 20 milligrams per deciliter.
   E. platelets greater than 300,000.

7. The basic underlying pathophysiologic disturbance in a patient with AIDS is
   A. infection with opportunistic organisms such as pneumocystis carinae.
   B. a cancer that affects the cell-mediated immune system.
   C. a decrease in number and function of T-4 lymphocytes.
   D. decrease in serum immunoglobulins, IGG and IGA.
   E. thrombocytopenia.
8. How many different species of bacteria are found in the vaginas of normal asymptomatic women when careful culturing is done?
   A. 2–3
   B. 6–10
   C. 12–15
   D. 17–20
   E. Greater than 30
9. The most specific test commonly used to detect AIDS is
   A. ELISA.
   B. Southern blot.
   C. immunocytochemistry.
   D. Northern blot.
   E. Western blot.
10. A young woman complains of a bad odor from the vaginal area after intercourse and during menses. She has very little discharge but it is irritating. The reason for the odor is most likely
    A. breakdown of blood or protein in semen.
    B. increased number of anaerobes.
    C. E. coli.
    D. normal vaginal secretions.
    E. release of amines in an alkaline milieu.
11. A 26-year-old woman complains of a vaginal discharge associated with itching and burning. The pH of the discharge is 5.5. Which of the following is the *least* likely diagnosis?
    A. Chlamydia cervicitis
    B. Gonorrhea cervicitis
    C. Yeast vaginitis
    D. Trichomonas vaginitis
    E. Bacterial vaginosis
12. A young woman has trichomonas vaginitis. The probability that her male sex partner also has the disease is about
    A. 5%.
    B. 20%.
    C. 40%.
    D. 60%.
    E. 80%.
13. Clue cells are often seen in the wet mount of the vaginal secretions of a patient with bacterial vaginosis. A clue cell is a/an
    A. WBC with phagocytized bacteria.
    B. epithelial squamous cell covered with bacteria.
    C. epithelial columnar cell covered with bacteria.
    D. WBC containing gram-negative paired cocci.
    E. squamous epithelium containing macrophages.
14. After candida albicans, the yeast most often found in the vagina is
    A. tricophyton rubrum.
    B. candida glabrata.
    C. microsporum canis.
    D. candida tropicalis.
    E. pityrosporum orbiculare.
15. A 21-year-old woman is seen in the Emergency Room with hypotension, fever, diarrhea, headache, myalgia, red eyes, and a skin rash. She states she has felt ill for 2 days and the symptoms are worse. She is sexually active and uses barrier contraception. She denies abdominal pain, vaginal discharge, or any drug ingestion except aspirin. Her periods are regular. Her last normal period began 4 days ago. The most likely diagnosis is
    A. Rocky Mountain spotted fever.
    B. scarlet fever.
    C. toxic shock syndrome.
    D. meningococcemia.
    E. leptospirosis.

DIRECTIONS: For each numbered item, select the one heading most closely associated with it. Each lettered heading may be used once, more than once, or not at all.

16–19. Match the causative organism with the disease or lesion.
   (A) Calymmatobacterium
   (B) Chlamydia
   (C) Spirochete
   (D) Mycobacterium
   (E) Hemophilus ducreyi
16. Gumma
17. Granuloma inguinale
18. Chancroid
19. Condyloma lata
20–23. Match the disease with the Figure. (See Figures 21-2 through 21-5 on pp.137-138.)
   (A) Primary herpes of the cervix
   (B) Molluscum contagiosum
   (C) Condyloma lata
   (D) Lymphogranuloma venereum
   (E) Invasive cancer

20. Figure 21-2
21. Figure 21-3
22. Figure 21-4
23. Figure 21-5
24–26. For each numbered item, indicate whether it is associated with
   A: Chlamydia
   B: GC
   C: Both
   D: Neither
24. Causes a mucopurulent cervicitis.
25. Cultured on agar media.
26. Treated with tetracycline.

DIRECTIONS: Each question contains four suggested answers, of which one or more is correct. Choose the answer
   A if 1, 2, and 3 are correct
   B if 1 and 3 are correct
   C if 2 and 4 are correct
   D if 4 only is correct
   E if all are correct

27. A 16-year-old patient presents during a menstrual period with hypotension, skin rash, fever, and myalgia. She is found to have staphylococci in her vaginal culture. Her mother wishes an explanation for her daughter's illness and a discussion of the treatment plan. You should tell her
   1. symptoms are due to staphylococcus aureus bacteremia.
   2. almost all cases are sexually transmitted.
   3. if she stops using tampons, the symptoms will almost always resolve.
   4. antibiotic treatment is necessary.

28. A 24-year-old woman has had several sexual contacts in the last 20 days, but no sexual contact for several months prior to this time. She presents with a small tender ulcer on her vulva of 3 days duration. She also has enlarged, slightly tender inguinal nodes. She has no other signs or symptoms. At this visit you should
   1. culture for HSV.
   2. obtain a serologic test for syphilis.
   3. perform a dark field study.
   4. biopsy for cancer.

29. Clinical patterns associated with active AIDS are
   1. lymphadenopathy.
   2. nonmechanical ileus.
   3. autoimmune thrombocytopenia purpura.
   4. severe muscle cramps.

30. A 35-year-old woman with flat warts of the cervix and vulva asks about etiology and risk of cervical and vulvar cancer. You can explain
   1. certain types of warts, namely 16, 18, and 31, are associated with an increased risk of dysplasia and carcinoma.
   2. genital condyloma acuminata is sexually transmitted with an incubation period of 1–8 months.
   3. diabetes mellitus, immunosuppression, and pregnancy predispose to an increased infection with human papilloma virus.
   4. condyloma acuminata occur only on genital epithelium and glabrous skin.

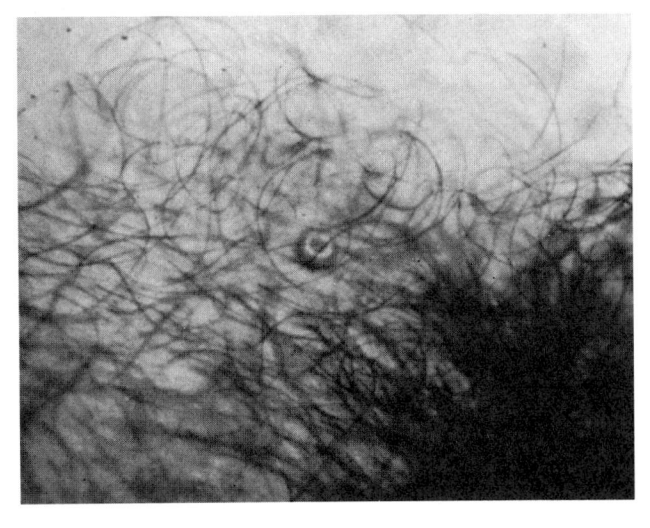

FIGURE 21-2.
(From Brown ST. In Holmes KK, Mårdh PA, Sparling PF, et al, eds: Sexually transmitted diseases. New York, McGraw-Hill, 1984, p. 394.)

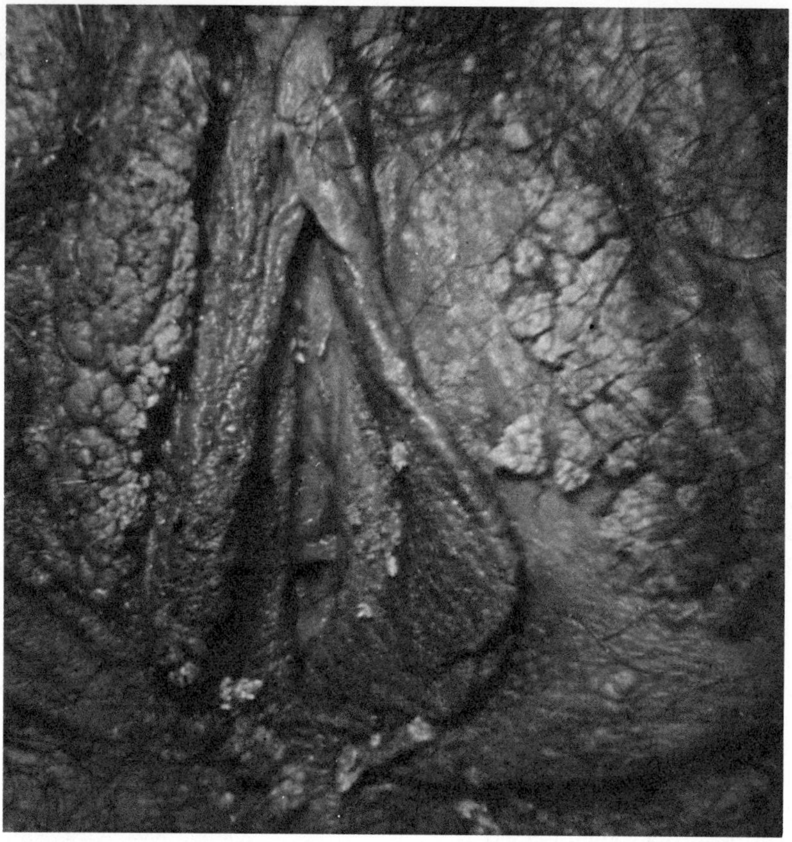

FIGURE 21-3.
(From Friedrich EG: Vulvar disease, 2nd ed. Philadelphia, W.B. Saunders Co., 1983, p. 25.)

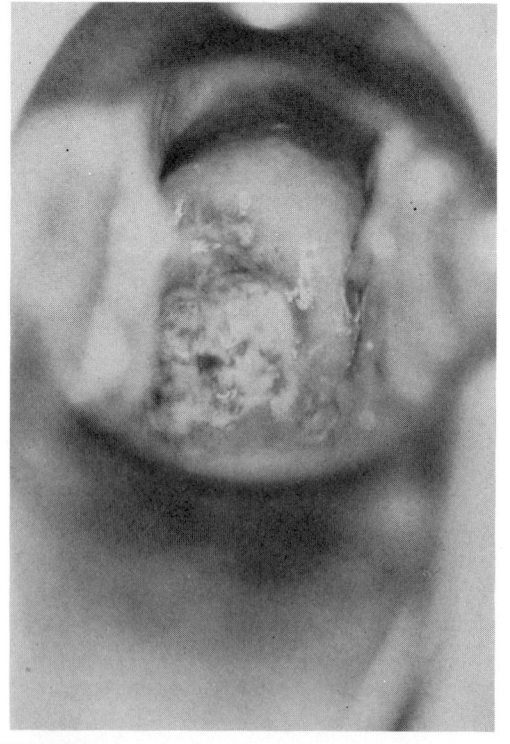

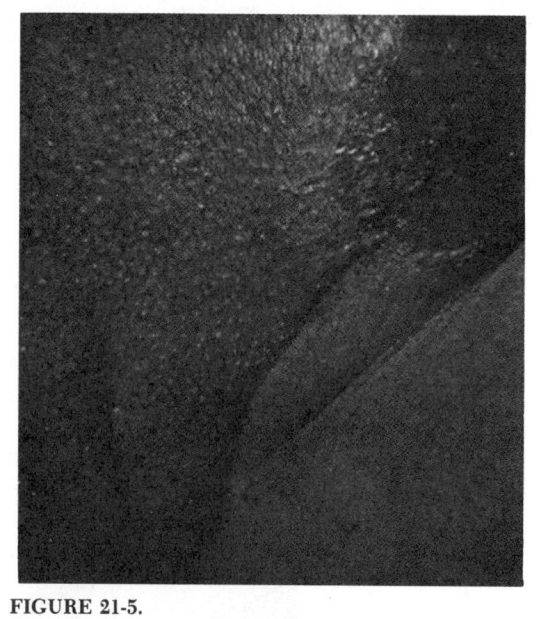

FIGURE 21-5.
(From Friedrich EG: Vulvar disease, 2nd ed. Philadelphia, W.B. Saunders Co., 1983, p. 229.)

FIGURE 21-4.
(From Kaufman RH, Faro S: Clin Obstet Gynecol 28:154, 1985.)

31. A woman with florid condyloma acuminata on the vulva desires their removal. Her PAP smears are negative. Methods of treatment include
    1. podophyllin.
    2. trichloracetic acid.
    3. surgery.
    4. cryocautery.
32. A 26-year-old woman complains of burning of the vulva, which has been present for 6 days and is increasing in severity. Differential diagnosis should include a
    1. primary vaginal infection.
    2. primary skin irritant.
    3. secondary skin infection.
    4. contact dermatitis.

ANSWERS

1. **E**, Pages 568–569. Fever and chills are usually a major feature in pyelonephritis, which also presents with increased bacteria and WBCs in the urine. Vulvovaginitis may be associated with dysuria, but careful history reveals the pain is external, away from the urethra, and due to urine contact on the tender vulva. Physical exam reveals vaginal discharge. Although cystitis may have symptoms similar to urethral syndrome, greater than 100 bacteria per ml are cultured from the urine. Cervicitis usually does not cause urinary symptoms unless there is concomitant infection of the urethra, which is often true with organisms such as gonorrhea or chlamydia. The acute urethral syndrome is defined by symptoms of dysuria and frequency and pyuria without significant numbers of bacteria in the urine.

2. **E**, Pages 588–589. The repetitive nature of the symptoms makes flu and measles unlikely. Weil's disease is the sequel of severe infection with leptospirosis, which is a rare condition and much more severe than the symptoms outlined. However, it is one of the differential diagnoses in cases of severe toxic shock syndrome (TSS). The premenstrual syndrome occurs prior to the menses. A mild form, or "forme fruste," of toxic shock syndrome is likely with the use of tampons. Vaginal cultures for staphylococcus aureus should be done and the use of tampons discontinued until such time as the bacteria is eradicated, and then worn for no longer than 6 hours.

3. **B**, Page 572. The distribution, with increased itching at night, makes scabies the most likely diagnosis. This diagnosis can be proven by an Indian ink test to identify the burrows, or by making a slide of the scrapings from the affected skin and using mineral oil to prevent loss of specimen. Allergies are unlikely to have a concomitant genital, wrist, and breast distribution and are often associated with hives. Molluscum contagiosum has classic umbilicated papules, and lice tend to be located in hair-bearing areas. Pityriasis rosea has a truncal and upper extremity distribution, often with a history of a herald patch.

4. **E**, Page 581 and Table 21-1 (from Droegemueller). Granuloma inguinale is due to a gram negative, nonmotile, encapsulated rod, calymmatobacterium granulomatis. The pathonomonic Donovan bodies are clusters of dark-staining, bipolar-appearing (safety pin) bacteria in large mononuclear cells. The disease is found in subtropical areas and is rare in the United States. Treatment is with tetracycline. See answer for questions 21–24.

5. **C**, Page 605. Approximately 85% of potentially culturable gonococcal cervicitis will be found by a single appropriately performed endocervical culture using a sterile cotton swab inserted in the endocervical canal and rotated long enough to fully moisten the cotton. You can increase the detection rate to 93% with the addition of a separate rectal culture. The important point to remember is that cultures are not infallible and do not detect every case of gonorrhea.

6. **D**, Page 589 and Table 21-3 (from Droegemueller). A patient with severe toxic shock syndrome usually has less than 860 lymphocytes per ml, pmns greater than 90%, platelets less than 150,000, a SGOT greater than 40 units per deciliter, and a BUN greater than 20 milligrams per deciliter. The last two are indicative of liver and kidney involvement, which occurs in severe disease. An elevated creatine phosphokinase is also frequently found due to muscle damage.

7. **C**, Pages 590–591. AIDS victims often acquire the disease from contact with homosexuals or shared IV drug needles. They may suffer infection with opportunistic bacteria, viruses, or parasites, develop thrombocytopenia, Kaposi's sarcoma, or have increased immunoglobulins. The basic problem is infection of the T lymphocytes with RNA human immunodeficiency virus. This causes a decrease in function of the T-4 lymphocytes, resulting in breakdown of cell-mediated immune responses that allow the secondary infections or Kaposi's sarcoma to occur.

8. **D**, Page 593. The most common bacteria in the vagina is the lacto bacillus found in 60–80% of normal women. Other facultative aerobes include diphtheroids, streptococcus, staphylococcus, gardnerella vaginalis, and E. coli. Anaerobes can be cultured in the vaginas of approximately 80% of normal women. These include peptostreptococcus, peptococcus, and bacteroides. Normal asymptomatic women harbor 17–29 species of bacteria. Candida is commonly included. The

quantity of the different species varies. Both anaerobes and aerobes are found in significantly increased amounts in patients with bacterial vaginosis.

9. **E**, Page 592. ELISA is a screening test for AIDS which has a significant number of false positives and negatives. Western blot is a method of detecting specific proteins within the human immunodeficiency virus (HIV). Southern blot and Northern blot use the same methodology to detect DNA and RNA, respectively. Immunocytochemistry involves using antibodies to find antigens within cells.

10. **E**, Page 594. Volatile amines are released in an alkaline media. The normal pH of the vagina is less than 4.5, but both blood and semen have a high pH (around 7.2–7.4). The amines are formed by anaerobic bacteria and become volatile, and therefore noticeable when the pH rises above the normal vaginal pH of 4.5. Addition of KOH to vaginal secretion volatilizes the amines also, and this forms the basis for the "sniff test," the fishy smell associated with bacterial vaginosis.

11. **C**, Pages 592–593. The normal pH of the healthy vagina is 3.8 to 4.2. If the pH is greater than 5.0, bacterial vaginosis, trichomonas, or some other bacteria infection is likely. A yeast infection or physiologic discharges are likely if the pH is normal. Testing the pH is quick and easy, and it divides symptomatic vaginal discharges into bacterial infections versus yeast and physiologic discharge quite well. It should be measured routinely in patients with complaints of vaginal discharge.

12. **E**, Pages 596–597 and Figure 21-6 (from Droegemueller). Trichomonas is found in 67–100% of male partners of women who have trichomoniasis. It is a sexually transmitted disease which requires a significant innoculum to establish a vaginal infection. Many vaginal infections are asymptomatic. Diagnosis is by saline wet mount. Treatment with met ronidazole is usually curative. Dosage may be either a 2 gram single dose, 250 mg every 8 hours times 7 days, or 500 mg b.i.d. times 7 days. The single dose is cheaper, has better compliance, and achieves nearly as good a cure rate for trichomonas.

13. **B**, Pages 594, 596 and Figure 21-20 (from Droegemueller). A clue cell is a squamous epithelial cell so heavily covered with numerous bacteria that its outline is obscured. These cells are found in high numbers in patients with bacterial vaginosis. Columnar cells are rarely seen in wet mounts. WBCs with intracellular gram-negative diplococci are indicative of gonococcal infection. Macrophages in the epithelium are seen on histologic specimens, not on wet mounts.

14. **B**, Page 599. Candida are found normally in 25% of women. They are an opportunistic pathogen and grow in the G.I. tract from the mouth to the anus, even more readily than in the vagina. Candida glabrata is occasionally found in the vagina and is said to cause burning rather than itching. It does not produce filaments. Therefore, spores only are found. It does not respond well to the imidizoles but may be treated with gentian violet. Trichophyton rubrum is the fungus that usually causes tenia cruris (jock itch) or tenia corporis. Microsporum canis causes tenia caputas and pityrosporum orbiculare causes tenia versicolor.

15. **C**, Pages 588–589. The onset with the period and symptoms make toxic shock syndrome the most likely of the diagnoses mentioned. She has hypotension, rash, fever and three organ symptom manifestations, thereby meeting the criteria for the diagnosis of toxic shock syndrome. However, one must not forget other diseases that cause similar symptoms, such as Rocky Mountain spotted fever, scarlet fever, meningococcemia, leptospirosis, measles, and Kawasaki's disease.

16–19. 16, **C**; 17, **A**; 18, **E**; 19, **C**; Pages 581–585. Chlamydia is well known to cause cervicitis, nonspecific urethritis, PID, and trachoma. It also causes lymphogranuloma venereum, which is not as common. Gumma and condyloma lata are lesions of secondary syphilis, which are not often seen, and not nearly so well known as the chancre of primary syphilis. Chancroid is a rare disease caused by hemophilus ducreyi, which may form the classic "school of fish" appearance of extracellular streptobacillary chains on gram smear. It is hard to remember the signs, symptoms, causative agents, diagnostic methods, and treatment of rare diseases; yet these rare manifestations should be reviewed regularly, as they are all in the differential diagnosis for genital lesions that are frequently seen, such as condyloma acuminata, herpes, or the less common, but very serious, vulvar carcinoma. Granuloma inguinale is caused by calymmatobacterium granulomatis and is very rare in the United States. It generally starts as an asymptomatic nodule, which then develops into a painless ulcer.

20–23. 20, **B**; 21, **C**; 22, **A**; 23, **D**; Pages 572–573 and 580–584. Visual identification of some vulvar lesions is easy, but confirmation by culture and/or biopsy is usually indicated. Molluscum contagiosum lesions appear umbilicated and have a central core of hyperkeratotic epidermis, which is easily expelled. Microscopically, it contains intracytoplasmic inclusions. Treatment is by curettage. Lymphogranuloma venereum is caused by chlamydia trachomatus, and in its secondary stage has enlarged lymph nodes which coalesce, forming skin depressions between groups of the inflamed nodes, yielding the groove sign. Fluctuant nodes may be aspirated for diagnosis. Treatment is 3 to 6 weeks of tetracycline or erythromycin.

Herpes simplex may form a necrotic ulcer of the cervix with remarkably few systemic symptoms. One must remember that HSV is likely in a young woman and obtain cultures for herpes virus. In such cases, if culture does not confirm the diagnosis, biopsy should be done to rule out cancer. A course of Acyclovir should be given for treatment of herpes. It will decrease the time and severity of symptoms, but does not affect the frequency of recurrences.

Condyloma lata are lesions of secondary syphilis. Other manifestations are a red, macular rash on the palms of the hands and soles of the feet. The flat papules of condyloma lata may form ulcers and may be mistaken for HSV and cancer. Treatment for syphilis is low dose intramuscular penicillin or oral tetracycline, given for 15–30 days depending on the stage of the disease. This lengthy treatment is necessary because of the low replication rate of treponema pallidum.

All of these lesions can be confused with cancer, and one should not be hesitant to biopsy a lesion if there is doubt. Perhaps the only exception to this is the fluctuant nodes of lymphogranuloma venereum, which tend to form draining sinuses after incision.

24–26. 24, **A**; 25, **B**; 26, **C**; Pages 604–606. Chlamydia, gonorrhea, and herpes simplex virus can all produce cervical mucopus. However, neither HSV- nor GC-positive cultures correlated significantly with mucopus when mucopus was defined as purulent endocervical discharge from which a gram stain shows equal to or greater than 10 WBCs per hpf. Gonorrhea grows well on modified Thayer-Martin agar, while chlamydia, being an obligate, intracellular organism, requires cell cultures. Chlamydia is treated with doxycycline, erythromycin, or trimethoprim-sulfamethoxizole, in both males and females. While penicillin derivatives are effective, gonorrhea is also sensitive to doxycycline or tetracycline.

27. **D** (4), Pages 588–589. The symptoms are due to absorption of an exotoxin produced by the staphylococcus aureus. Blood cultures are rarely positive. The use of tampons allows the staphylococcus to grow and excrete the exotoxin, which is then absorbed through the vaginal mucosa. Sexual transmission is not a common factor, as staphylococcus can commonly be cultured from the vaginas of many sexually inactive women. Treatment with an anti-staphylococcal antibiotic will prevent recurrent episodes, which occur in approximately 1/3 of untreated women even if they stop using tampons. Regardless, the 16-year-old should be encouraged to stop using tampons or at least change them every 6 hours during the day and use sanitary napkins at night.

28. **B** (1, 3), Pages 584–585. In a woman with this history, the primary possibility is herpes simplex virus, though the differential must include syphilis along with several less common possibilities such as chancroid, granuloma inguinale, and cancer. An HSV culture would be indicated, as would a dark field study. A serologic test for syphilis could be obtained in case she had prior syphilis, but it is too soon to have developed a positive test from her recent exposure. It takes 4 to 6 weeks for a positive serologic test for syphilis to develop. Cancer is unlikely in this age group, but could be ruled out by biopsy if the lesion is not healed or markedly improved within two weeks.

29. **B** (1, 3), Page 591. Four clinical presentations are associated with active AIDS. These are lymphadenopathy, thrombocytopenia purpura, Kaposi's sarcoma, and multiple opportunistic infections. The mildest form is the lymphadenopathy, which may persist for months or years. Muscle cramps are not a common clinical syndrome found in AIDS.

30. **A** (1, 2, 3), Pages 573, 575–576. Condyloma acuminata is a sexually transmitted disease with an incubation which averages 3 months with a range of 1–8 months. It is caused by human papilloma virus which can infect any mucous membrane and has been found in the rectum, bladder, and respiratory tract. The virus appears to grow more rapidly in patients who have some immune suppression, including pregnancy and diabetes. Certain types, particularly 16, 18, and 31, are associated with genital carcinoma. Other types are associated with other malignancies.

31. **E** (All), Pages 573, 575–577. Several therapeutic modalities for warts are available. For recently developed florid condyloma acuminata (wart), podophyllin and trichloracetic acid work quite well. If the warts are larger, surgical excision, cryocautery, and laser are more effective. However, none of these modalities destroy the viable viral DNA in the basal cells, or virons in the epithelium, which are located distant from the florid wart. Therefore, close observation and followup is required. Frequent recurrence is common.

32. **E** (All), Page 588. The vulva is often irritated by primary vaginal infections, which are the most common cause of the above symptoms. However, allergens such as soap and perfumes, contact toxins (such as poison oak and ivy, which are primary skin irritants), and secondary skin infections which occur after a primary insult should be remembered as causes of this frequent complaint.

CHAPTER 22

Upper Genital Tract Infections

DIRECTIONS: Select the one best answer or completion.

1. Given a patient with a tuboovarian complex discovered at the time of surgery, which organism associated with acute pelvic inflammatory disease is most likely to be cultured?
   A. Group D enterococcus
   B. Mixed anaerobes
   C. Chlamydia trachomatis
   D. Neisseria gonorrhea
   E. Escherichia coli

2. A 17-year-old nulliparous patient has bilateral lower abdominal pain, a fever of 38 degrees centigrade, and a tender left adnexa which feels thickened. Cervical culture is positive for Chlamydia trachomatis. Assuming a correct diagnosis of acute PID, the best treatment is
   A. outpatient treatment with IM cefoxitin and oral doxycycline.
   B. oral doxycycline alone.
   C. IM procaine penicillin.
   D. hospitalization with parenteral doxycycline and cefoxitin.
   E. hospitalization with parenteral cefoxitin alone.

3. Empiric antibiotic protocols used to treat acute pelvic inflammatory disease should cover a wide range of bacteria which includes all of the following *except*
   A. Neisseria gonorrhea.
   B. Chlamydia trachomatis.
   C. Bacteroides species.
   D. Peptococcus species.
   E. Clostridium species.

4. What percentage of laparoscopically confirmed acute pelvic inflammatory disease will be associated with the clinical triad of fever, elevated erythrocyte sedimentation rate, and adnexal tenderness?
   A. 5–10
   B. 15–20
   C. 25–30
   D. 35–40
   E. 45–50

5. Which of the following contraceptive methods does not *lower* the relative risk of incurring a sexually transmitted disease?
   A. Nonoxynol 9 (spermicidal jelly or cream)
   B. Intrauterine device
   C. Condoms
   D. Oral contraceptives
   E. Diaphragm

6. The diagnosis of acute pelvic inflammatory disease, when using clinical criteria alone, is incorrect in approximately
   A. 15% of patients.
   B. 35% of patients.
   C. 50% of patients.
   D. 75% of patients.
   E. 95% of patients.

7. Bacteriologic and immunologic studies suggest the most prevalent sexually transmitted organism causing upper genital tract disease in the United States is
   A. human immunodeficiency virus (HIV).
   B. herpes simplex.
   C. Neisseria gonorrhea.
   D. Chlamydia trachomatis.
   E. Mycoplasma hominis.

8. Which facultative organism is most likely to contribute to the formation of an acute tuboovarian complex?
   A. Chlamydia trachomatis
   B. Neisseria gonorrhea
   C. Mycoplasma hominis
   D. Escherichia coli
   E. Clostridium species

DIRECTIONS: For each numbered item, select the one heading most closely associated with it. Each lettered heading may be used once, more than once, or not at all.

9–11. (A) Chlamydia trachomatis
      (B) Neisseria gonorrhea
      (C) Mycoplasma hominis
      (D) Hemophilus gardnerella

9. Cultured from the fallopian tube in up to 20% of all women with acute PID.

10. Progression to upper tract disease largely via parametria rather than through tubal lumen.

11. Fifteen percent of women with cervical infection will develop acute pelvic inflammatory disease.
12–14. (A) Recurrent acute PID
    (B) Chronic pelvic pain
    (C) Death
    (D) Infertility
12. Will occur at a rate four times greater in patients treated for PID.
13. Occurs in up to 10% of patients with tuboovarian abscess.
14. Will occur in 25% of patients treated for PID.

DIRECTIONS: For each numbered item, indicate whether it is associated with
A. only (A).
B. only (B).
C. both (A) and (B).
D. neither (A) nor (B).

15–17. (A) Doxycycline IV; cefoxitin IV
    (B) Clindamycin IV: gentamicin IV
    (C) Both
    (D) Neither
15. Positive Neisseria gonorrhea culture from cervix only.
16. Seven centimeter abscess, fever, negative cervical culture.
17. Bilateral adnexal tenderness, low grade temperature, positive gonorrhea culture.
18–20. (A) Acute PID associated with Chlamydia trachomatis
    (B) Acute PID associated with Neisseria gonorrhea
    (C) Both
    (D) Neither
18. Five to ten percent associated with Fitz-Hugh–Curtis syndrome (perihepatic inflammation).
19. Causative organism may be harbored in the endosalpinx for more than 4 weeks.
20. More than two-thirds of patients will have temperature elevation of greater than 38 °C.
21–23. (A) Ectopic pregnancy
    (B) Chronic pelvic pain
    (C) Both
    (D) Neither
21. At least a fourfold increase in patients with acute PID.
22. Directly related to alterations in endosalpinx caused by acute PID.
23. Related to colonization of endosalpinx by anaerobic bacteria.

DIRECTIONS: Each question contains four suggested answers, of which one or more is correct. Choose the answer

A if 1, 2, and 3 are correct
B if 1 and 3 are correct
C if 2 and 4 are correct
D if 4 only is correct
E if all are correct

24. Oral contraceptives protect against the development of sexually transmitted diseases by
    1. altering bacterial flora of the vagina.
    2. changing the cervical mucus.
    3. causing a plasma cell infiltrate in the endosalpinx.
    4. decreasing the duration of menstruation.
25. Acute pelvic inflammatory disease caused by Neisseria gonorrhea
    1. evokes an antibody response in the majority of patients.
    2. disrupts tubal mucosa by direct cytotoxicity.
    3. is resistant to penicillin when it acquires a resistance factor plasmid.
    4. is associated with an elevated erythrocyte sedimentation rate.
26. True statements regarding the pathogenesis of acute pelvic inflammatory disease (PID) include:
    1. It is an ascending infection from the flora of the cervix and vagina.
    2. It is associated with menstruating women.
    3. It is polymicrobial.
    4. It is more common in women using oral contraceptives.
27. Components of pelvic inflammatory disease (PID) may include
    1. endometritis.
    2. salpingitis.
    3. oophoritis.
    4. parametritis.
28. A 28-year-old woman presents with a 4 month history of intermittent intermenstrual bleeding, dull midline lower abdominal pain, and postcoital spotting. Indicated diagnostic tests include
    1. endometrial culture.
    2. endocervical culture.
    3. endometrial biopsy.
    4. hysteroscopy.
29. Nonpuerperal endometritis
    1. represents an intermediate state of ascending infection.
    2. results from canalicular spread of organisms.
    3. is associated with elevated serum antibody levels to Chlamydia trachomatis.
    4. is more common in multiparous women than in nulliparous women.

ANSWERS

1. **B**, Pages 634–635. Abscesses caused by acute pelvic inflammatory disease contain a mixture of anaerobes and facultative or aerobic organisms. The environment of an abscess cavity results in a low level of oxygen tension. Therefore, anaerobic organisms predominate and have been reported to be present in between 60 and 100% of cases.

    The clinical implications are important in deciding rational antibiotic treatment. Basic investigations have discovered that clindamycin penetrates the human neutrophil, and it is possible that this property facilitates the elevated level of clindamycin within the abscess. This drug is also stable in the abscess environment, which is not true of many other antibiotics. This serves as the basis for using clindamycin and an amino-glycocide in the treatment in this entity. Metronidazole is also an effective alternative to clindamycin for anaerobic infections and has been shown in some studies to be present in higher levels within abscess cavities. If there is poor response to the above combination or if enterococcus is recovered in cultures, it is important to add a broad-spectrum penicillin such as ampicillin.

2. **D**, Pages 631–633. This question addresses a number of factors having to do with optimal treatment of acute pelvic inflammatory disease. Especially important in this patient are a number of factors, including her young age, demonstrable fever, and the presence of a palpable inflammatory thickening. Outpatient therapy does not provide high enough levels of appropriate antibiotics to successfully penetrate a developing tuboovarian complex. (See criteria for hospitalization in Droegemueller, page 632.) The presence of the Chlamydia trachomatis mandates treatment with doxycycline, and the presence of a palpable inflammatory thickening implicates other opportunistic organisms as pathogens. Cefoxitin is an excellent antibiotic for peptococcus and peptostreptococcus as well as E. coli. An alternative to this regimen would include parenteral clindamycin and an aminoglycocide. This combination has an advantage of providing better coverage for anaerobic infections and facultative gram-negative rods.

    One must keep in mind that neither regimen is ideal for all patients. The clinician needs to be ready to change the antibiotic regimen depending on patient response and bacteriologic results.

3. **E**, Page 630. Empirical antibiotic protocols should cover a wide range of bacteria, including Neisseria gonorrhea, Chlamydia trachomatis, anaerobic rods and cocci, gram negative aerobic rods, gram positive aerobes, and mycoplasma species. Clostridium species are rarely implicated in acute tuboovarian disease, and therefore treatment for this group of organisms is not indicated initially. Selection of one antibiotic protocol over another will often depend on the clinical history and combinations of findings such as those shown in Table 22-16 (from Droegemueller).

    Unfortunately, recent epidemiologic studies have shown that most women with acute pelvic inflammatory disease are treated as outpatients and have received only a single antibiotic regimen. Of these, less than one-third of the patients receive tetracycline to treat possible chlamydial infection. This underscores the need for thorough knowledge of the bacteriology of acute pelvic inflammatory disease as a polymicrobial infection.

4. **B**, Page 625. Historically, the diagnosis of acute pelvic inflammatory disease was not established unless the patient had the triad of fever, elevated erythrocyte sedimentation rate, and adnexal tenderness or a mass. Only 17% of laparoscopically identified cases have this classic triad. It is apparent that the disorder (PID) has historically been made to fit the criteria established for it. Usually, in clinical practice the criteria should fit the disease.

5. **B**, Page 622 and Table 22-7 (from Droegemueller). On arbitrary risk rating scales in which the risk of developing acute pelvic inflammatory disease in sexually active women not using contraception is assigned a score of 1, the corresponding risk among women wearing an intrauterine device is 2 to 4, among women using oral contraceptives 0.3, and among women using a barrier method, including spermicidal preparations, 0.4.

    Nonoxynol 9, the material found in spermicidal preparations, is both bactericidal and virucidal, and laboratory tests have demonstrated its effectiveness against all sexually transmitted diseases including human immunodeficiency virus (HIV).

6. **B**, Page 625. Patients with acute pelvic inflammatory disease present with a wide range of nonspecific clinical symptoms. Since the diagnosis is usually based on clinical criteria, there is both a high false-positive rate and a high false-negative rate. Laparoscopic studies of women with a clinical diagnosis of acute pelvic inflammatory disease suggest that this diagnosis is in error in over one-third of patients. Of this approximately 35%, 20% have no identifiable intra-abdominal or pelvic disease, and approximately 15% have other entities such as ectopic pregnancy, acute appendicitis, or torsion of the adnexa.

7. **D**, Page 620. Chlamydia trachomatis is an intracellular, sexually transmitted bacterial pathogen. This organism has recently become more prevalent than gonorrhea. From 20% to

40% of sexually active women have antibodies against C. trachomatis. From 10% to 30% of women with acute pelvic inflammatory disease who do not have cultures positive for chlamydia have evidence of acute chlamydial infection by serial antibody testing.

Although considered a sexually transmitted organisms, herpes is generally not associated with acute upper tract infection, and human immunodeficiency virus is considered a systemic illness rather than an infection limited to the upper gynecologic tract.

Mycoplasma hominis appears in direct tubal cultures in approximately 15% of women with acute inflammatory disease and the gonococcus is cultured less than 15% of the time in women with upper tract disease.

8. **D**, Page 630 and Table 22-15 (from Droegemueller). The choice of antibiotic therapy is based on knowledge of the bacterial flora which may be present in both the upper and lower genital tract. Certain groups of bacteria are known to exist in the genital tract under normal circumstances and become pathogenic only in the face of antecedent inflammation. This would include a group of bacteria such as streptococcus species, staphylococcus species, hemophilus species, and most commonly Escherichia coli. Other bacteria are known to be primarily transmitted through sexual contact, such as Chlamydia trachomatis and Neisseria gonorrhea. These are less commonly recovered from tubal cultures, in part due to the difficulty in recovering these organisms directly from the fallopian tube or cul-de-sac aspirate. Rarely, Clostridium species and Actinomyces (both anaerobes) may contribute to upper genital tract infections.

9–11. 9, **A**; 10, **C**; 11, **B**; Pages 617, 621. This series of questions addresses the subject of the bacteriology of acute pelvic inflammatory disease.

When contemplating therapy for acute pelvic inflammatory disease, the clinician needs to be aware of certain bacteriologic phenomena. Approximately 20% of all women with acute salpingitis have tubal cultures positive for chlamydia. Neisseria gonorrhea and Chlamydia trachomatis coexist in the same individual between 25 and 40% of the time. Therefore, treatment of patients who have positive cultures for one or the other of these organisms should include treatment for both organisms.

Approximately 15% of women with cervical cultures positive for Neisseria gonorrhea subsequently develop acute pelvic inflammatory disease. However, only 50% of women with endocervical cultures positive for Neisseria gonorrhea at the time of acute pelvic inflammatory disease will have the same organism cultured from the fallopian tubes. If this is the only organism cultured from the fallopian tube or cul-de-sac aspirate, patients will usually respond readily to treatment.

Although Mycoplasma hominis and Ureaplasma urealyticum are obtained from the majority of young, sexually active women, their roles in the pathogenesis of acute pelvic inflammatory disease are unclear. These organisms are recovered infrequently from the fallopian tube or cul-de-sac aspirates in patients with acute pelvic infection. Experimental evidence suggests that the route of spread for mycoplasmas is via the parametria rather than across the mucosal surfaces. This may help to explain the low success rate of direct tubal cultures.

Whereas gonorrhea remains in the fallopian tubes for at most a few days in untreated patients, chlamydia may remain in the fallopian tubes for months following initial colonization of the upper genital tract.

12–14. 12, **B**; 13, **C**; 14, **A**; Pages 614, 635–636. Before antibiotic therapy the mortality associated with acute pelvic inflammatory disease was 1% of all patients. Although the rate of death is lower with modern treatment, it has been estimated that there still is one death every other day in the United States directly related to pelvic inflammatory disease. Most of these deaths result from rupture of a tuboovarian complex, which carries with it a mortality rate of between 5 and 10%.

Recurrent pelvic inflammatory disease is experienced by approximately 25% of patients. Younger women become reinfected twice as often as older women.

The number of ectopic pregnancies has doubled over the past 10 years and is directly related and proportional to the increase in sexually transmitted diseases. Pathologic studies estimate that approximately one-half of ectopic pregnancies occur in oviducts damaged by previous salpingitis.

The chance that women will develop chronic pelvic pain following acute salpingitis is four times greater than the risk for control subjects.

Acute pelvic infection is one of the major causes of female infertility. Epidemiologic studies estimate that between 4 and 13% of women are infertile or have an operative procedure performed because of prior acute pelvic inflammatory diseases.

The direct and indirect monetary costs of pelvic inflammatory disease are estimated to be in the billions of dollars in the United States each year. The long-term *sequelae* of ectopic pregnancy, chronic pelvic pain, and infertility cannot be measured and are considered major public health hazards.

15–17. 15, **D**; 16, **B**; 17, **A**; Pages 632–633. This question addresses issues pertaining to optimum treatment for patients with acute pelvic inflammatory disease. Patients without evidence of upper tract disease who have positive screening cultures only may be treated with outpatient oral antibiotics. In this case, the presence of Neisseria gonorrhea warrants such treatment. Usually, when Neisseria gonorrhea is cultured, the CDC recommends that patients should receive penicillin or some equivalent as well as doxycycline since there is a high association with infection by chlamydia as well as by Neisseria gonorrhea.

In the presence of an abscess or tuboovarian complex, one assumes the presence of anaerobic organisms and/or facultative gram-negative rods. Therefore, treatment which includes parenteral clindamycin and an amino-glycocide is preferable. Appropriate cervical cultures are often negative in this situation despite upper tract disease.

In a patient with the presence of demonstrable upper tract disease but in the absence of a palpable abscess, doxycycline followed by a broad-spectrum agent such as cefoxitin is adequate since there is no evidence for the need to penetrate an abscess cavity.

The clinician should remember that the guidelines provided by the Centers for Disease Control are generally accepted and apply in most situations. Treatments must be individualized in cases that are refractory to treatment or in cases where culture results dictate the need for additional antibiotic therapy.

18–20. 18, C; 19, A; 20, D; Page 628. Five to ten percent of women with acute pelvic inflammatory disease caused by either Chlamydia trachomatis or Neisseria gonorrhea develop symptoms of perihepatic inflammation—the Fitz-Hugh–Curtis syndrome. This condition is often mistakenly diagnosed as either pneumonia or acute cholecystitis. The symptoms include right upper quadrant pain, pleuritic pain, and tenderness in the right upper quadrant. It develops from transperitoneal or vascular dissemination of the organisms causing acute pelvic inflammatory disease.

Whereas the gonococcus survives no more than a few days in the endosalpinx of untreated patients, chlamydia may remain in the fallopian tubes for months following initial colonization of the upper genital tract.

Only one out of three women with acute pelvic inflammatory disease presents with a temperature greater than 38°C, as demonstrated laparoscopically confirmed cases of acute pelvic inflammatory disease.

21–23. 21, C; 22, A; 23, D; Pages 616–617. Acute pelvic inflammatory disease can be directly related to medical *sequelae* in 25% of patients. This includes a rate of ectopic pregnancy which is increased six to tenfold, and a fourfold increase in chance of developing chronic pelvic pain. In the United States each year 26,000 ectopic pregnancies and 90,000 new cases of chronic abdominal pelvic pain are directly related to pelvic inflammatory disease. There are no data to suggest that alterations in tubal architecture caused by infection contribute to chronic pelvic pain, but there is a definite association with an increase of ectopic pregnancy. Neither entity is directly related to species-specific anaerobic colonization of the endosalpinx. The term chronic pelvic inflammatory disease should not be used since the majority of cases with *sequelae* of chronic pelvic infection are bacteriologically sterile, including hydrosalpinx. Chronic pelvic pain may exist with minimal visual anatomic changes and in the absence of positive endosalpingeal cultures.

24. C (2, 4), Page 622. Women using oral contraceptives have two infection-preventing effects: (1) the decrease in incidence of upper tract disease is believed to be secondary to thicker cervical mucus produced by the progestin component of oral contraceptives, and (2) the decrease in duration of menstrual flow theoretically creates a shorter interval for bacterial colonization of the upper tract. Women using oral contraceptives have a lower incidence of acute PID and a milder form of upper tract genital infection if PID does occur.

25. E (All), Page 619. A number of observations have been made in patients with acute pelvic inflammatory disease caused by Neisseria gonorrhea.
   1. Immunologic studies have demonstrated that an antibody against the outer membrane protein of the gonococcus develops in approximately 70% of women following severe pelvic infection.
   2. The gonococcus produces an intense inflammatory reaction in the tubes, which causes the tubal lumen to swell with necrotic debris and purulent material. This is in contradistinction to chlamydia, which disrupts the tubal mucosa by immunopathologic mechanism rather than direct cytotoxicity.
   3. Penicillinase-producing N. gonorrhea organisms were first identified ten years ago, and it is assumed that a resistance factor plasmid enables the gonococcus to produce an enzyme which destroys penicillin.
   4. The erythrocyte sedimentation rate is a *nonspecific* test which may be elevated in any type of inflammatory process, including autoimmune phenomena. It should not be relied upon as a *specific marker* in patients with acute pelvic inflammatory disease, but can be relied upon as a nonspecific factor.

26. **A** (1, 2, 3), Page 616. Factors associated with the pathogenesis of acute pelvic inflammatory disease (PID) include that it represents an ascending infection from bacteria in the vagina or cervix in 99% of the cases; that it is rare in women without menstrual periods; and that it involves a mixture of aerobic and anaerobic bacteria which appear clinically as a single complex infection. More than 20 species of microorganisms have been cultured from direct aspiration of purulent material from infected fallopian tubes. Usually the inciting organism is one of the more common sexually transmitted bacteria such as chlamydia or gonorrhea. Subsequent upper tract disease is often associated with coliform organisms and/or anaerobic organisms which become involved in an opportunistic fashion.

The incidence of PID is less common in oral contraceptive users, presumably because of the alteration of cervical mucus and decreased amount of menstrual blood flow.

Pelvic inflammatory disease is the most common serious infection of women between the ages of 16 and 25, and the morbidity it produces exceeds that of all other infections in this age group.

27. **E** (All), Page 615. The term pelvic inflammatory disease is a generic term and may refer to inflammation caused by infection in any part of the upper genital tract. Although PID usually implies salpingitis, the endometrium, ovaries, myometrium, and parametrium (broad ligaments and uterine serosa) may be involved. The term is often misused to imply sexually transmitted diseases only. Likewise, chronic pelvic inflammatory disease is a term that has largely been abandoned because of the long term *sequelae* of acute infection, such as hydrosalpinx and adhesions, are bacteriologically sterile. With the exception of infection by extremely rare diseases such as tuberculosis or actinomycosis, pelvic infections are not chronic.

28. **A** (1, 2, 3), Page 615. In a patient of this age who presents with a history of intermenstrual bleeding, dull lower midline abdominal pain, and postcoital spotting, one should be suspicious of an endocervical or endometrial inflammatory process. The classic symptom of chronic endometritis is intermenstrual vaginal bleeding. The diagnosis of chronic endometritis is established by endometrial biopsy and culture. Likewise, endocervical culture should be done, since the two entities can coexist and since chronic endometritis may well result from endocervicitis.

The histologic findings of chronic endometritis are inflammatory reactions of monocytes and plasma cells in the endometrial stroma. This may be associated with lymphoid follicles and stromal necrosis. Treatment consists of oral tetracycline, 2 grams a day, or doxycycline, 100 mg twice daily for 10 days.

29. **A** (1, 2, 3), Page 615. Nonpuerperal endometritis is an obscure chronic infection of the lining of the uterus. Although research is scant, it probably represents an intermediate state of ascending infection which is spread through the canaliculi which connect the lower genital tract to the upper genital tract. There is a positive correlation between serum antibody levels against both Microplasma hominis and Chlamydia trachomatis and the prevalence of nonpuerperal endometritis. The organisms commonly found with this entity are similar to those found in the endocervical canal; no association with parity has been made.

CHAPTER 23: Preoperative Management

DIRECTIONS: Select the one best answer or completion.

1. The part of the preoperative evaluation that is most apt to reveal medically important information is the
   A. medical history and physical exam.
   B. medical history and laboratory evaluation.
   C. physical examination and laboratory evaluation.
   D. history and nursing evaluation.
   E. physical and nursing evaluation.

2. Of the following, the cephalosporin with the longest half-life is
   A. cephalothin.
   B. cephazolin.
   C. cefoxitin.
   D. cefotaxime.
   E. moxalactam.

3. The overall mortality rate from nonradical hysterectomy is
   A. 1 in 10,000.
   B. 6 in 10,000.
   C. 12 in 10,000.
   D. 18 in 10,000.
   E. 24 in 10,000.

4. You have ordered an IVP on a 48-year-old woman who is scheduled for surgery for a large uterine fibroid. She denies allergies. She asks about the risk of death from an IVP. You can correctly respond
   A. 1 per 1000.
   B. 1 per 10,000.
   C. 1 per 100,000.
   D. 1 per 1,000,000.
   E. Nonexistent in nonallergic people.

5. A 35-year-old woman with heart disease, who has difficulty walking one block without becoming short of breath, is in need of emergency laparotomy for suspected ectopic. According to the DRIPPS American Society of Anesthesiology risk classification, she is class
   A. 1.
   B. 2.
   C. 3.
   D. 4.
   E. 5.

6. Which of the following hypertensive medications should be discontinued prior to a surgical procedure?
   A. Beta blockers
   B. Diuretics
   C. Clonidine
   D. Calcium channel blockers
   E. MAO inhibitors (Monoamine oxidase inhibitors)

7. The usual dose for heparin as prophylaxis against postsurgical thromboembolism is
   A. 5000 units IM every 12 hours.
   B. 10,000 units IM every 12 hours.
   C. 5000 units IM every 8 hours.
   D. 10,000 units subcutaneously every 8 hours.
   E. 5000 units subcutaneously every 12 hours.

8. A 37-year-old obese female with stage 1B carcinoma of the cervix is scheduled for a radical hysterectomy and node dissection. She has been on birth control pills for contraception, and has a history of varicose veins. Which of the following factors place her at the greatest risk for postoperative thromboembolism?
   A. Obesity
   B. Carcinoma of the cervix
   C. Varicose veins
   D. Age
   E. Estrogen use

9. A 42-year-old diabetic woman is on 28 units of insulin each day and has fasting blood sugars between 105 and 180 milligrams per deciliter. She also has stress urinary incontinence and wants a surgical repair. You should
   A. schedule the surgery as usual for next week.
   B. refuse to operate at all.
   C. set up appointments to evaluate and control her diabetes better.
   D. admit her to the hospital for diabetic control.
   E. increase her insulin 5 units a day and schedule the surgery.

10. An otherwise healthy 29-year-old woman with a tender pelvic mass is scheduled for exploratory laparotomy. She has no urinary or bowel symptoms. Which of the following lab tests is not indicated?
    A. Pregnancy test
    B. Hematocrit
    C. Coagulation tests
    D. Urinalysis
    E. Blood type and screen

11. A 23-year-old healthy female is being evaluated for exploratory laparotomy for a possible unruptured ectopic pregnancy. She has no cardiac symptoms. A mid-systolic click over the mitral area is heard with no other extraneous sounds or murmurs.
    A. Surgery should not be performed.
    B. Surgery should be postponed until cardiac workup can be done.
    C. Prophylactic antibiotics for subacute bacterial endocarditis should be given before surgery.
    D. A cardiac surgeon should stand by during the exploratory laparotomy.
    E. None of the above.

12. An asymptomatic patient undergoing hysterectomy for leiomyomata is most apt to have postoperative complications because of significant abnormalities of the
    A. G.I. system.
    B. central nervous system.
    C. cardiovascular system.
    D. musculoskeletal system.
    E. respiratory system.

13. You are planning a hysterectomy and bilateral salpingo-oophorectomy on a patient with a mitral valve replacement. The current recommended protocol for antibiotic prophylaxis for bacterial endocarditis is
    A. 250mg of penicillin VK, orally every 6 hours.
    B. cephalothin, 1 gram every 8 hours times 3 doses.
    C. tetracycline, 500mg, and metronidazole, 1 gram, 1 hour before surgery.
    D. ceftriaxone, 250mg IM every 6 hours times 3 doses.
    E. ampicillin, 2 grams, and gentamicin, 1.5 mg per kilogram, 1 hour before surgery.

14. A 35-year-old woman who smokes heavily has severe stress incontinence with coughing. She is scheduled for surgical repair. For the best results in the postoperative course, she should be told
    A. to stop smoking the day before surgery.
    B. to stop smoking 5 days before surgery.
    C. to stop smoking 10 days before surgery.
    D. to stop smoking 4 weeks before surgery.
    E. that stopping smoking will not make any difference.

15. Which of the following characteristics of a patient results in the greatest risk for pulmonary complications if she has surgery?
    A. Body weight greater than 30% of ideal
    B. Smoking
    C. Asthma
    D. Myocardial infarction within 3 months
    E. Uncontrolled diabetes mellitus

16. Two days after a vaginal hysterectomy a patient, who otherwise is doing very well, complains of a continuing pain in her left knee. It hurts when flexed and has pain on pressure in the lateral joint area. The most likely etiology is
    A. septic arthritis from bacteremia.
    B. anterior cruciate ligament tear.
    C. gouty arthritis.
    D. improper positioning during surgery.
    E. thrombophlebitis.

DIRECTIONS: Each question contains four suggested answers of which one or more is correct. Choose the answer
A if 1, 2, and 3 are correct
B if 1 and 3 are correct
C if 2 and 4 are correct
D if 4 only is correct
E if all are correct

17. The purposes of performing a preoperative evaluation on a patient include:
    1. education of the patient and her family.
    2. evaluation of physical and mental health.
    3. allaying fears and anxieties.
    4. avoiding unanticipated findings at the time of surgery.

18. A healthy 38-year-old woman is scheduled for a vaginal hysterectomy. Which of the following statements regarding giving her prophylactic antibiotics are true?
    1. The antibiotic *must* be present in the tissue before the surgery.
    2. There is no need to kill all the bacteria in the operative site.
    3. Third-generation cephalosporins are the best prophylactic antibiotics.
    4. Prophylactic antibiotics are more cost-effective with vaginal hysterectomy than with abdominal hysterectomy.

19. From a patient's point of view, a major operation is one that
    1. removes a major body organ.
    2. involves opening the abdomen.
    3. has to be done in the hospital.
    4. is performed on her.

20. *Mechanical* cleansing of the bowel prior to surgery is accomplished by
    1. enemas (Fleets).
    2. volume lavage (Go Lytely).
    3. laxatives (Dulcolax).
    4. nonabsorbable antibiotics (neomycin).
21. A 58-year-old patient who is scheduled for total abdominal hysterectomy and bilateral salpingo-oophorectomy is on several medications. Which of the following should be discontinued several days to several weeks prior to the procedure?
    1. Thyroxin
    2. Cortisol
    3. Warfarin
    4. MAO inhibitors (Nardin)
22. A 28-year-old woman has been scheduled for exploratory surgery to evaluate an anterior pelvic cystic mass palpated in clinic. Prior to the procedure a bowel prep and bladder catheterization was performed. On exam under anesthesia (EUA) no mass is palpated. Possible explanations are
    1. abdominal muscle guarding was mistaken for a mass.
    2. an ovarian cyst has ruptured.
    3. a loop of bowel was mistaken for an adnexal cyst.
    4. the full bladder was confused with the cyst and is now emptied.
23. A 63-year-old woman with a long smoking history is scheduled for exploratory laparotomy. Tests of pulmonary function that should be obtained are
    1. chest X-ray.
    2. arterial PO_2.
    3. vital capacity.
    4. FEV_1 (Forced Expiratory Volume at 1 second).
24. You wish to decrease the risk of thromboembolic disease in a healthy 60-year-old woman who is on oral replacement estrogen and is scheduled for an anterior vaginal repair. You should
    1. discontinue her replacement estrogen.
    2. order prophylactic heparin.
    3. order elastic wraps from foot to thigh for 3 days postoperatively.
    4. ambulate her early.
25. A 38-year-old patient calls you two days before her total abdominal hysterectomy for leiomyomata, which was scheduled 2 weeks ago. She states she has just developed a cold and wants to know what to take for her runny nose and cough. She denies chills or fever and is known to be otherwise healthy. You should
    1. meet her in the hospital for an emergency examination.
    2. cancel her surgery.
    3. have her come in for a CBC, urinalysis, and throat culture.
    4. prescribe antibiotics.
26. A hypertensive 63-year-old woman with procidentia had a myocardial infarction 2 months ago. She has also had angina for several years. The procidentia is becoming ulcerated and is creating care problems. She wishes a surgical repair. You can correctly inform her that
    1. stable angina without myocardial infarction is not a contraindication to surgery.
    2. she should discontinue her beta blocker antihypertensive medication prior to surgery.
    3. a myocardial infarction within 3 months of surgery greatly increases the risk of recurrence perioperatively.
    4. once the operation is over her immediate postoperative risk is not increased.

ANSWERS

1. **B**, Page 644. A careful history is the most valuable portion of any evaluation, but its importance tends to be overlooked. Instead, laboratory tests or imaging techniques giving numerical or written data are often overemphasized by both the patient and the physician. An adequate history should include questions regarding the major organ systems, medications, allergies, habits, family and social history. A thoroughly performed history and physical examination form a rational basis upon which further laboratory assessment and other diagnostic aids can be obtained.
2. **E**, Page 653 and Table 23-4 (from Droegemueller). The half-life of a medication determines how long that drug will be active. Of the first and second generation cephalosporins, moxalactam has the longest half-life (120 minutes) and cephazolin has the next longest (100 minutes). Cephazolin reaches high peak serum levels (80 micrograms per ml after a 1 gram dose), but has rather high protein binding (80%, which leaves 20% free in the tissues). Moxalactam is only 50% protein bound.
3. **C**, Page 648. The rate of death from hysterectomy is 12 per 10,000. This is important when you counsel patients about the procedure in order to obtain informed consent. If the patient has other medical or surgical problems, the risk increases. For example, women with cancer have a death rate of 38 per 10,000 from hysterectomy, while those with benign disease have a rate of only 6 per 10,000. When obtaining informed consent, discussion should cover the general risks of anesthesia, hemorrhage, infection, damage to other organs, death, and failure to achieve the desired

result in each case. In addition, specific risks inherent in the specific procedure contemplated should be reviewed.
4. **C, Page 656.** Five to eight percent of women will have an allergic reaction to the contrast medium used in performing an IVP. This is often an allergy to the iodine in the contrast. Of these, approximately one to two percent will be life-threatening, with an estimated mortality of 1 in 100,000. An IVP should be done for significant reasons such as large pelvic masses or pelvic malignancies, but should not be obtained routinely.
5. **C, Page 649.** The DRIPPS anesthesia risk classification is shown in Table 3. This patient with severe, but not incapacitating disease, would be a class 3. Because of the emergency nature of the surgery, her anesthetic risk is doubled.

TABLE 3 Dripps-American Society of Anesthesiologists Classification

Class	Description
1	A normal healthy patient
2	A patient with mild-to-moderate systemic disease
3	A patient with severe systemic disease with limited activity but not incapacitated
4	A patient with incapacitating, constantly life-threatening systemic disease
5	A moribund patient not expected to survive 24 hours with or without operation

Adapted from New classification of physical status. Anesthesiology 24:111, 1963.
From Jewell ER, Persson AV: Preoperative evaluation of the high-risk patient. Surg Clin North Am 65:4, 1985.

6. **E, Page 660.** Antihypertensive medications should be maintained during surgery. MAO inhibitors should be stopped 2 or more weeks prior to surgery, as they can augment effects of sympathetic amines to produce severe increases in blood pressure. Sympathetic amines are given to prevent hypotension during surgical procedures. There is a concomitant release of catecholamines from the stress of surgery. It is best not to have any drugs such as MAO inhibitors which may result in more labile response of blood pressure.
7. **E, Page 664.** The dose of heparin for protection against postoperative thromboembolism is 5000 units subcutaneously every 12 hours starting just before surgery and continuing until the patient is fully ambulatory. Heparin should never be given IM, nor should other medications be given IM when a patient is on heparin because of the high risk of hematoma formation from needle trauma to the muscle.
8. **B, Page 653.** All of the factors such as obesity, carcinoma of the cervix, varicose veins, age, and use of birth control pills increase her risk of thromboembolism. However, the greatest risk in the patient is the malignancy. Adding to her high risk are the problems of longer surgery, immobilization after surgery, and risk for postoperative infection. Ideally, the birth control pills should be stopped for at least 4 weeks prior to the surgery. She would be a candidate for minidose heparin as prophylaxis against thrombosis.
9. **C, Pages 658–659.** No elective surgery should be scheduled for this patient until her diabetes has been evaluated and is under better control. Her cardiovascular, renal, and neurologic systems should be evaluated by appropriate tests. Maintenance of postprandial serum glucose at less than 140 milligrams per ml should be achieved and controlled at that level over several weeks before elective surgery is scheduled. Frequent monitoring of diet, exercise, insulin, and blood sugars is necessary to maintain good control.
10. **C, Page 646.** The hematocrit, urinalysis, blood typing, and screening should be obtained prior to any major surgery. Urinalysis rarely changes management, but is cheap and may reveal asymptomatic bacteruria or unknown diabetes. Anemia should be ruled out. Knowledge that compatible blood is available in your facility before surgery is important. Coagulation tests are not indicated routinely, but should be obtained if there is a history of bleeding in either the patient's personal or family history. A pregnancy test should be obtained in any sexually active woman who does not have a regular menstrual history. In this case the possibility of an ectopic pregnancy should be considered. A barium enema and IVP are other tests that need not be done routinely unless the history and physical findings so dictate.
11. **E, Page 661.** Mitral prolapse with no evidence of other cardiac disease does not contraindicate surgery, nor does it require prophylactic antibiotics although some authorities suggest that they be given. If used, ampicillin, 2 grams IM or IV, and gentamicin, 1.5 milligrams per kilogram IM, should be given an hour before surgery.
12. **E, Page 657.** Mild COPD is a frequent finding, especially in obese patients or patients who smoke. Anesthesia, postoperative pain, abdominal distention, and relative immobility combine to produce symptomatic atelectasis in many patients, and this is intensified in those with pre-existing pulmonary disease. Such patients need definite preoperative instructions in deep breathing, coughing, movement, and pulmonary ventilatory exercises to prevent severe pulmonary complications.
13. **E, Page 666.** The dose for bacterial endocarditis prophylaxis is ampicillin, 2 grams, and gentamicin, 1.5 milligrams per kilogram, 1 hour before

surgery. The risk of endocarditis is low, but the morbidity is high if it occurs, and therefore the antibiotics should be given. If the patient is allergic to penicillin, vancomycin, 1 gram IV, may be substituted for the ampicillin.

14. **D, Page 657.** Smoking causes a six fold increase in risk of postoperative pulmonary complications. Smoke deposits particulate matter in the lungs and paralyzes respiratory cilia, thus preventing normal removal of these particles. Coughing is increased. This places additional stress on the surgical repair. Therefore, it is best if the patient can stop smoking for a prolonged time, but even her willingness to stop smoking for a few days will decrease sputum production and be beneficial in the postoperative course.

15. **B, Pages 657–659.** Common conditions can cause a marked increase in surgical risk. Obesity greater than 30% of average doubles the risk of surgery. Current smoking increases the risk of pulmonary complications sixfold even if the amount smoked is small. Asthma increases the risk of pulmonary complications fourfold. Diabetes and cardiovascular disease may cause problems because of increased cortisol, catecholamines, glucagon, and ADH released by the patient during the perioperative period, not to mention the potential stress of changing blood volumes or possible infections that may occur. Diabetics also have poor wound healing and an increased infection rate. A myocardial infarction within three months will increase the mortality rate from recurrent MI 30% if noncardiac surgery is performed during this time.

16. **D, Page 662.** Pressure on the joint by the stirrup or by a surgeon leaning on the supported leg is most likely. Without heat or fever, a septic process is unlikely. The location and timing are wrong for thrombophlebitis. The position is also wrong for an anterior cruciate ligament tear, and this would be an unusual site for gout. Remember to check for pressure points after positioning any patient for surgery.

17. **E (All), Pages 644–645, 647.** Patient education is necessary to obtain an informed consent. The patient should know both what can and cannot be expected from a procedure. The evaluation of the physical and mental health of the patient is incumbent on the health care team prior to any surgical procedure. Allaying the fears and anxieties of the patient is equally important. If all these have been successfully accomplished, the surgeon is unlikely to encounter surprises either during surgery or afterward, and the patient is not likely to have expectations from the results of the surgery that are different from what actually occurs.

18. **C (2, 4), Pages 651–652.** There is no need to kill all the bacteria in the operative site, but it is necessary to reduce their numbers. Prophylactic antibiotics are more cost-effective with vaginal hysterectomy than with abdominal hysterectomy. Antibiotics should be present in the tissue within at least three hours of the tissue injury in order to provide effective prophylaxis. Usually the course is started just prior to surgery. The best antibiotic for prophylaxis has yet to be determined. However, the usual antibiotics are first or second generation cephalosporins or ampicillin or tetracycline. These are given in a single dose or a three-dose regimen. Further prolongation does not add to their prophylatic effectiveness.

19. **E (All), Page 643.** Patients are understandably concerned about any procedure that is performed on them. An adequate informed consent must be obtained. This implies a recognition of the risks and benefits of the procedure. Any surgical procedure entails some risk that is borne by the patient, and she has a right to understand it and regard the surgery as a major event. Even a relatively less dangerous procedure may have severe consequences, either in its performance or its findings. For example, a D&C may lead to the diagnosis of endometrial cancer, so a patient is apt to be quite anxious. Recognition of, and empathy for, the patient's concerns are parts of the art of medicine. Patients should have help to alleviate their fears and anxieties.

20. **A (1, 2, 3), Pages 655–656.** Enemas cause direct mechanical cleansing of the bowel while laxatives work by stimulating bowel peristalsis to evacuate the contents. Go Lytely is a volume lavage given orally which causes diarrhea without significant fluid or electrolyte shifts. Antibiotics do not result in mechanical cleansing, but do cause marked decrease in the number of bacteria found in the gut, thereby decreasing the probability of infection if the bowel is opened during the procedure.

21. **D (4), Page 649.** MAO should be stopped. Anticoagulants and corticosteroids may be continued with adjustment in type and/or dosage prior to and during surgery. If anticoagulation is needed, it is better to use heparin than coumadin. Cortisol may be increased if a patient is on adrenal suppressive doses for other systemic disease. Thyroid replacement should be given until the day of surgery in its usual dose.

22. **E (All), Page 662.** Most pelvic surgeons have found at least once that suspected pathology has disappeared, or that previously unsuspected pathology was present when they did an examination under anesthesia (EUA) just prior to surgery. Therefore this examination should be routinely performed.

23. **E** (All), Page 658. In an older patient with a positive history or physical examination suggestive of respiratory problems, an extensive evaluation of the pulmonary function is warranted. Vital capacity should be greater than 50% of expected, and PO_2 should be greater than 65 millimeters of mercury. The FEV_1 should be greater than 75% of expected, and the chest X-ray should be normal. If any of these findings are abnormal, further evaluation and treatment should be done before any elective surgery is undertaken.

24. **D** (4), Page 654. This healthy woman is going to have a short procedure that has no high risk factors dictating the use of subcutaneous doses of heparin for prophylaxis. Replacement estrogen is not associated with increased thrombosis. However, a younger woman on birth control pills should stop them several weeks before major elective surgery. The birth control pills decrease the concentration of coagulating inhibitors (antithrombin) and elevate several clotting factors. Elastic wraps to go above the knee are often counterproductive in that they exert a tourniquet effect at the joint. If used, they must be monitored very closely. Early ambulation is one of the best preventive measures.

25. **C** (2, 4), Page 657. Elective surgery should not be performed during or immediately after an upper respiratory infection. A waiting period of 10 or more days is appropriate to decrease the risk of pulmonary complication. There is no need to perform an emergency examination or do lab work that you would not normally do for a common cold. Decongestants are a reasonable choice to decrease the symptoms in this otherwise healthy woman. She can be seen if the symptoms do not resolve in a short period of time.

26. **B** (1, 3), Pages 660–661. Angina of recent occurrence (within 3 months) is a high risk factor, but stable angina is not. The recent myocardial infarction is of serious concern. Patients with recent myocardial infarctions should wait at least 6 months before any elective surgical procedure is done. The risk of repeat myocardial infarction persists for several days postoperatively and about one-third occur on the third or fourth postoperative day. Therefore, the patient should be followed closely in the immediate postoperative period. Discontinuing the beta blocker may be harmful. It should be continued through the perioperative period.

Chapter 24

Postoperative Complications

DIRECTIONS: Select the one best answer or completion.

1. The initial management of moderate superficial thrombophlebitis at the site of an intravenous catheter includes all of the following *except*
   A. heat.
   B. elevation.
   C. rest.
   D. ibuprofen.
   E. heparin.

2. The most cost-efficient modality in preventing and treating atelectasis is
   A. chest physical therapy.
   B. bedside incentive spirometer.
   C. intermittent positive pressure breathing.
   D. aerosol therapy.
   E. bronchoscopy.

3. On the fifth postoperative day a patient has a fever of 102°F but does not feel bad. She does not appear so sick as her temperature would imply. She has been on intravenous Keflin for a suspected urinary tract infection for 5 days. The most likely diagnosis is
   A. atelectasis.
   B. urinary tract infection.
   C. wound infection.
   D. drug fever.
   E. pneumonia.

4. Of the following, the blood component that *does not* carry with it the risk of hepatitis is
   A. packed cells.
   B. frozen plasma.
   C. cryoprecipitate.
   D. platelet concentrate.
   E. Factor VIII concentrate.

5. The most likely sign of pulmonary emboli is
   A. tachycardia.
   B. tachypnea.
   C. rales.
   D. cyanosis.
   E. accentuation of pulmonic closure.

6. The most accurate method for detecting deep vein thrombophlebitis is
   A. physical examination.
   B. venography.
   C. fibrinogen ^{125}I scan.
   D. Doppler ultrasound.
   E. impedance plethysmography.

7. Of the symptoms listed, the *least* common in cases of documented pulmonary embolus is
   A. dyspnea.
   B. chest pain.
   C. apprehension.
   D. hemoptysis.
   E. cough.

8. A 35-year-old patient has just undergone an uneventful abdominal hysterectomy for leiomyomata. Eight hours after surgery, her hematocrit is reported to be 27%. Vital signs are stable and her physical examination is unremarkable. Her preoperative hematocrit was 37%. There was a 500 cc blood loss at surgery and anesthesia records indicated that she was given 2000 cc of D5 Ringers' Lactate as intravenous fluid. Her urine output has been 30–70 cc per hour. You should
   A. repeat the hematocrit in 12–24 hours.
   B. perform a pelvic examination.
   C. transfuse with two units of packed red blood cells.
   D. order a pelvic ultrasound.
   E. perform an exploratory laparotomy.

9. The test with the greatest accuracy in detecting pulmonary emboli is
   A. pulmonary angiography.
   B. ventilation-perfusion lung scan.
   C. arterial blood gas determination.
   D. EKG.
   E. chest X-ray.

DIRECTIONS: For each numbered item, select the one heading most closely associated with it. Each lettered heading may be used once, more than once, or not at all.

10–11. A. Pelvic cellulitis
B. Granulation tissue
C. Prolapsed fallopian tube
D. Lymphocyst
E. Ovarian abscess

10. Consequence of pelvic node dissection.
11. Fatal intraperitoneal rupture.

DIRECTIONS: For each numbered item, indicate whether it is associated with
A only (A)
B only (B)
C both (A) and (B)
D neither (A) nor (B)

12–14. A. Atelectasis
B. Pneumonia
C. Both
D. Neither

12. Predisposing factors include nasogastric suction, obesity.
13. Characterized by fever, tachypnea.
14. Chest x-ray may show patchy infiltrate.

15–17. A. Heparin therapy
B. Thrombolytic (streptokinase–urokinase) therapy
C. Both
D. Neither

15. Indicated for nonmassive pulmonary emboli.
16. Continued for 10 days.
17. May be used long-term instead of warfarin.

18–21. A. Vesicovaginal fistula
B. Ureterovaginal fistula
C. Both
D. Neither

18. Intermittent urine loss more typical than constant loss.
19. IV indigo carmine causes staining of a vaginal tampon.
20. Transurethral methylene blue instillation causes staining of a vaginal tampon.
21. Surgical repair delayed at least two months.

22–25. A. Postoperative ileus
B. Postoperative obstruction
C. Both
D. Neither

22. Progressively severe crampy, abdominal pain.
23. Nausea and vomiting.
24. Absent bowel sounds.
25. Air-fluid levels on abdominal X-ray.

DIRECTIONS: Each question contains four suggested answers, of which one or more is correct. Choose the answer

A if 1, 2, and 3 are correct
B if 1 and 3 are correct
C if 2 and 4 are correct
D if 4 only is correct
E if all are correct

26. A 35-year-old patient, 3 hours following a total abdominal hysterectomy for large leiomyomata, develops increasing tachycardia and decreasing blood pressure. Initial management should include
  1. insertion of a Foley catheter.
  2. insertion of a Swan-Ganz catheter.
  3. infusion of 1 ml Crystalloid solution, 3 ml for each ml of estimated blood loss.
  4. immediate exploratory surgery.

27. Early signs of hypovolemia due to postoperative intraperitoneal hemorrhage include
  1. shoulder pain.
  2. tachycardia.
  3. muscle rigidity.
  4. decreased urine output.

28. A 47-year-old patient, three weeks after a vaginal hysterectomy and posterior repair, complains of ten days of involuntary passage of gas and small amounts of fecal material from the vagina, and a foul-smelling vaginal discharge. On physical examination, a 1/2 cm dark red area of what appears to be granulation tissue is seen in the lower 1/3 of the posterior vagina. At this point you would
  1. place the patient on a low-residue diet.
  2. schedule the patient for repair after completion of a bowel prep.
  3. perform a preoperative proctoscopy.
  4. perform a preoperative barium enema.

29. Factors which contribute to the development of wound infection include
  1. obesity.
  2. use of cautery.
  3. presence of a hematoma.
  4. increased duration of preoperative hospitalization.

30. Postoperative factors contributing to the development of atelectasis include
  1. incisional pain.
  2. bulky abdominal dressings.
  3. immobility.
  4. anorexia.

31. Causes of shock include
  1. cardiac failure.
  2. sepsis.
  3. an anaphylactic reaction.
  4. hemorrhage.

32. You are called on the phone by the nurse about an obese 40-year-old patient who underwent a total abdominal hysterectomy 18 hours ago. She reports that the vital signs are temperature 38°, BP 80/40, pulse 110, respirations 30. The nurse raises the possibility of postoperative atelectasis. Those vital signs that support her hypothesis include
   1. temperature.
   2. pulse.
   3. respiratory rate.
   4. blood pressure.

33. You are planning to perform a total abdominal hysterectomy/bilateral salpingo-oophorectomy on a 50-year-old markedly obese, insulin-dependent diabetic patient for symptomatic leiomyomata. Methods to reduce the risk of deep vein thrombophlebitis in this patient include:
   1. subcutaneous low dose heparin.
   2. intra- and postoperative intermittent leg compression.
   3. intravenous dextran.
   4. oral warfarin.

34. True statements concerning the postoperative use of urinary tract catheters include:
   1. Foley catheterization promotes earlier spontaneous voiding than suprapubic catherization.
   2. Suprapubic catheters are more comfortable than Foley catheters.
   3. Prophylactic antibiotics are recommended if urinary catheters are used.
   4. Infections are more common after Foley catheter use than after intermittent straight catheterization.

35. Three days after uneventful total abdominal hysterectomy/bilateral salpingo-oophorectomy, a 40-year-old patient is found to have a hematocrit of 20%. Her preoperative hematocrit was 34%. Blood loss at surgery was estimated at 700 cc. Vital signs are stable. She has mild lower abdominal tenderness with a 5 cm tender fluctuant midline mass at the apex of her vaginal cuff. Given the most likely diagnosis, you would
   1. order a BE.
   2. order an IVP.
   3. plan an exploratory laparotomy.
   4. begin a transfusion of packed red blood cells.

36. A 30-year-old patient develops a fever to 38° in the first 48 hours after vaginal hysterectomy. Based on the timing of the onset of fever, *unlikely* causes of the fever include
   1. pneumonia.
   2. cuff cellulitis.
   3. phlebitis.
   4. urinary tract infection.

37. The etiology of wound dehiscence is associated with
   1. an incision through an area of previous incision.
   2. use of catgut suture.
   3. wound infection.
   4. vertical abdominal incision.

38. *Sequelae* of deep vein thrombophlebitis include
   1. chronic edema.
   2. pain on exercise (claudication).
   3. skin ulceration.
   4. muscle atrophy.

ANSWERS

1. **E**, Page 677. Superficial thrombophlebitis is most commonly associated with intravenous catheters. Although the inflammation does not necessarily cease when the catheter is removed, it is recommended that this be done as soon as the diagnosis is made. Mild cases of superficial thrombophlebitis should be treated with rest, local heat, and elevation. A nonsteroidal anti-inflammatory agent such as ibuprofen may be used in cases that are more severe. The use of heparin and antibiotics is reserved for the rare case of proximal progression of inflammation.

2. **B**, Page 672. The basis for preventing atelectasis consists of simple activities that are, unfortunately, more difficult for the postop patient. These include taking deep breaths, walking, coughing, turning from side to side, and not lying supine. If necessary, an incentive spirometer can be used effectively to prevent or treat atelectasis. If these techniques do not clear the atelectasis, the patient should then be managed with chest physical therapy, intermittent positive pressure breathing, or aerosol therapy. Bronchoscopy may be required to remove large mucus plugs.

3. **D**, Page 670. Drug fever is often a diagnosis of exclusion. It may be suspected if eosinophilia is discovered or if the patient feels and looks better than the temperature course might suggest. Presumptive evidence of drug fever is a fever that disappears when a drug is discontinued.

4. **D**, Page 674 and Table 24-2. Platelet concentrate is the only component listed that does not expose the recipient to the risk of hepatitis. It can, however, cause Rh isoimmunization if the blood types are not compatible. Packed cells, frozen plasma, cry-

oprecipitate, and Factor VIII concentrate do carry the risk of hepatitis.

5. **B**, Page 684. In a national study of documented pulmonary emboli conducted by Blinder and Coleman,* tachypnea was found over 90% of the times, rales were discovered 58%, tachycardia 44%, cyanosis 20%, and accentuation of pulmonic closure 53%. Shock and syncope are associated with massive pulmonary emboli.

6. **B**, Page 680. Although signs and symptoms of deep vein thrombophlebitis depend on the severity and extent of the process, 50% of patients are asymptomatic. Physical examination of the legs results in false positive findings 50% of the time. In cases where signs and symptoms suggest deep vein thrombophlebitis, the diagnosis should be confirmed with an imaging technique. Venography is the most accurate current method for detecting deep vein thrombophlebitis. The diagnostic accuracy is 95% for peripheral disease and 90% for iliofemoral thrombophlebitis. Scanning with fibrinogen ^{125}I correlates 90% with venography. The test is not diagnostic above mid-thigh. Doppler ultrasound and impedance plethysmography are noninvasive screening methods with less diagnostic accuracy.

7. **D**, Page 684. Signs and symptoms of pulmonary embolus are nonspecific. Chest pain, dyspnea and apprehension are the most common symptoms. In a national study conducted by Blinder and Coleman (see Answer 5), only 30% of patients with documented pulmonary embolus had hemoptysis. Cough was found in 53%.

8. **A**, Page 670. A patient's hematocrit should be checked twice during the postoperative course. Significant intraperitoneal or retroperitoneal blood loss can occur without apparent changes of vital signs, physical examination, or urine output. Because of physiologic release of aldosterone and antidiuretic hormone in response to the stress of surgery, the hematocrit on the first postoperative day may be misleading, reflecting changes in fluid status rather than hemorrhage. A drop of 4 to 5 points in the hematocrit usually reflects blood loss of 500 cc. Most healthy patients can easily tolerate a hematocrit of 24–25. In the patient described, repeating the hematocrit would be the most reasonable action.

9. **A**, Page 685. Pulmonary angiography is the most definitive test in the detection of emboli. Because of potential morbidity (5%) and mortality (0.2%) associated with angiography, the ventilation-perfusion lung scan is the first imaging technique usually used to diagnose a pulmonary embolus. A negative scan essentially rules out an embolus. Findings on blood gas determination, chest X-ray, and EKG are helpful but not diagnostic.

10. **D**, Pages 697–699. A lymphocyst is a local collection of lymphatic fluid found most frequently following pelvic node dissections. Small cysts regress spontaneously while larger ones require intermittent aspiration or insertion of an indwelling catheter.

11. **E**, Pages 697–699. An ovarian abscess is a potentially fatal complication of a vaginal hysterectomy. If the diagnosis is not made, intraperitoneal rupture may ensue. Initial therapy is parenteral broad-spectrum antibiotics, although most patients require surgical removal of the affected adnexa.

12–14. 12, **C**; 13, **C**; 14, **C**; Pages 672–673. It is critical to be able to differentiate postoperative atelectasis from pneumonia. The two are commonly associated, and the treatments are the same except for the addition of parenteral antibiotics for the patient with pneumonia. Patients who are obese or who have nasogastric suction are at risk for both conditions. Atelectasis and pneumonia both typically present with fever and tachypnea. An important difference is that pneumonia also typically presents with productive, purulent sputum. If a chest X-ray is performed, a patchy infiltrate is compatible with either condition.

15–17. 15, **A**; 16, **A**; 17; **D**; Pages 585, 683. The management of most cases of pulmonary emboli is with full-dose intravenous heparin. One method of administration is to give an initial loading dose of 5000 IU, followed by hourly infusion of 1000–1500 IU. Thrombolytic (streptokinase–urokinase) therapy is reserved for cases of massive embolus only. A thrombolytic agent is used only in the first 24 hours of therapy. Heparin is continued for 7–10 days. All patients with pulmonary emboli should have warfarin therapy for 3–6 months. Neither heparin nor thrombolytic therapy is indicated for long-term therapy.

18–21. 18, **B**; 19, **C**; 20, **A**; 21, **C**; Pages 687–688. The classic symptom of a vesicovaginal fistula is painless and almost continuous loss of urine. If this loss is intermittent and related to position, a ureterovaginal fistula should be suspected. Intravenous injection of 1–2 ml of indigo carmine will result in the blue staining of a vaginal tampon both in cases of ureterovaginal fistula and a vesicovaginal fistula. If a vesicovaginal fistula is suspected, methylene blue is instilled into the bladder. A tampon is placed in the vagina. The tampon will be discolored blue if a vesicovaginal fistula exists, but not in the presence of a

---

*Blinder RA, Coleman RE: Evaluation of pulmonary embolism. Radiol Clin North Am 23:392, 1985.

ureterovaginal fistula. The repair of both vesicovaginal and ureterovaginal fistulas should be delayed at least two months after the initial operation either to allow possible spontaneous healing or to maximize the integrity and health of the surgical area after it has completely healed.

22–25. 22, **B**; 23, **C**; 24, **A**; 25, **C**; Pages 689–692. A dynamic ileus probably is a result of poorly coordinated motor activity of the small intestine. It is not easily differentiated from small bowel obstruction because an ileus is often associated with a partial small bowel obstruction. The patient with an ileus is uncomfortable, but it is the patient with an obstruction that suffers from progressively severe, crampy abdominal pain. Patients with either an ileus or a small bowel obstruction have nausea and vomiting. Bowel sounds are hypoactive or absent with an ileus, whereas in obstruction peristaltic rushes and high-pitched tinkles are common. Air-fluid levels on abdominal X-ray may occur in either ileus or obstruction. In the former, they occur infrequently and if so, at the same levels. In the latter, air-fluid levels are common and demonstrate a step-ladder appearance—multiple air-fluid levels throughout the small intestine with an absence of gas in the colon and rectum.

26. **A** (1, 2, 3), Pages 674–675. The goals in initially managing the patient who has developed presumed postoperative hemorrhage should be replacement of circulating blood volume and establishment of cellular perfusion and oxygenation. Crystalloid solution should be infused rapidly, with 3 ml being used for each 1 ml of blood loss. In order to monitor the rapid changes of fluid status, a Swan-Ganz catheter should be inserted if rapid changes in fluid status and blood pressure continue. Similarly, a Foley catheter is used in all cases to monitor urinary output. Exploratory surgery should be promptly performed if there is evidence of postop bleeding, but only after adequate volume replacement has been accomplished.

27. **C** (2, 4), Pages 673–674. Tachycardia and decreased urine output are two early signs of hypovolemia due to hidden internal bleeding. Tachycardia is caused by the body's adrenergic response to hemorrhage, and the decreased urine output is caused by poor perfusion of the kidneys. Both shoulder pain and muscle rigidity of the abdominal wall are late signs of intraperitoneal hemorrhage and are not due to hypovolemia.

28. **B** (1, 3), Pages 692–693. The patient described presents with the classic symptoms (involuntary loss of gas and stool, a foul-smelling vaginal discharge) of a rectovaginal fistula. It is more commonly associated with obstetric rather than gynecologic complications. Initial therapy includes low-residue diet and Lomotil. One in four will heal spontaneously. If corrective surgery must be performed, a 2–3 month delay is appropriate. Preoperative evaluation should include visualization of the entire vagina and sigmoidoscopy of the rectal mucosa to discover if there is more than one opening. A barium enema or flexible endoscopy is needed if there is suspicion of the coexistence of inflammatory bowel disease.

29. **E** (All), Page 693. There are many factors which contribute to the development of wound infection. Most significant are local factors, which include the presence of foreign bodies, necrotic tissue, hematomas, dead space, use of cautery, and decreased tissue perfusion. Systemic factors include malnutrition, obesity, diabetes, liver disease, immunosuppression, age, and increased duration of preoperative hospitalization.

30. **A** (1, 2, 3), Pages 671–672. Atelectasis develops in 10% of women who undergo pelvic surgery. It is the most common cause of postoperative fever. Pain, the supine position, and abdominal distension deter the patient from taking deep inspirations. Deep breaths normally expand all areas of the lung, thus preventing atelectasis. Similarly, immobility and binding around the abdomen and chest cause the patient to breath at lower lung volumes, thus predisposing to atelectasis. Obesity, smoking, age greater than 60 years, prolonged operative time, and coexisting medical problems such as cardiac disease and pulmonary infection all predispose patients to postoperative atelectasis. Anorexia *per se* is not known to be the direct cause of atelectasis.

31. **E** (All), Page 673. Shock is a condition in which circulatory insufficiency prevents adequate vascular perfusion of vital organs. The etiology of shock includes cardiac failure, sepsis, an anaphylactic reaction, and hemorrhage. Shock due to postoperative hemorrhage is usually seen within the first few hours of surgery. These cases are due primarily to inadequate hemostasis. In general, it takes a reduction of approximately 20% of the blood volume to produce shock in a woman of reproductive age.

32. **A** (1, 2, 3), Page 672. The classic triad of atelectasis is fever, tachypnea, and tachycardia, presenting in the first 72 postoperative hours. These findings must, however, be evaluated along with the other clinical factors. In the case described, marked hypotension of 80/40 in an obese patient would suggest consideration of other causes, such as postoperative bleeding.

33. **A** (1, 2, 3), Pages 681–683. Prophylaxis against deep vein thrombophlebitis for high risk

patients such as the 50-year-old obese, diabetic patient described can be accomplished with subcutaneous heparin, intravenous dextran, or intermittent pneumatic compression. Embolex (dihydroergotamine mesylate plus heparin) has also been shown to be effective; however, because of its listed contraindications of sepsis, hypertension, and atherosclerotic heart disease (ASHD), it would probably not be appropriate in the obese, diabetic patient described since she might also have ASHD and hypertension. Oral warfarin is used in the treatment of deep vein thrombosis or pulmonary embolus after a week of heparin therapy and is not appropriate for prophylactic use.

34. **C** (2, 4), Page 687. Compared with intermittent straight catheterization and suprapubic catheterization, the use of a Foley catheter delays spontaneous voiding, is more uncomfortable, and predisposes the patient to urinary tract infection. Although systemic prophylactic antibiotics do decrease the initial incidence of infection, the effect is short-lived only. The use of prophylactic antibiotics also promotes the emergence of antibiotic-resistant bacteria. As a result, antibiotics are not recommended for catheterized patients unless they are immunocompromised. In fact, catheter-related infections are not treated with antibiotics unless the patient is febrile.

35. **D** (4), Page 676. The patient described has probably developed a postoperative cuff hematoma. The hematoma is usually the result of slow, venous oozing and is self-limiting. Even if the hematoma is not infected, a low-grade fever is common because of inflammation surrounding the hematoma. The diagnosis of a retroperitoneal hematoma is usually possible by physical exam. Only rarely are radiologic studies needed. One might consider ordering an IVP if the position of the hematoma suggests that a ureter might be obstructed. Surgical management is usually not recommended unless there is evidence of persistent blood loss. If needed, surgery is usually via the extraperitoneal route.

36. **E** (All), Page 669 and Table 24-1 (from Droegemueller). Only 20% of postoperative fevers are directly related to infection. It is not unusual for a hysterectomy patient to have a mild temperature elevation during the first 72 postoperative hours with no identifiable infection. Atelectasis is the cause of over 90% of fevers presenting in the first 48 hours. Pneumonia, cuff cellulitis, phlebitis, and urinary tract infection tend to cause fever after the first 48 hours.

37. **A** (1, 2, 3), Pages 694–696. Wound dehiscence usually implies disruption of the abdominal wound through the fascia but not through the peritoneum. Wound infection is present in half of women with a wound disruption. As stronger synthetic absorbable sutures have replaced catgut, the incidence of dehiscence has decreased. There appears to be little effect on the incidence of dehiscence whether a vertical or horizontal incision had been made. Important mechanical factors predisposing to disruption are conditions that increase the tension on the incision line, such as abdominal distension and chronic lung disease. Other factors include obesity, the patient's age, malignant disease, prior radiation, and whether the incision was made through a previous incision. A mass closure utilizing through-and-through monofilament nylon is a commonly used abdominal closure for incisions which have broken down. An alternative closure is the Smead-Jones closure.

38. **A** (1, 2, 3), Page 678. Deep vein thrombophlebitis is the process of venous thrombosis formation occurring in any deep vein due to blood coagulation and fibrin formation in the presence of venous stasis. In addition to pulmonary embolus, major *sequelae* of deep vein thrombophlebitis include chronic venous insufficiency resulting in damage to the valves of deep veins. This produces shunting of blood to superficial veins, skin ulceration, pain on exercise, and chronic edema. Deep vein thrombophlebitis has not been shown to be associated with muscle atrophy.

PART FOUR: GYNECOLOGIC ONCOLOGY

CHAPTER 25: Principles of Radiation Therapy and Chemotherapy in Gynecologic Cancer

DIRECTIONS: Select the one best answer or completion.

1. The cell is most sensitive to radiation damage in which growth phase?
   A. Mitosis
   B. Phase of protein synthesis
   C. Phase of DNA duplication
   D. Phase of RNA synthesis
   E. Resting phase

2. Three months ago, a 60-year-old woman completed a nine course treatment with Cytoxan, *cis*-platinum, and adriamycin for Stage III serous cystadenocarcinoma of the ovary. At "second look" operation 1 year after the onset of treatment, there is no microscopic or macroscopic evidence of the disease. What is this response best called?
   A. Cure
   B. Complete remission
   C. Objective response
   D. Stabilization
   E. Partial remission

3. Energy (such as that used to treat cancers) transmitted from a source to a target area
   A. converges as it approaches the target tissue.
   B. diverges as it approaches target tissue.
   C. travels parallel as it approaches target tissue, that is, neither converges nor diverges.
   D. converges or diverges dependent upon the energy source.
   E. is transmitted as a wave form.

4. Each of the following improves the effectiveness of a chemotherapeutic agent **except** a
   A. small original tumor burden.
   B. more frequent administration of chemotherapeutic agent.
   C. higher dose of chemotherapeutic agent.
   D. smaller percentage of cells in G_0 (resting) phase.
   E. decreased mitotic activity of tumor cells.

5. The major advantage of high energy particulate radiation, such as accelerated neutrons, is that it
   A. can kill the cell directly.
   B. has low linear energy transfer (LET).
   C. is most effective in well-oxygenated tissue.
   D. can be administered from both external and internal sources.
   E. does not decrease proportional to the distance traveled.

DIRECTIONS: For each numbered item, select the one heading most closely associated with it. Each lettered heading may be used once, more than once, or not at all.

   (A) Interferon
   (B) BCG (bacillus Calmette-Guerin)
   (C) Dinitrochlorobenzene (DCNB)
   (D) Active specific immunotherapy
   (E) Passive immunity

6. Nonspecific immunotherapy used to activate both cell mediated and humoral antibody.
7. Radiated tumor cells used to produce a vaccine.
8. Prevents cancer cell division by augmenting natural killer cells.
9. Extracts of "transfer factor" confers immunologic memory to patient's lymphocytes.

   (A) Doxorubicin (Adriamycin)
   (B) Cyclophosphamide (Cytoxan)
   (C) Methotrexate
   (D) Vincristine
   (E) *Cis*-platinum

10. Positively charged alkyl groups react with negatively charged portion of DNA.
11. Plant alkaloid that attacks the cell spindle during mitosis.
12. Enzymatic inhibitor in synthesis of purine nucleotides.
13. May cause cardiomyopathy.

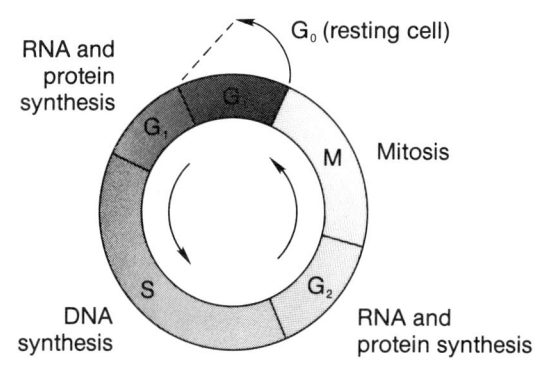

Principles of Radiation Therapy and Chemotherapy in Gynecologic Cancer 161

FIGURE 25-1.
Phases of the cell.

(From Droegemueller W, Herbst AL, Mishell DR, Stenchever MA: Comprehensive gynecology. St. Louis, The C.V. Mosby Co., 1987.)

(A) Mitosis (M)
(B) Resting cell (G₀)
(C) Protein synthesis (G₂)
(D) DNA synthesis (S)

14. Phase of cell cycle resistant to cytotoxic drugs.
15. Phase most affected by antimetabolites (methotrexate).
16. Phase most affected by vinca alkaloids (vincristine).

DIRECTIONS: For each numbered item, indicate whether it is associated with

A only (A)
B only (B)
C both (A) and (B)
D neither (A) nor (B)

(A) Isodose curve A
(B) Isodose curve B
(C) Both
(D) Neither

17. More likely to treat deep pelvic nodes in a woman 5 feet 2 inches tall, weighing 240 lbs.
18. High doses more likely to cause skin damage.
19. Could be used to treat 3 cm central recurrence of epidermoid carcinoma of cervix.

(A) Brachytherapy
(B) Teletherapy
(C) Both
(D) Neither

20. Dose delivered to the cancer by inverse square law.

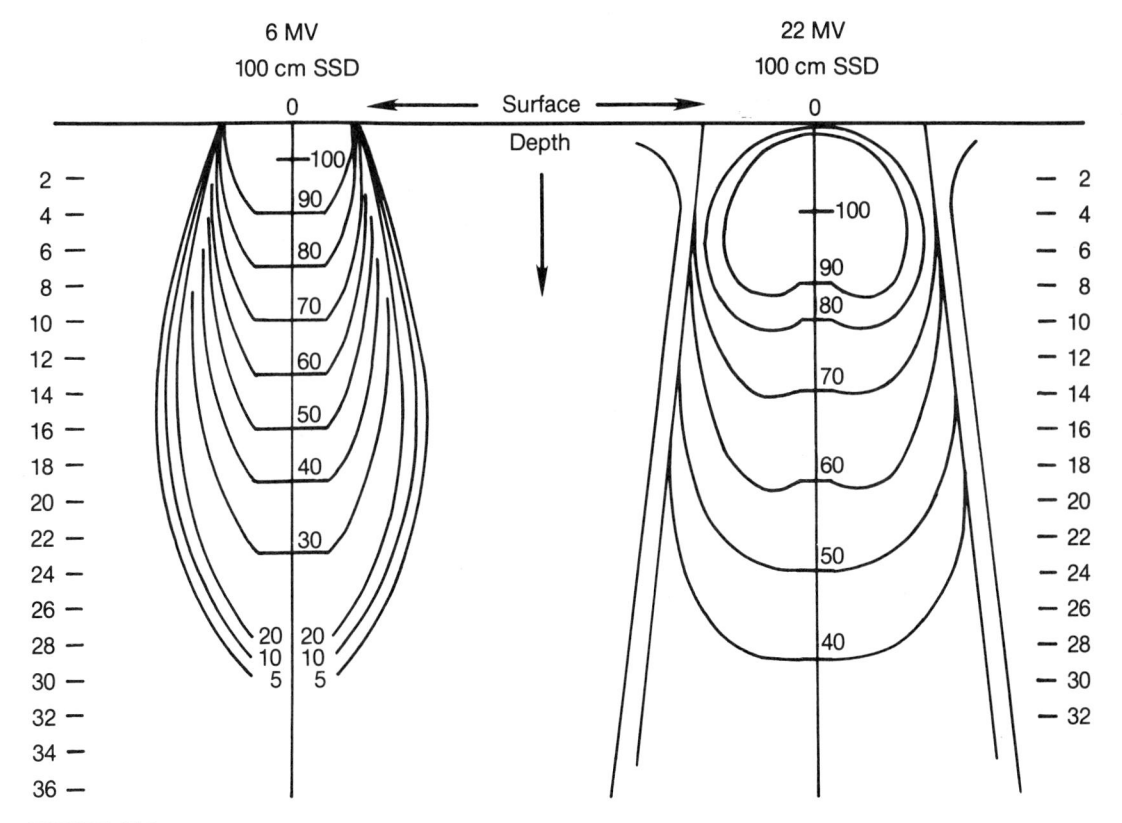

FIGURE 25-2.
Comparison of isodose curves and depth-dose distribution for 6 MV and 22 MV beatrons.
(Redrawn from DiSaia PJ, and Creasman WT: Clinical gynecologic oncology, 2nd ed. St. Louis, The C.V. Mosby Co, 1984.)

21. Uses radioisotope with defined half-life of radionuclides.
22. Uses concept of Source Axis Distance (SAD).

DIRECTIONS: Each question contains four suggested answers of which one or more is correct. Choose the answer
- A if 1, 2, and 3 are correct
- B if 1 and 3 are correct
- C if 2 and 4 are correct
- D if 4 only is correct
- E if all are correct

23. Tumor growth stimulates the host immune system and specifically has been shown to activate
    1. T-lymphocytes.
    2. B-lymphocytes.
    3. macrophages.
    4. tumor-specific antigens.
24. Which are characteristics of *growth fraction* (GF) of a given tumor?
    1. Determines doubling time
    2. Faster in smaller tumors
    3. Faster after chemotherapy
    4. Slower in metastatic lesions
25. Ionizing radiation causes cell death by
    A. directly altering the localized host immune response.
    B. producing free hydroxyl radicals.
    C. causing an increase in the oxygen tension of the target tissue.
    D. leading to the formation of peroxide in tissues.
26. Which are advantages of multiple chemotherapeutic regimens over single-agent regimens?
    1. Intervention at different phases in the cell cycle.
    2. Better response against larger tumors.
    3. Helps to prevent emergence of resistant cells.
    4. Total treatment time is shortened.
27. Which factors increase the rate of radiation-related complications?
    1. Decreased intestinal motility from postoperative adhesions.
    2. Large tumor requiring expanded radiation.
    3. Decreased vascularity to normal tissues resulting from prior surgery.
    4. Concomitant chemotherapy.
28. Which are characteristics of electromagnetic ionizing radiation (photons of x-rays and gamma rays) used for tumor therapy?
    1. No mass
    2. No electrical charge
    3. Energy is proportional to frequency
    4. Produced in discrete quanta
29. An important principle guiding the total dose of irradiation and the number of fractions by which that dose is administered is/are
    1. distance of energy source to target tissue.
    2. the type of tumor being irradiated.
    3. the age of the patient.
    4. the mitotic activity of the tumor cells.
30. Which factors contribute to the resistance of large tumors to chemotherapy?
    1. Increased DNA synthesis
    2. Heterogeneous cell population
    3. Increased RNA synthesis
    4. Lower growth fraction

ANSWERS

1. **A,** Page 714. During mitosis the cell is most sensitive to radiation. Thus rapidly dividing cells are the most radiosensitive. Dividing radiation into a number of smaller doses (fractionation) allows for effective treatment of the tumor without increasing the complications of radiation to the normal surrounding tissues which have a rapid turnover such as the bone marrow and intestine.
2. **B,** Page 722. In assessing the effect of chemotherapeutic agents, a number of definitions are used to describe the response of the tumor being treated. A cure implies a permanent absence of disease for a period of 5 years or longer. A complete remission is total disappearance of the tumor for at least 1 month. An objective response is a 50% or greater reduction in the size of the tumor for at least 1 month. Stabilization is used to indicate that the disease has not changed in size. The phrase *partial remission* is no longer used in lieu of the term *objective response*.
3. **B,** Page 713. Regardless of the source of electromagnetic or photon radiation, the transmitted energy from the source diverges as the distance it travels from the source increases. This divergence causes a decrease in energy, and the relationship is described by the inverse square law. For example, the dose of radiation 2 cm from a point source is only one fourth the value of the dose at 1 cm.
4. **E,** Pages 720–721. One of the reasons chemotherapy appears to affect cancer tissue more than normal tissue is that malignant tumor cells have a higher growth fraction in comparison to normal cells. The ability of a chemotherapeutic agent to destroy a greater number of cancer cells more effectively is enhanced if the agent can be given more frequently or in larger doses per unit time. However, dose and frequency are limited by tolerance of normal tissue. A higher percentage of cells in the G_0 or resting phase will limit chemotherapeutic effectiveness. Increased, not decreased, mitotic activity of tumor cells will render them more susceptible to successful chemotherapy.

5. **A**, Page 714. With particulate radiation using heavy particles such as neutrons, the ionization is known as high linear energy transfer. That is, the rate of energy loss as it traverses a unit length of tissue is greater than with photon irradiation. This form of radiation produces high energy recoil protons which kill the cell directly upon impact and are independent of oxygenation. Currently, systems are being developed that use neutron generators as a form of external beam therapy. This type of energy cannot be generated by internal sources. Even though this is a high energy source, the principle of the inverse square law still applies with this type of radiation.

6–9. 6, **B**; 7, **D**; 8, **A**; 9, **E**; Pages 726–727. A number of approaches have been taken to augment the immune response to human tumors. Most of these remain investigational, but the clinician should be aware that it is this field of tumor biology which shows the most promise for successful cancer treatment.

Interferon has been found to prevent cancer cell division by augmenting the action of natural killer cells. By preventing the replication of cancer cells, the treatment should gradually lead to tumor regression, especially if used as an adjunctive treatment.

Active specific immunotherapy involves the use of tumor cells and their antigens to produce specific tumor immunity. These cells are usually modified by chemotherapy or radiation and grown in media to produce a vaccine. Passive immunity may be conferred through transferring specific immunity using extracts of lymphocytes sensitized to tumor antigens. These "transfer factors" may lead to a type of adoptive immunotherapy by transfer of "immunologic memory" to the patient's own lymphocytes.

Another method involves the use of nonspecific immunotherapy which involves the use of adjuvant agents, usually of a microbiologic origin. These are used to simulate cell-mediated and humoral immunity as well as to activate macrophages. The most commonly cited example of this is the use of BCG. This agent produces a marked proliferation of lymphocytes, but its use as effective therapy in gynecologic malignancies has not yet been identified.

10–13. 10, **B**; 11, **D**; 12, **C**; 13, **A**; Pages 723–726, Table 25-3 (from Droegemueller). This series of questions addresses characteristics of commonly used cytotoxic agents in gynecologic malignancy. They represent different classes of drugs with generally different mechanisms of action. Although a single drug characteristic out of context may not seem important, a general knowledge of the classes of cytotoxic agents is important when determining rational therapy for gynecologic malignancy.

The alkylating agents, of which chlorambucil and cyclophosphamide are examples, interfere directly with DNA replication and function. Cross-linking of DNA also occurs. These agents may be administered either intravenously or orally, and they are particularly toxic to bone marrow.

Vinblastine and vincristine are plant alkaloids. They attack the cell during mitosis and cause toxic destruction of the mitotic spindle. However, this can result in synchronization of the cell cycle for those cells surviving therapy, and therefore these agents are often given as part of a combination treatment to cause a greater sensitivity to other agents. There is little bone marrow suppression with this group of drugs, but they can be severely neurotoxic.

Methotrexate has been used longer than any of the above chemotherapeutic agents and is an enzyme inhibitor. Metabolic transfer of one carbon unit is prevented, thereby inhibiting the synthesis of thymidylic acid as well as different purine nucleotides. Side effects of this treatment may be overcome by administration of folinic acid (citrovorum factor) which replenishes the tetrahydrofolate.

The antitumor antibiotics most commonly used in gynecologic malignancy are doxorubicin (Adriamycin) and Actinomycin D. Myelosuppression occurs regularly with both of these agents, and they are often used as part of multiple agent protocols. Adriamycin in particular can cause cardiomyopathy, and cardiac function is often monitored by ultrasound evaluation or radionuclide scans. Other agents include the heavy metal derivatives, such as *cis*-platinum, and hormones such as progestin derivates.

14–16. 14, **B**; 15, **D**; 16, **A**; Pages 720, 724. This series of questions refers to the use of chemotherapy relative to its mechanism of action in the cell replication cycle. Knowledge of cell kinetics is important in understanding the rational use of various chemotherapeutic agents. Knowledge of cell type, size of tumor, and previous treatment are all important in determining chemotherapeutic agents.

A problem with larger tumors is that they contain a higher proportion of cells in the resting or G_0 phase of the cell cycle. These cells are resistant to cytotoxic drugs and may become a source of future growth when they leave the G_0 phase to enter the cell replication cycle. Thus smaller tumors, those with a higher growth fraction, and those with a shorter doubling time are the most sensitive to cytotoxic agents.

Antimetabolites prevent metabolic transfer of one carbon unit and inhibit the synthesis of DNA. An example is Methotrexate. Plant alkaloids attack the cell during the M phase and cause toxic destruction of the mitotic spindle and thus arrest mitosis.

These examples should illustrate that knowledge of cell kinetics is important, especially when determining combination chemotherapeutic agents and their effects on different phases of the cell cycle.

17–19. 17, **B**; 18, **A**; 19, **C**; Page 716. An isodose curve is a line that connects points in the tissue that receive equivalent doses of irradiation. Figure 25-2 contrasts the isodose curves for 6 and 22 MV machines. For the 6 MV machine the maximum dose is near the surface, with a more rapid fall off in the deeper tissues, while in the 22 MV machine the maximum dose is well beneath the surface. Thus at any given depth, the higher dose of radiation can be achieved with the 22 MV, sparing the effects of radiation on the skin. These high-energy machines are particularly useful for treating deep tumors and for treating obese patients. Either of these sources could be used for treating a central recurrence. This choice is dependent on factors such as the size of the patient and the size of the field being treated. Larger fields contain more scattered radiation, which leads to greater dose at a given depth. Thus, the radiation dose delivered to a point within the tumor is affected by the energy source, the depth of the tumor beneath the surface, and the size of the field undergoing irradiation.

20–22. 20, **C**; 21, **A**; 22, **B**; Pages 714–715. In general, two techniques are used in radiation treatment: brachytherapy (internal) and teletherapy (external). Both of these radiation techniques rely on the principle of the inverse square law to determine treatment doses of radiotherapy.

Since brachytherapy refers to the radiation source being placed within or adjacent to the target tissue, these systems use radioisotopes with defined half-lives. Examples include interstitial needles, afterloading systems placed in the vagina and cervix, and the intraperitoneal installation of radioactive liquids.

Since teletherapy refers to the placement of the radioactive source at a distance from the patient, consideration of the source-to-tumor distance is important in determining overall dosage and avoiding unnecessary damage to normal tissues. With the use of different angles and ports of treatment, the concept of source axis distance (SAD) has been introduced; it denotes the distance from the radiation source to the central axis of the machine rotation. Treatment ports are arranged around this axis to optimize tumor dose and minimize damage to normal tissues.

23. **A** (1, 2, 3), Page 725. It has been shown that many experimental animal tumors are able to elicit an immune response. However, specific antigens unique to a given gynecologic tumor have not been identified as yet. It appears that tumor growth stimulates the major cells of the immune system, including the T-lymphocyte, B-lymphocyte, and macrophages. T-lymphocytes confer cell-mediated immunity, B-lymphocytes are responsible for antibody production and humoral immunity, and macrophages provide direct action against tumor cells.

24. **A** (1, 2, 3), Page 720. The proportion of cells actually involved in proliferation of the tumor is known as the growth fraction (GF). It is this proportion which determines doubling time of a given tumor. In general, smaller tumors and metastatic lesions grow more rapidly than larger tumors. Increased growth rate also appears to be operative following the administration of cytotoxic agents. These agents reduce the mass of the tumor, but cell replication then appears to proceed at a faster rate.

25. **C** (2, 4), Page 713. Radiation biology principles that cause cell death include ionizing radiation, which dislodges orbital electrons from the atoms of the medium or tissue through which they pass. This produces secondary electrons and free hydroxyl radicals, which damage the cell and the normal DNA replication process. In addition, free hydroxyl radicals may react with molecular oxygen to form peroxide in the tissues. This adds to the lethal effects of radiation.

Although there may be a change in the host immune response based on extensive radiation therapy, there is no known change in local immune response of the target tissues. Further, whereas oxygen is important for the tissue effects of photon irradiation, the oxygen tension of target tissue is not increased. In fact, since cancerous tissue frequently has decreased oxygenation, the effects of photon irradiation in these relatively hypoxic areas are often diminished.

26. **E** (All), Page 722. The potential to treat simultaneously different cell lines within the tumor has led to the development of multiple-agent chemotherapy, which is more effective than single agents. Such combination therapy appears to enhance activity against larger tumors and to prevent the emergence of resistant cells because fewer cells are in phases that are not affected (for example, the resting phase). The use of combination drugs, therefore, will reduce duration of chemotherapy.

27. **E** (All), Page 719. All of the listed factors will contribute to an increasing rate of complications in irradiated patients. After surgery with decreased bowel motility, relatively fixed intestinal structures receive a higher than normal dose of radiation. To treat a large tumor adequately, the field to be irradiated must be large; this will result in increased dosages to the deep tissues and may increase the dose to normal tissues beyond tolerance. Decreased vascularity as a result of radical pelvic surgery often makes the bladder and lower bowel more susceptible to radiation damage. Concomitant chemotherapy will contribute to a higher rate of complications due to its cellular destruction and interference with host immune response.

Generalizations regarding tissue tolerance in relation to the total dosage must be regarded as approximations. These factors and many more influence late effects that radiation has on normal tissue.

28. **E** (All), Pages 712–713. One form of ionizing radiation is electromagnetic, which refers to x-rays or gamma rays. These sources of energy have no mass and no electrical charge. They are produced in discrete quanta or photons, and their energy is proportional to their frequency; that is, higher energies are transmitted at a higher frequency of electromagnetic radiation. Since the frequency of a photon is inversely proportional to the wavelength, electromagnetic radiation with shorter wavelengths has a higher frequency and thus higher energy. Examples of these types of energy sources used to treat tumors include both external beam therapy and radiation caused by decay of radioactive isotopes. Examples of the use of isotopes are internal systems, such as cesium applicators.

29. **E** (All), Page 714. Another major principle is that a given dose of radiation kills a constant fraction of the number of cells irradiated. In other words, each dose kills the same percentage of remaining cells as the previous dose. Although the other choices listed, such as distance from energy source to target tissue, type of tumor, and mitotic activity of the tumor, may alter the overall dose of radiation, the dose principle applies once a given total dosage is calculated for an individual patient.

30. **C** (2, 4), Page 720. Although some tumors may have their origins in a single (stem) cell, clinically evident malignancies are composed of a heterogeneous population of cells with different cell cycle lengths and varying growth fractions. Larger tumors are more likely to contain cells resistant to a single cytotoxic agent. An additional problem with larger tumors is their lower growth fraction, meaning a larger proportion of cells in their resting or G_0 phase of the cell cycle. These cells are more resistant to cytotoxic drugs. As a larger proportion of these cells are in the resting phase, during which there is decreased DNA and RNA synthesis, they do not respond to chemotherapy.

Chapter 26: Intraepithelial Neoplasia of the Cervix

DIRECTIONS: Select the one best answer or completion.

1. A 35-year-old patient has had two pap smears that were consistent with severe dysplasia and a colposcopically-directed biopsy showing CIN I. The ECC (endocervical curettage) is negative. The management of choice is
   A. repeat the pap smear every 3 months.
   B. conization.
   C. repeat the colposcopy and directed biopsy.
   D. cryocautery.
   E. laser ablation.

2. The difference between leukoplakia and acetowhite epithelium is
   A. Acetowhite epithelium is white and leukoplakia is not.
   B. Leukoplakia appears white without acetic acid.
   C. Leukoplakia is a clinical description and acetowhite epithelium is a histological description.
   D. Leukoplakia is precancerous and acetowhite epithelium is not.
   E. Acetowhite epithelium is a clinical diagnosis and leukoplakia is a histologic diagnosis.

3. What is the frequency of developing cervical cancer of a woman who marries a man whose first wife had carcinoma of the cervix, compared to the frequency in a woman whose husband's first wife did not have carcinoma of the cervix?
   A. 0.3
   B. 0.5
   C. 1.0
   D. 2.0
   E. 3.0

4. What is the purpose of a routinely processed endocervical curettage?
   A. Identify which part of the cervical canal has cancer.
   B. Rule out endocervical human papilloma virus infection.
   C. Ascertain with high reliability whether a neoplasm exists in the endocervical canal.
   D. Document chlamydial cervicitis.
   E. Accurately detect tubal or ovarian carcinoma.

5. Of the following, which factor is currently felt most likely to be significant in causing cervical cancer?
   A. Herpes simplex virus (HSV)
   B. Human papillomavirus (HPV)
   C. Cytomegalovirus (CMV)
   D. Diethylstilbestrol (DES)
   E. Birth control pills (BCP)

6. A 32-year-old woman has a colposcopically-directed excisional biopsy revealing a single focus of microinvasive carcinoma with clear margins. An ECC is negative. She should have
   A. no further treatment.
   B. a cervical conization.
   C. a vaginal hysterectomy.
   D. a radical hysterectomy.
   E. cryocautery.

7. You are performing cryotherapy on a patient with a negative ECC and an adequate colposcopy after multiple directed cervical biopsies have diagnosed CIN II. The best technique is
   A. single 1-minute freeze.
   B. single 3-minute freeze.
   C. single 5-minute freeze.
   D. double 1-minute freeze.
   E. double 3-minute freeze.

8. A 24-year-old gravida 1 woman has had cervical conization for CIN III. On pathologic review, the proximal margins of the cone were involved with CIN III. The patient wants to retain her child-bearing capability. What is the best immediate course of action?
   A. Total abdominal hysterectomy
   B. Radical hysterectomy
   C. Laser treatment
   D. Repeat the cervical conization
   E. Follow with pap smears and colposcopies

9. To what depth do endocervical crypts extend in the cervix?
   A. 1 to 2 mm
   B. 3 to 4 mm
   C. 5 to 7 mm
   D. 8 to 10 mm
   E. 1.5 cm
10. A 24-year-old woman at 10 weeks of gestation is found to have an abnormal pap smear consistent with CIN III. What should immediate therapy include?
    A. Conization
    B. Suction D&C
    C. Repeat the pap smear
    D. Hysterectomy
    E. Colposcopy and biopsy

DIRECTIONS: For each numbered item, select the one heading most closely associated with it. Each lettered heading may be used once, more than once, or not at all.

11-13. Choose the most appropriate interval between pap smears for the following patients:
   (A) Annually.
   (B) Annually until two negative tests, then stop.
   (C) Every 3 to 5 years.
   (D) Every 6 to 8 years.
   (E) Testing may be stopped.
11. A sexually active 14-year-old female.
12. A 42-year-old female who had a hysterectomy 1 year ago for CIN III.
13. A 33-year-old female who had a hysterectomy 1 year ago for leiomyomata.
   (A) The area between the squamous epithelium of the cervical portio and the columnar epithelium of the endocervix
   (B) A colposcopic pattern that contains white epithelium with stippling due to blood vessels seen on end
   (C) A name for cells with perinuclear cavitation
   (D) A colposcopic pattern that reveals acetowhite areas outlined by blood vessels
   (E) The native squamous epithelium
14. Punctation
15. Mosaic
16. Koilocytes
17. Transformation zone
   (A) Figure 26-1
   (B) Figure 26-2
   (C) Figure 26-3
   (D) Figure 26-4
   (E) Figure 26-5
18. Cervical intraepithelial neoplasia (CIN I)
19. Cervical intraepithelial neoplasia (CIN III)
20. Moderate dysplasia of the cervix (CIN II)
21. Invasive squamous cell carcinoma of the cervix

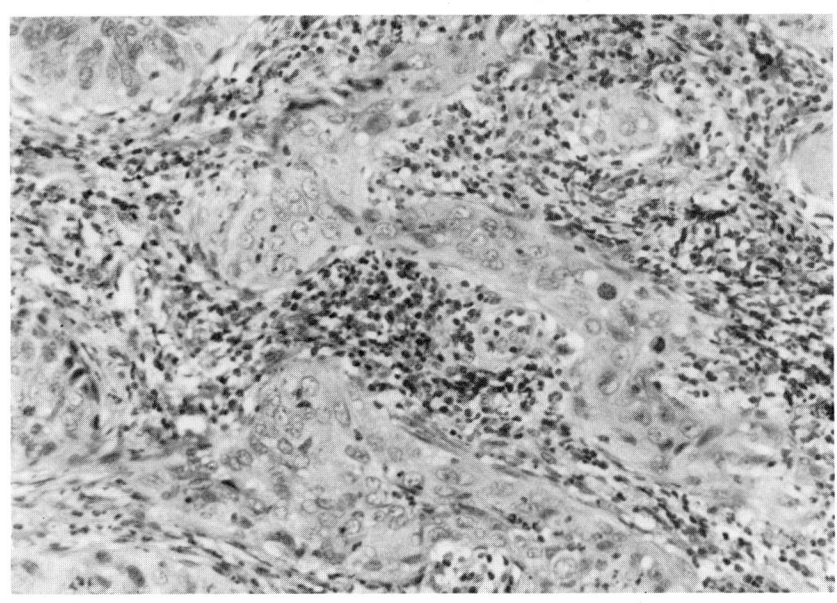

FIGURE 26-1.
(From Droegemueller W, Herbst AL, Mishell DR, Stenchever MA: Comprehensive gynecology, St. Louis, The C.V. Mosby Co, 1987.)

FIGURE 26-2.
(From Droegemueller W, Herbst AL, Mishell DR, Stenchever MA: Comprehensive gynecology, St. Louis, The C.V. Mosby Co, 1987.)

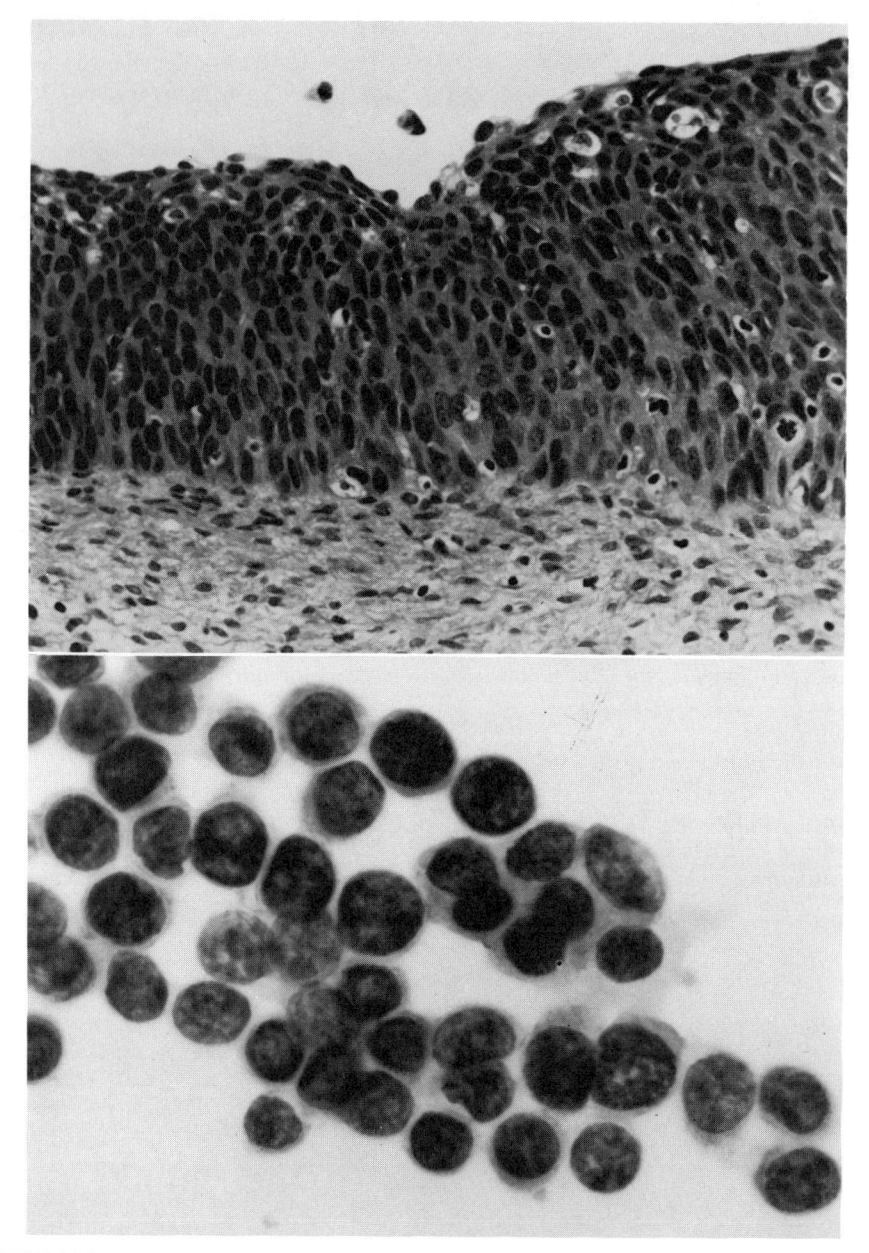

DIRECTIONS: For each numbered item, indicate whether it is associated with

A only (A)
B only (B)
C both (A) and (B)
D neither (A) nor (B)

  (A) Cervical intraepithelial neoplasia (CIN)
  (B) Human papillomavirus (HPV) infection

(C) Both
(D) Neither

22. Stains acetowhite on colposcopy
23. A cause of atypia on pap smears
24. Koilocytosis
25. Dysplasia of the cervical squamous epithelium.

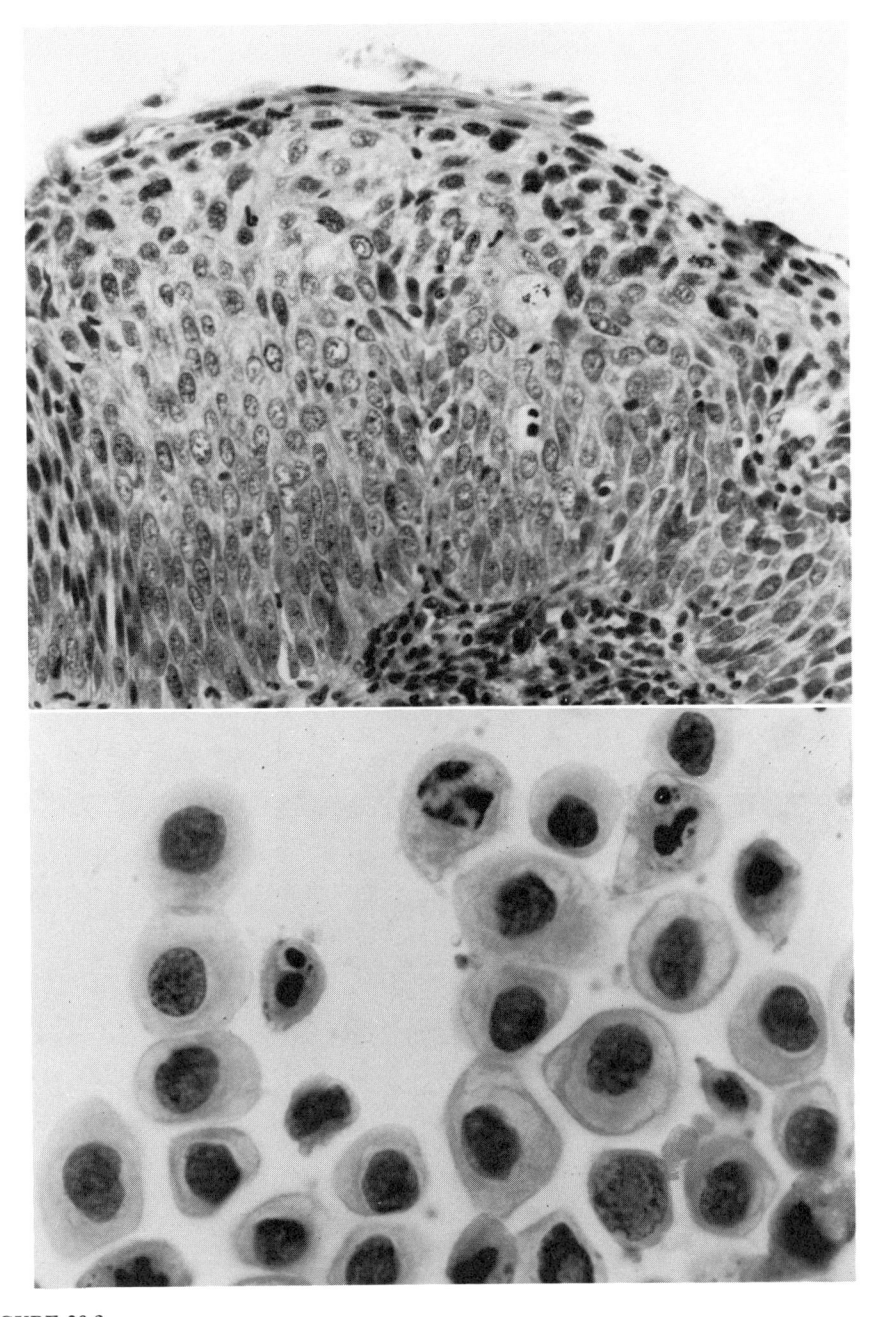

FIGURE 26-3.
(From Droegemueller W, Herbst AL, Mishell DR, Stenchever MA: Comprehensive gynecology, St. Louis, The C.V. Mosby Co, 1987.)

DIRECTIONS: Each question contains four suggested answers of which one or more is correct. Choose the answer
- A if 1, 2, and 3 are correct
- B if 1 and 3 are correct
- C if 2 and 4 are correct
- D if 4 only is correct
- E if all are correct

26. Which factors are known to increase the risk of squamous cell carcinoma of the cervix?
    1. Multiple sexual partners
    2. Smoking
    3. Immunosuppression
    4. Intrauterine DES exposure

27. Suspicious findings for significant dysplasia on colposcopy include
    1. wide, irregular intercapillary distances.
    2. irregular surface pattern.
    3. opaque acetowhite color.
    4. large, abnormal transformation zone.

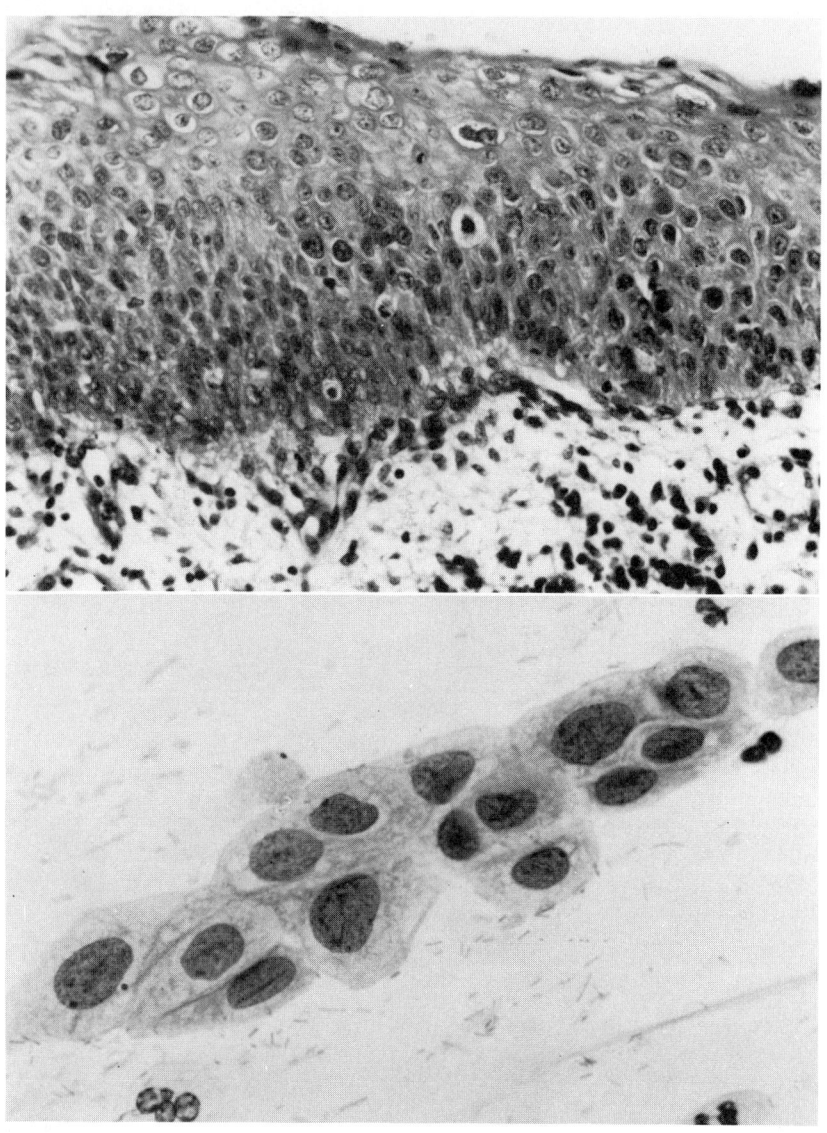

FIGURE 26-4.
(From Droegemueller W, Herbst AL, Mishell DR, Stenchever MA: Comprehensive gynecology, St. Louis, The C.V. Mosby Co, 1987.)

28. Which factors help identify dysplastic cervical lesions that are most likely to progress to more severe lesions?
    1. Initial degree of dysplasia
    2. Associated viral type
    3. Amount of nuclear DNA content
    4. Findings on colposcopic examination
29. Which are requirements for adequate colposcopy?
    1. ECC
    2. Demonstration of white epithelium
    3. Demonstration of leukoplakia
    4. Visualizing the entire transformation zone
30. A patient with extensive CIN III is diagnosed by multiple colposcopically-directed biopsies and a negative ECC. All abnormal areas were completely visualized. How may this patient be treated?
    2. Laser ablation
    3. Conization
    4. Electrocautery
31. A 30-year-old woman with a pap smear consistent with CIN II and an ECC showing dysplasia is being counseled regarding cervical conization as treatment. She asks the risks of conization. You should tell her that she may develop
    1. cervical stenosis.
    2. bleeding.
    3. infertility.
    4. incompetent cervix.

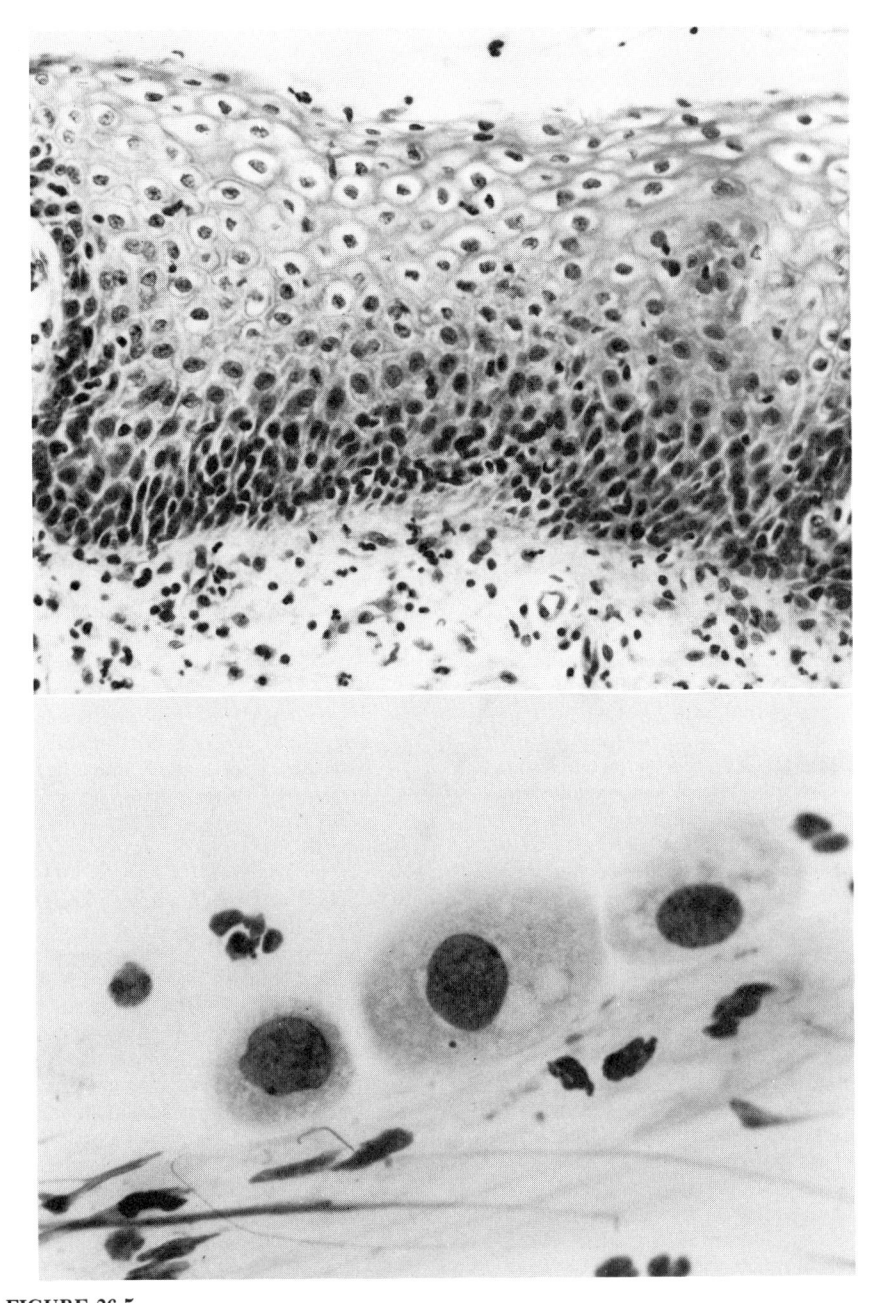

FIGURE 26-5.
(From Droegemueller W, Herbst AL, Mishell DR, Stenchever MA: Comprehensive gynecology, St. Louis, The C.V. Mosby Co, 1987.)

ANSWERS

1. **B,** Pages 755, 757. Specific indications for cervical conization are: 1) unsatisfactory colposcopy; 2) positive ECC; 3) cells on pap smear that are not adequately explained by histology on biopsy; 4) microinvasive cancer; 5) clinical uncertainty regarding the presence of invasive disease. It has also been suggested that conization should be done in patients over the age of 50 if a biopsy diagnosis of carcinoma in situ is made because of the incidence of unsuspected invasion is high beyond this age. The purpose of conization is to rule out invasive cancer.

2. **B,** Page 729. Leukoplakia and acetowhite epithelium are both clinical descriptive terms. Leukoplakia is white before the application of acetic acid, while acetowhite epithelium looks normal initially and becomes white after application of acetic acid. Neither term defines a precancerous lesion. The histology of either one may be precancerous, but not necessarily so.

3. **E**, Page 738. Epidemiologic studies indicate that women whose husbands' first wives had carcinoma of the cervix are at three times the risk of developing cervical cancer when compared to women whose husbands' first wives did not have cervical cancer. This supports the hypothesis that a factor causing cervical cancer may be sexually transmitted. Some other factors that increase the risk of cervical cancer are related to sexual activity, such as multiple sex partners and venereal disease.

4. **C**, Page 746. The endocervical curettage (ECC) is designed to find whether or not endocervical neoplasia exists. It can detect dysplasia, squamous carcinoma, and adenocarcinoma. An ECC should be done whenever a biopsy is taken from the cervix. The ECC cannot identify which part of the cervical canal has cancer, rule out endocervical human papilloma virus infection, or document chlamydial cervicitis. Although cells from ovarian or other upper abdominal carcinoma can be found on either pap smears or ECC specimens, neither of these modalities provides an accurate way of making the diagnosis of upper genital tract or other abdominal carcinoma.

5. **B**, Pages 738–741. Of all the options including the herpes simplex virus, cytomegalovirus, diethylstilbestrol, and birth control pills, only human papillomavirus (HPV) is highly associated with cervical cancer, especially HPV types 16, 18, 31, and 33. Infection with HPV has been shown to precede invasive cervical carcinoma by approximately 27 years. Cervical cancer may develop within 3 years after infection with types 16 and 18. Type 16 has been reported in a large number of cervical cancers. Women with HPV on pap smear are at increased risk of developing cancer, as compared to those women who do not have evidence of HPV on pap smears. None of this proves a cause and effect relationship.

6. **B**, Pages 750–751. A biopsy diagnosis of microinvasive cancer of the cervix requires conization to rule out invasive disease. A radical hysterectomy may be too much treatment if no invasion exists, and a vaginal hysterectomy is too little treatment if it does. Cryocautery should not be done for this lesion. Further study and appropriate treatment are mandatory depending upon the eventual diagnosis. If the cone is negative and she desires more children, the conization can be considered treatment at this time.

7. **E**, Pages 752–753. A double 3-minute freeze will cure approximately 90% of CIN lesions in which the initial evaluation is adequate, as it was in this patient. The double freeze will destroy most of the transformation zone in cervical crypts. However, close follow-up with a pap smear every 6 months for 1 or 2 years, followed by annual pap smears, is needed to assure that the dysplastic process has been eliminated. These women should always have pap smears done at least annually.

8. **E**, Page 757. Studies have shown that even with positive margins on a cervical conization, up to 70% of these patients have no recurrence at 5 years. With careful follow-up, which includes endocervical pap smears, most of these patients may retain their fertility.

9. **C**, Pages 754, 762. Endocervical crypts can be involved with dysplasia. Therefore, the base of such crypts should be sampled or destroyed when treating CIN. The crypts may extend as far as 5 to 7 mm beneath the surface of the cervical epithelium, and therefore diagnostic or therapeutic procedures for CIN should extend to that depth.

10. **E**, Pages 758, 760. There is no need to terminate the pregnancy for CIN. The first step is evaluated by an experienced colposcopist with biopsy if indicated. Often the transformation zone and endocervical canal can be better seen because of eversion during pregnancy. If no invasive cancer is found, the patient may delivery vaginally. Conization would be done only if there is suspicion of invasion by either cytology or colposcopy that is not confirmed on biopsy. This is a rare situation.

11–13. 11, **A**; 12, **A**; 13, **C**; Pages 744–745; Table 26-2 (from Droegemueller). Different reports give different intervals at which pap smears are recommended. However all agree that young, sexually active women should have annual smears until at least two smears are negative. Most also state that high risk women should continue to have annual smears. High risk women are those who began sexual intercourse at an early age, have had multiple sexual partners, or have had abnormal pap smears, HPV or HSV infections in the past. A woman who has had a hysterectomy for dysplastic disease remains at high risk for dysplasia or carcinoma at the vaginal apex. Women who had hysterectomy for benign disease should still have pap smears, but the interval between them can safely be extended to 3 to 5 years. The pelvic exam done in conjunction with obtaining a pap smear in any woman is also a good clinical screening tool for such entities as vaginitis, cervicitis, ovarian tumors, and other pelvic pathology. It also brings the patient in for other health maintenance measures such as mammography.

14–17. 14, **B**; 15, **D**; 16, **C**; 17, **A**; Page 729. Mosaicism, punctation, and transformation zone are terms used to describe colposcopic findings. Respectively, they refer to a colposcopic pattern with acetowhite areas outlined by blood vessels, a pattern that contains stippling due to blood vessels seen on end in acetowhite areas, and the expanse of epithelium at the junction between the squamous epithelium of the cervix and the columnar epithelium of the endocervix. Koilocytes are caused by infection with human papillomavirus and are cells with perinuclear cavitation (Figure 26-9 from Droegemueller). The native squamous epithelium is the original squamous epithelium found on the portio of the cervix and in the vagina.

18–21. 18, **E**; 19, **C**; 20, **D**; 21, **A**; Pages 730–731. The concept of dysplastic changes of the cervical epithelium progressing to invasive carcinoma is well established. Various terms have been used to describe the histology of the dysplastic changes in the cervix. Cervical intraepithelial neoplasia (CIN) is designated as I, II, or III. CIN I and II are described as having the same histologic findings as mild and moderate dysplasia, respectively. CIN III refers to the same histologic patterns found in either severe dysplasia or carcinoma in situ. As the treatment for severe dysplasia or carcinoma in situ is the same, the term CIN III has been used to describe both of these entities. As degrees of CIN or dysplasia lie on a continuum, the distinctions may be interpreted differently by different observers, especially at the less severe end of the spectrum.

22–25. 22, **C**; 23, **C**; 24, **B**; 25, **A**; Pages 731, 741–742. Both CIN and some HPV (Human papillomavirus) stain acetowhite with application of acetic acid. Both may result in atypical cells appearing on the pap smear. For these reasons, colposcopically-directed biopsies must be taken to rule out dysplasia when abnormal findings are reported on pap smear or seen with the colposcope. It is difficult, if not impossible, to rule out the presence of dysplasia by pap smear or colposcopy only.

Koilocytes are specific for HPV. They may be found in areas of dysplasia (CIN) as well, but they imply a concomitant HPV infection. If dysplastic cells occur through the entire thickness of the cervical epithelium, the diagnosis is carcinoma in situ, which is included in the diagnosis of CIN III. CIN III may also be associated with HPV infection. In cases of obvious dysplasia, the presence or absence of HPV infection is disregarded for purposes of therapy.

26. **A** (1,2,3), Pages 737–739. Multiple sex partners and immunosuppression have been implicated epidemiologically with an increased incidence of cervical carcinoma. In some studies, birth control pill use has not been found to increase the risk of cervical carcinoma independent from the risk associated with increased sex partners, whereas in other studies, it appears to be a risk factor. Smoking appears to increase the relative risk of cervical carcinoma by 1.5. Intrauterine DES exposure is not yet proven to increase the risk of carcinoma of the cervix, although concern exists over this possibility.

27. **E** (All), Page 746. On colposcopic examination, the main criteria used to detect the most severe lesions are the vascular pattern, the distance between capillaries, the sharpness of the borders, the intensity of the color, and the size of the abnormal transformation zone.

28. **A** (1, 2, 3), Pages 741–742. The more severe dysplasias are more likely to progress to carcinoma in situ or invasive carcinoma, as are dysplasias with cells having aneuploid amounts of DNA. Also, certain HPV types (16, 18, 31, and 33) are most often associated with more advanced dysplasias and also with those that are more likely to progress. Colposcopy can identify the lesion, but cannot predict its propensity to progress.

29. **D** (4), Pages 746–747, 750. Colposcopy is used to detect abnormality and to determine the best site for biopsy. To do this adequately, the entire transformation zone must be seen. White epithelium and leukoplakia may define abnormalities, but do not define whether the colposcopic exam was adequate or inadequate. An ECC is usually done to complete the evaluation of the patient, but is not in itself required for adequate colposcopy.

30. **E** (All), Pages 752–755. The purpose behind the treatment of CIN is to completely eradicate the dysplastic epithelium. Electrocautery, laser, cold knife conization, or cryocautery can all eradicate the dysplasia. Conization has the advantage of complete removal and provision of a histologic specimen. The techniques employed must be done properly and long-term follow-up is required. The chance of developing new sites of CIN is greater in this patient than in the general population because she has demonstrated a propensity to develop CIN.

31. **E** (All), Page 758. The risks of any surgical procedure include anesthesia, infection, hemorrhage, damage to surrounding organs, and failure to achieve the desired result. With cervical conizations, specific complications are incompetent cervix, infertility, and cervical stenosis. These are not common complications but should be outlined while counseling the patient.

CHAPTER 27

Malignant Disease of the Cervix

DIRECTIONS: Select the one best answer or completion.

1. A patient with a diagnosis of a stage IIa adenocarcinoma of the cervix would have the greatest chance for survival with an initial treatment of
   A. combined radiation and surgery.
   B. surgery.
   C. radiation.
   D. chemotherapy.
   E. surgery and immunotherapy.

2. A 49-year-old woman has had squamous cell carcinoma of the cervix diagnosed by biopsy. On examination under anesthesia she is found to have a tumor in the upper third of the vagina and the parametria. IVP reveals obstruction of the left ureter. In which stage is her tumor now?
   A. Ib
   B. IIa
   C. IIIa
   D. IIIb
   E. IV

3. Which of the following procedures is most reliable in detecting parametrial spread of cervical cancer?
   A. Flat plate of the pelvis
   B. IVP
   C. CT scan
   D. Pelvic lymphangiography
   E. Pelvic examination

4. A 52-year-old patient who had a supracervical hysterectomy in the past now has stage IIb carcinoma of the cervix. Which is the best treatment choice?
   A. External radiation
   B. Intracavitary radiation
   C. Radical surgery
   D. Chemotherapy
   E. Trachelectomy

5. A 60-year-old woman presents with a firm nodule above her left clavicle. Her history reveals slight weigh loss and mild vaginal spotting for 6 months. She has not had a physical examination or pap smear for many years. On pelvic exam she has a large bulky cervix with firm induration extending to the pelvic side walls. A biopsy of the cervix reveals invasive squamous cell carcinoma. Chest x-ray and IVP are normal. What is the next major step in her management?
   A. External radiation to 50 Gy
   B. Total abdominal hysterectomy and bilateral salpingo-oophorectomy
   C. Radical hysterectomy and pelvic lymph node dissection
   D. 500 mg hours of cervical brachytherapy
   e. Scalene node biopsy

DIRECTIONS: For each numbered item, select the one heading most closely associated with it. Each lettered heading may be used once, more than once, or not at all.

6–9. Match the patient with the most likely 5-year survival:
   (A) 8%
   (B) 31%
   (C) 57%
   (D) 70%
   (E) 78%

6. A 28-year-old woman with stage I carcinoma of the cervix.

7. A 42-year-old woman with invasive carcinoma discovered in an operative specimen after a vaginal hysterectomy for prolapse.

8. A 42-year-old woman with stage III carcinoma of the cervix.

9. A 28-year-old woman with stage II carcinoma of the cervix discovered during the second trimester of pregnancy

10–12. Match the description with the most likely source:
   (A) Vulvar
   (B) Cervical
   (C) Endometrial
   (D) Ovarian
   (E) Vaginal

10. Female genital tract cancer causing the greatest number of deaths

11. Most common female genital tract-type cancer

12. The genital tract cancer whose frequency is steadily decreasing as a result of population screening

DIRECTIONS: For each numbered item, indicate whether it is associated with

A only (A)
B only (B)
C both (A) and (B)
D neither (A) nor (B)

(A) Brachytherapy
(B) Teletherapy
(C) Both
(D) Neither

13. Form of radiation therapy
14. Employs colpostats
15. Flecher-Suit applicator
16. A surgical procedure which severs nerves to prevent pain

(A) Endophytic cervical carcinoma
(B) Exophytic cervical carcinoma
(C) Both
(D) Neither

17. Barrel-shaped cervix
18. Associated with early abdominal bleeding and staining
19. Primary path of distant spread is through lymphatics to regional lymph nodes

(A) Radical hysterectomy
(B) Total hysterectomy
(C) Both
(D) Neither

20. Includes surgical removal of the paraaortic nodes
21. Includes surgical removal of the pelvic nodes
22. Includes surgical removal of the ovaries

(A) Point A
(B) Point B
(C) Both
(D) Neither

23. Arbitrary reference points used in calculating dosage of pelvic irradiation.
24. Located on the lateral pelvic sidewall
25. Receives 85 Gray of total radiation dosage in standard therapy for invasive carcinoma.

(A) Complication of radical hysterectomy for cervical cancer
(B) Complication of radiation treatment for cervical cancer
(C) Both
(D) Neither

26. Urinary fistula
27. Bladder dyssynergia
28. Shrinkage of vaginal apex
29. Hemorrhagic cystitis

DIRECTIONS: Each question contains four suggested answers of which one or more is correct. Choose the answer

A if 1, 2, and 3 are correct
B if 1 and 3 are correct
C if 2 and 4 are correct
D if 4 only is correct
E if all are correct

30. In the treatment of carcinoma of the cervix Stage Ib or IIa, what is/are the major advantage(s) of surgery?
    1. Preservation of the ovaries
    2. Exploration of the abdomen
    3. Less vaginal fibrosis
    4. Better cure rate
31. Compared to squamous cell carcinoma, adenocarcinoma of the cervix
    1. is less apt to be cured by radiation therapy.
    2. is increased in younger women with prior DES exposure.
    3. is more frequently found in older women.
    4. has a better prognosis.
32. A prognosis for a patient with invasive carcinoma of the cervix is related to
    1. tumor size.
    2. depth of invasion.
    3. tumor type.
    4. tumor grade.
33. Which of the following statements regarding recurrent carcinoma of the cervix is true?
    1. Carcinoma recurs after 6 months.
    2. Half of all recurrences are in the pelvis.
    3. Treatment depends on tumor site and prior therapy.
    4. Currently chemotherapeutic regimens which include *cis*-platinum are the most effective.

ANSWERS

1. **A**, Pages 781, 790. Recent reports suggest that patients with early stages of adenocarcinoma of the cervix have a better survival if treated with partial irradiation by local implants of radium in the cervix and vagina followed by radical surgery. The approach of radiation followed by surgery is also used in stage Ib barrel-shaped squamous cells carcinoma of the cervix. Radiation alone is used in more advanced cases of carcinoma of the cervix.
2. **D**, Pages 768, 777. The stage is defined by the greatest extent of tumor spread which in this case is the ureteral obstruction as demonstrated by the IVP. Currently, in contrast to ovarian carcinoma, the staging of cervical cancer is done by physical exam and a few spe-

cialized tests such as IVP and chest x-ray. Once the stage is so determined, it does not change even if operative findings show that it is further or less advanced than determined by the initial clinical staging. The staging criteria for cervical cancer should be committed to memory.

3. **E, Page 782.** The CT scan may be superior to the IVP for defining the extent of cervical carcinoma because it is more likely to detect obstructed ureters and enlarged pelvic nodes that are suspicious for a metastasis. Therefore, from a cost benefit standpoint, an IVP is an adequate screen for stages I–IIa, but a CT scan should be utilized for more advanced disease. The pelvic examination, however, remains the most accurate method for detecting parametrial spread.

4. **A, Page 791.** Supracervical hysterectomies are not often done now but were common several years ago. Although radical surgery may be considered for stage I or IIa disease, stage IIb presents a more advanced tumor than is amenable to surgical therapy. Brachytherapy is difficult because the uterine fundus is removed, and this makes it difficult to place intracavitary radiation sources. Therefore, external radiation is the best choice. Chemotherapy as an initial or secondary treatment for carcinoma of the cervix is not satisfactory and trachelectomy is inadequate treatment.

5. **E, Page 783.** A patient with large supraclavicular nodes, weight loss and proven invasive carcinoma of the cervix is apt to have metastases via the pelvic and paraaortic nodes to the supraclavicular node. The presence or absence of metastases should be evaluated before any form of major therapy is begun, because the presence of a positive supraclavicular node would change both the prognosis and therapy.

6–9. **6, E; 7, D; 8, B; 9, C; Page 780.** Although individual reports may give somewhat different figures, the worldwide statistics from FIGO in 1985 showed a 5-year survival for stage I carcinoma of the cervix to be approximately 78%, stage II approximately 57%, stage III approximately 31%, and stage IV 7.8% (see Table 4). Patients with carcinoma of the cervix in pregnancy have the same survival, stage for stage, as patients who are not pregnant. Overall survival of early carcinoma discovered inadvertently after hysterectomy performed for another reason is approximately 70%, whether either additional surgery or adjunctive radiation therapy is employed.

10–12. **10, D; 11, C; 12, B; Page 768.** Endometrial carcinoma is the most frequent of the genital tract cancers but causes relatively fewer deaths than either ovarian or cervical cancer because it is often found and treated early. Ovarian cancer is less common, but because of its silent early course, it is often not discovered until it has already metastasized. The incidence of cervical carcinoma has been decreasing, in part, because of early detection of dysplastic lesions by routine pap smears.

13–16. **13, C; 14, A; 15, A; 16, D; Pages 767, 768, 786.** Brachytherapy and teletherapy are both forms of radiation therapy. With brachytherapy, the radiation source is placed close to the tumor employing interstitial needles, intracervical tandems, or vaginal ovoid applicators. A Fletcher-Suit applicator is a specific vaginal ovoid applicator to deliver brachytherapy. With teletherapy, the radiation source is at a distance from the patient and is usually called external therapy. Surgery severing the lateral spinothalamic tract to prevent pain is called a cordotomy.

17–19. **17, A; 18, B; 19, C; Page 777.** Cervical carcinoma can develop as an ulcer, a cauliflowerlike growth on the outside of the cervix, or a silent, penetrating tumor growing into the cervical stoma. The ulcer or cauliflower (exophytic) type tends to present with irregular bleeding, while the internally growing tumor

TABLE 4 Carcinoma of the Cervix Uteri: Distribution by Stage and Five-Year Survival Rates*

Stage	Patients Treated*		5-Year Survival	
	No.	%	No.	%
I	10,791	33.3	8,430	78.1
II	11,599	35.8	6,610	57.0
III	8,623	26.6	2,671	31.0
IV	1,377	4.3	107	7.8
No stage	9	0.0	4	—
TOTAL	32,428	100.0	17,843	55.0

Modified from Pettersson F, et al: Nineteenth annual report on the results of treatment in gynecological cancer. Stockholm, International Federation of Gynecologists and Obstetricians, 1985.
*Patients treated in 1976 to 1978.

(endophytic) is asymptomatic for a long time during which metastases often occur. The endophytic tumor often causes a large, bulky barrel-shaped cervix.

The most common mode of spread of all cervical cancer is through the cervical lymphatics into regional nodes. Blood-borne metastases occur much less frequently.

20–22. 20, **D**; 21, **D**; 22, **D**; Pages 767, 783–784. A radical hysterectomy removes the uterine cervix, upper vagina, and paracervical-parametrial tissue. A total hysterectomy removes the entire uterus (cervix and fundus). Neither removes the tubes, ovaries, or the pelvic lymph nodes. If any of these structures are removed, the surgery is identified by stating what is done (for example, bilateral salpingo-oophorectomy, pelvic lymphadenectomy, paraaortic node dissection). Many patients do not understand the difference between these two procedures. Before surgery, the patients should know exactly what is to be done. This requires time for careful counseling to assure that the patient understands.

23–25. 23, **C**; 24, **B**; 25, **A**; Page 787. See Figure 27-1. Points A and B are defined positions in the pelvis used for calculating radiation dosage. Point A is 2 cm cephalad to the vaginal fornix and 2 cm lateral to the cervical canal. Point B is 3 cm lateral to point A. Because point A is closer to the source of brachytherapy, it receives a higher dose of ionizing radiation (approximately 85 Gray) than point B (approximately 50 to 60 Gray) during standard radiation therapy for invasive cervical carcinoma.

26–29. 26, **C**; 27, **A**; 28, **B**; 29, **B**; Pages 786–787, 789–790. Surgical complications usually occur soon after the operation and include genital urinary fistula (less than 1%), bladder dysfunction, and a loss of sensation that is usually temporary. Radiation complications can occur during treatment or at any later date, although most are within 1 or 2 years. Ulcerations of the vagina and cervix may occur. Postradiation cystitis may cause frequency dysuria and bleeding. Fibrosis of the vagina and/or the ureters may be major problems for sexual and urinary function, respectively. Urinary fistulas can occur but with modern treatment are quite uncommon. They occur most frequently in cases where there has been bulky tumor involvement near the bladder. Bowel fistula, diarrhea, and rectal bleeding also may occur and are more common than urinary complications. The risk of radiation complication increases with increased radiation dose, and as the frequency of cure increases, the rate of complication from the radiation also increases.

30. **A** (1, 2, 3), Page 783. In young women, the preservation of ovarian and sexual function is very important and the ability to sample nodes for spread is also a distinct advantage in determining the need for further treatment. These are all advantages of surgery. However,

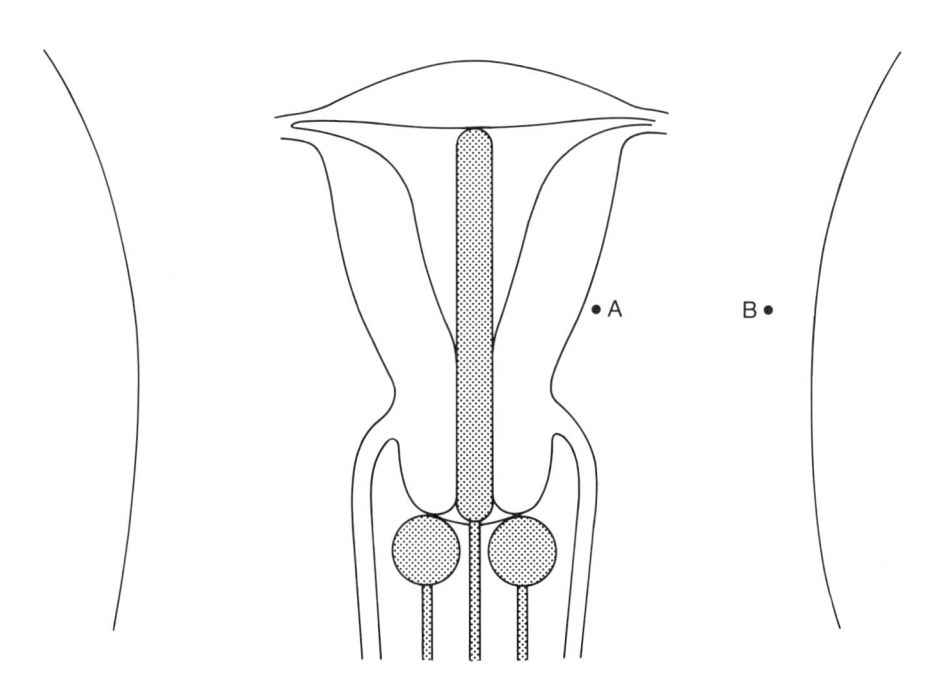

FIGURE 27-1.
Points A and B with central stem (tandem) and 2 ovoids in place.
(From Droegemueller W, Herbst AL, Mishell DR, Stenchever, MA: Comprehensive gynecology, St. Louis, The C.V. Mosby Co, 1987.)

the cure rate is similar for surgery and irradiation in Stage Ib and IIa cervical carcinoma.

31. **A** (1, 2, 3), Page 781. Women with adenocarcinoma of the cervix tend to be nulliparous, older, and more often diabetic than women with squamous cell cervical carcinoma. Cervical clear cell adenocarcinoma is rare, but the incidence is increased in women with prior DES exposure in utero. Adenocarcinoma generally has a worse prognosis than comparable stages of squamous cell carcinoma.

32. **A** (1, 2, 3), Pages 779–781. Cervical cancer prognosis has been definitely related to tumor size (worse as it gets bigger), depth of invasion (worse as the depth increases), and type (worse with adenocarcinoma than with squamous cell carcinoma). However, tumor grade has an inconsistent relationship with the prognosis in patients with cervical cancer.

33. **E** (All), Pages 792–794. The definition of recurrence of cervical cancer is that it reappears 6 months or more after the time of therapy. If the tumor reappears within 6 months, it is considered a persistence. Approximately 50% of recurrences will be in the pelvis. The site of the tumor and the prior mode of therapy determine the type and extent of treatment. For example, if the primary tumor was treated with radiation, the recurrence is central in the pelvis, and no distant metastases are found, then an exenterative surgical procedure can be done. In carefully selected patients, the cure rate can be as high as 50%. However few patients with recurrent carcinoma of the cervix qualify for exenterative therapy. Chemotherapy of recurrent cervical cancer is not very effective, but the best results occur with multiple-agent regimens that include *cis*-platinum.

CHAPTER 28: Neoplastic Diseases of the Uterus

DIRECTIONS: Select the one best answer or completion.

1. A 68-year-old woman complains of vaginal spotting. On examination she has an atrophic vagina, a clean cervix with a closed os, and a normal-sized uterus. No masses are felt. A pap smear is obtained from the exocervix. If this patient has endometrial carcinoma, in what percent of cases will the obtained pap smear detect it?
   A. 10%
   B. 25%
   C. 50%
   D. 75%
   E. 90%

2. A 53-year-old woman has a D&C for postmenopausal bleeding. The pathology report states she has a malignant glandular epithelium with areas of squamous metaplasia in the endometrium. What is the most likely diagnosis?
   A. Adenocarcinoma
   B. Adenoacanthoma
   C. Adenosquamous carcinoma
   D. Atypical adenematous hyperplasia
   E. Endolymphatic stromal myosis

3. A 63-year-old has a D&C for abnormal vaginal bleeding. On review of the pathology from the D&C, you see the following pattern (Figure 28-1). Many sections appear similar and no mitotic figures are seen. What is the diagnosis?
   A. Clear cell adenocarcinoma
   B. Cellular leiomyoma
   C. Cystic endometrial hyperplasia
   D. Malignant mixed müllerian tumor
   E. Atypical adenomatous hyperplasia

4. A 36-year-old woman has had a D&C for irregular bleeding. It reveals adenomatous hyperplasia without atypia. What can you tell the patient?
   A. Most (greater than 50%) will progress to carcinoma within 8 to 12 years.
   B. Treatment should be hysterectomy.
   C. Induction of ovulation is contraindicated.
   D. Progestin will usually promote monthly withdrawal.
   E. Repeat endometrial sampling is not necessary.

5. A 60-year-old woman has a prior diagnosis of endometrial hyperplasia. She has not yet been treated. Which of the following techniques is best to screen her for persistent or progressive disease?
   A. Pap smear
   B. Endometrial brushing
   C. Endometrial washings
   D. Endocervical aspiration
   E. Office vacuum curettage

6. A 47-year-old woman has a poorly differentiated endometrial carcinoma and a uterine cavity that measures 10 cm in depth. The endocervix has invasive endometrial carcinoma, but no other structure is involved. What is the stage of her endometrial cancer?
   A. Ia
   B. IIb
   C. II
   D. III
   E. IV

7. Of the following rare primary tumors of the endometrium, which has the worst prognosis?
   A. Clear cell adenocarcinoma
   B. Papillary serous carcinoma
   C. Secretory carcinoma
   D. Mucinous carcinoma
   E. Squamous cell carcinoma

8. Of the following situations, which one is most highly associated with positive lymph nodes in a patient with endometrial carcinoma?
   A. Grade 1
   B. Grade 2
   C. Invasion through two thirds of the myometrium
   D. 2-month duration of bleeding
   E. Grade 2 and invasion to the outer third of the myometrium

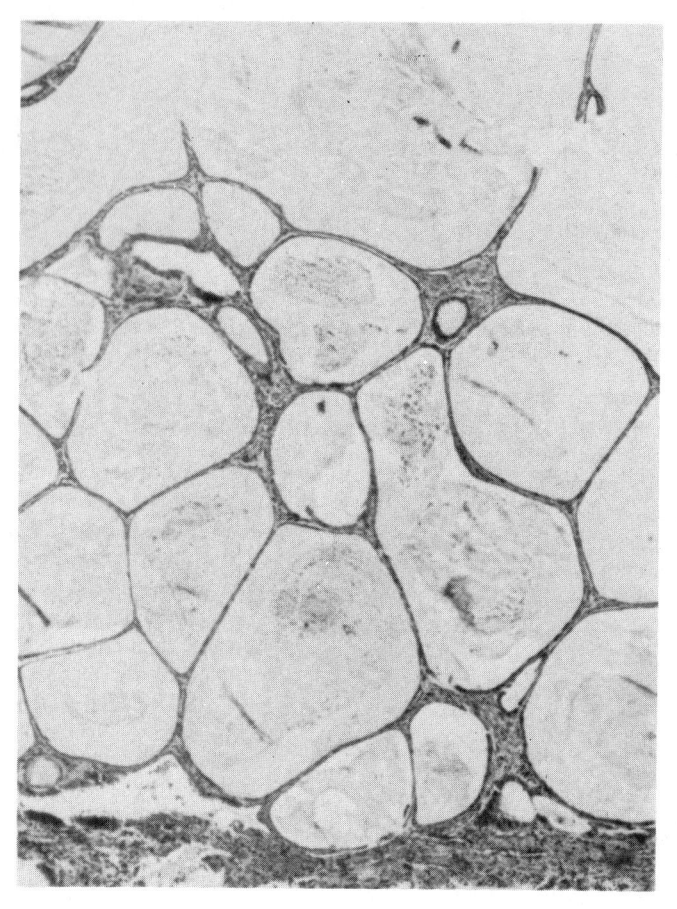

FIGURE 28-1.
(From Christopherson WM and Gray LA: In Coppleson M, ed: Gynecologic oncology, Edinburgh, Churchill-Livingstone, 1981.)

9. Which is the most common malignancy of the female genital tract?
   A. Endometrial carcinoma
   B. Cervical carcinoma
   C. Tubal carcinoma
   D. Vulvar carcinoma
   E. Ovarian carcinoma
10. Which tumor is most likely to respond to progesterone therapy?
    A. Stage III carcinoma of the cervix
    B. Stage III ovarian carcinoma
    C. Stage III endometrial carcinoma
    D. Stage III vulvar carcinoma
    E. Stage III vaginal carcinoma
11. An otherwise healthy 54-year-old white woman has an adenocarcinoma of the endometrium proven by D&C. The clinical examination reveals a mass in the left adnexal area. The side walls of the pelvis are free of tumor. Assuming the staging is correct, which is the best treatment among the following choices?
    A. Pelvic and whole abdomen irradiation to 50 Gy.
    B. Total abdominal hysterectomy and bilateral salpingo-oophorectomy with pelvic node sampling
    C. Radical hysterectomy and lymphadenectomy
    D. Total abdominal hysterectomy and bilateral salpingo-oophorectomy with postoperative external irradiation
    E. Multiple-agent chemotherapy, including progestins
12. Of the following cytotoxic chemotherapeutic agents, which would be *least* likely used in a patient who had persistence or recurrence of Stage III endometrial adenocarcinoma?
    A. Cyclophosphamide (Cytoxan)
    B. Doxorubicin HCL (Adriamycin)
    C. *cis*-platinum (Platinol)
    D. 5-FU (Adrucil)
    E. Mitomycin (Mutamycin)

13. A 57-year-old woman has homologous uterine sarcoma. What is the current recommended primary treatment?
    A. Radiation
    B. Chemotherapy
    C. Surgery
    D. Surgery and chemotherapy
    E. Surgery and irradiation
14. Ninety percent of adenocarcinomas of the endometrium that recur do so within approximately
    A. 1 year.
    B. 3 years.
    C. 5 years.
    D. 10 years.
    E. 20 years.
15. Which is the most common sarcoma of the uterus?
    A. Endometrial stromal sarcoma
    B. Rhabdomyosarcoma
    C. Liposarcoma
    D. Endolymphatic stroma myosis
    E. Leiomyosarcoma
16. A 56-year-old patient is found to have both an endometrial adenocarcinoma and a rhabdomyosarcoma of the uterus. The tumor would be best described as a
    A. heterologous sarcoma.
    B. endometrial stromal sarcoma.
    C. homologous sarcoma.
    D. carcinosarcoma.
    E. malignant mixed müllerian tumor.

DIRECTIONS: For each numbered item, select the one heading most closely associated with it. Each lettered heading may be used once, more than once, or not at all.

17–19. Match the following women with the most appropriate treatment:
    (A) No further treatment
    (B) Provera 10 mg daily
    (C) Clomid 50 mg on days 1–5
    (D) Megace 40-320 mg per day
    (E) Hysterectomy
17. A 28-year-old with benign endometrial hyperplasia found on D&C
18. A 58-year-old with atypical adenomatous endometrial hyperplasia
19. A 30-year-old anovulatory woman who wants a pregnancy now but who has mild atypical adenomatous endometrial hyperplasia

20–24. Match the following photomicrographs with the appropriate diagnosis.
    (A) Figure 28-2
    (B) Figure 28-3
    (C) Figure 28-4
    (D) Figure 28-5
    (E) Figure 28-6
20. Adenomatous hyperplasia
21. Papillary serous carcinoma
22. Atypical adenomatous hyperplasia
23. Adenoacanthoma
24. Adenocarcinoma of the endometrium

DIRECTIONS: Each question contains four suggested answers of which one or more is correct. Choose the answer
    A if 1, 2, and 3 are correct
    B if 1 and 3 are correct
    C if 2 and 4 are correct
    D if 4 only is correct
    E if all are correct

25. A 46-year-old woman complains of irregular periods and some spotting between periods not associated with coitus. General examination is within normal limits. The vagina and uterus have no evidence of abnormalities or lesions. You suggest an office D&C to evaluate the endometrium. Which of the following are true statements?
    1. The procedure requires regional anesthesia.
    2. Oral prostaglandin synthetase inhibitors may decrease uterine cramping.
    3. Endometrial polyps and small subserous fibromas are easily detected by office D&C.
    4. Suction curettage yields good samples.
26. During her routine annual examination, a 58–year-old woman asks about the risk of developing uterine cancer. True statements include:
    1. The incidence of cancer of the endometrium is greatest between 55 and 65.
    2. Polycystic ovarian disease is a risk factor.
    3. Late menopause is a risk factor.
    4. Hypertension is a risk factor.

182 Gynecologic Oncology

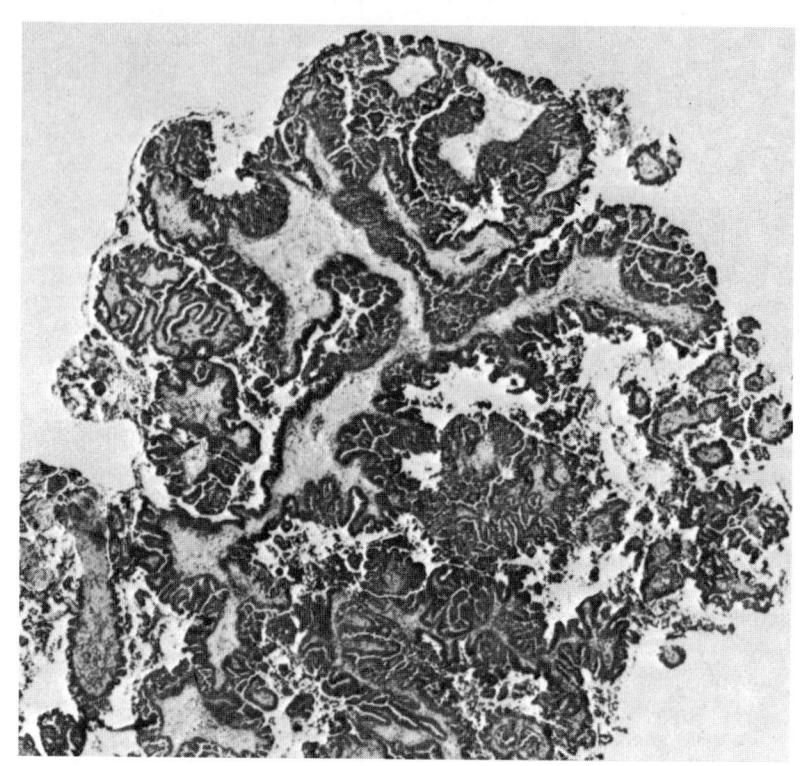

FIGURE 28-2.
(From Hendrickson M, Ross J, Eifel P, et al: Am J Surg Pathol 6:93, 1982.)

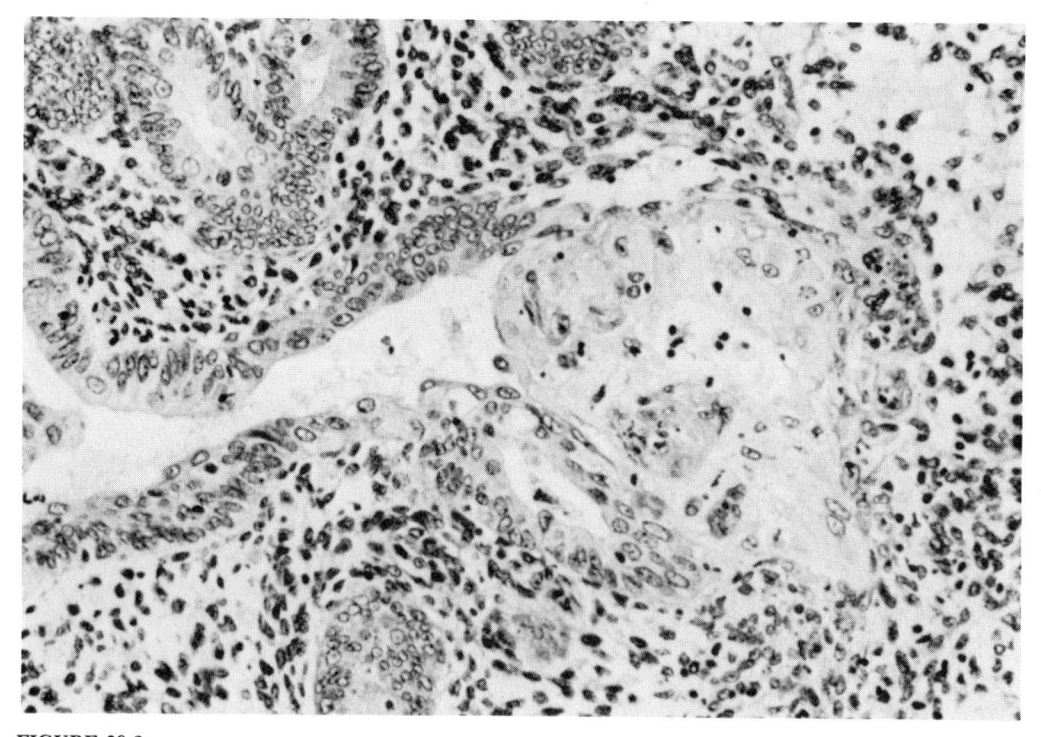

FIGURE 28-3.
(From Gompel C, Silverberg SG: Pathology in gynecology and obstetrics, 3rd ed. Philadelphia, J.B. Lippincott Co, 1985.)

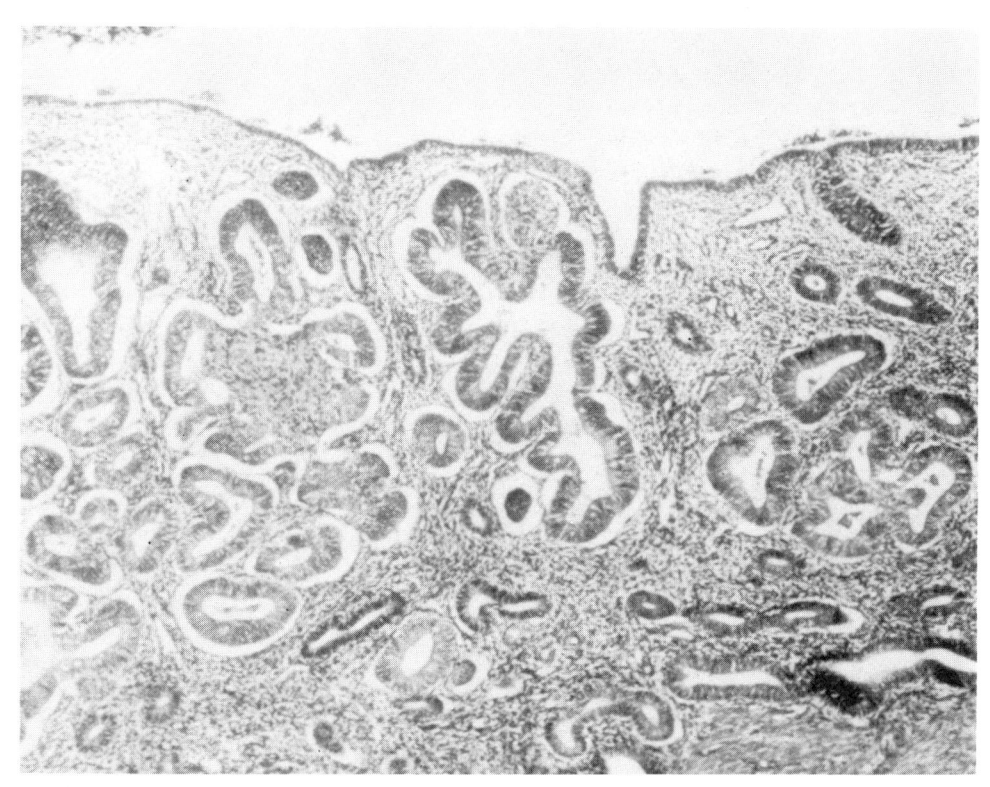

FIGURE 28-4.
(From Christopherson WM, Gray LA: In Coppleson M, ed: Gynecologic oncology, Edinburgh, Churchill-Livingstone, 1981.)

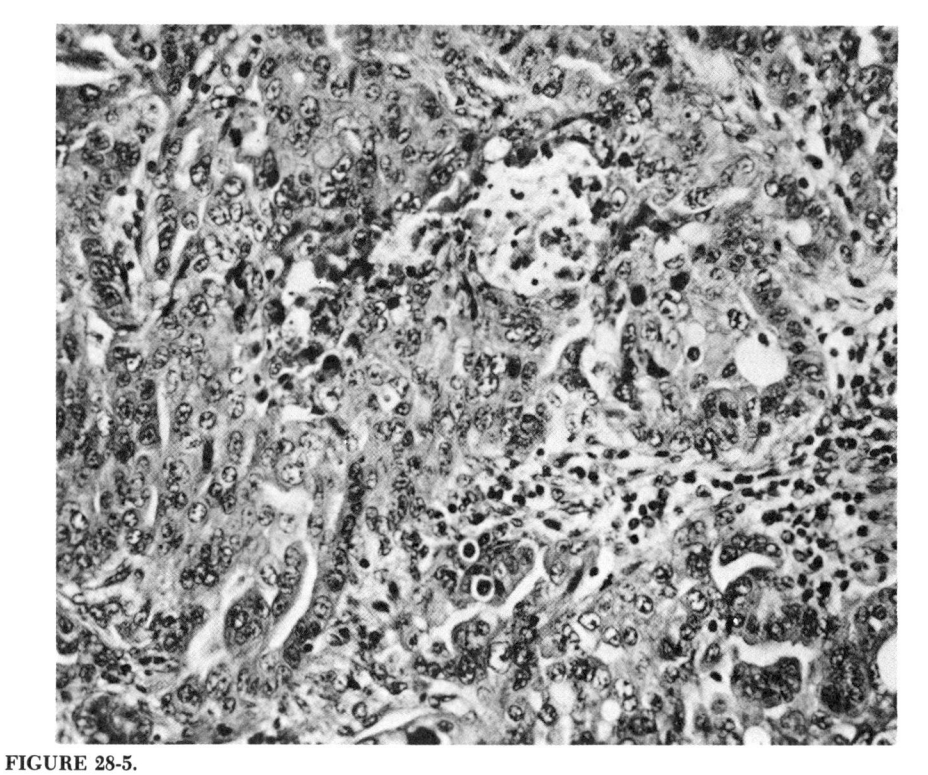

FIGURE 28-5.
(From Kurman RJ, Norris HJ: In Blaustein A, ed: Pathology of the female genital tract, 2nd ed. New York, Springer-Verlag, 1982.)

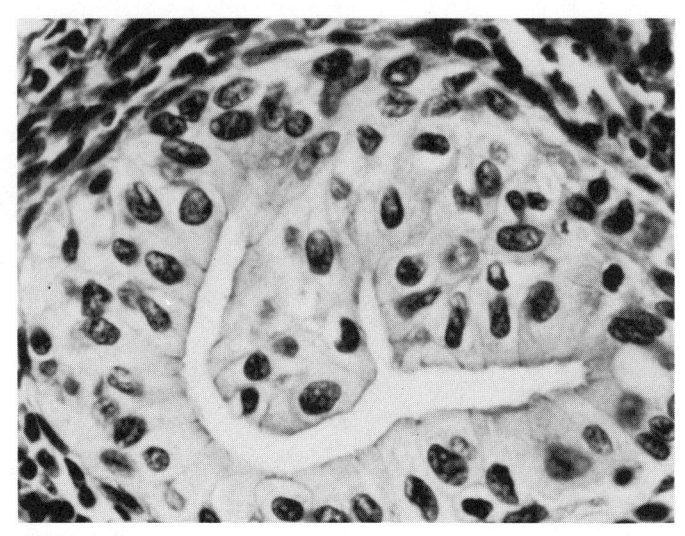

FIGURE 28-6.
(From Welch WR, Scully RE: Hum Pathol 8:503, 1977.)

27. A 53-year-old woman has metastatic endometrial carcinoma. Modes of spread include
    1. round ligament lymphatics.
    2. tubal lymphatics.
    3. infundibulopelvic ligament lymphatics.
    4. broad ligament lymphatics.
28. Which factors affect the prognosis of a patient with endometrial cancer?
    1. Age
    2. Race
    3. Stage
    4. Obesity
29. Which modalities are used in the initial treatment for Stage II adenocarcinoma of the endometrium?
    1. Surgery
    2. Brachytherapy
    3. External Irradiation
    4. Progesterone
30. In which of the following cases of endometrial adenocarcinoma should paraaortic and pelvic node sampling be done?
    1. Stage I, grade 2
    2. Stage I, grade 3
    3. Stage II
    4. Stage I, grade 1

ANSWERS

1. **C,** Page 809. A pap smear has a false negative rate of about 20% for cervical cancer and at least a 50% false negative rate for endometrial cancer. To rule out endometrial cancer, one must thoroughly sample the endometrium by curettage, preferably with separate samples from the endometrium and the endocervix. Approximately 14% of patients with postmenopausal bleeding will have that symptom due to endometrial carcinoma.

2. **B,** Page 800. Malignant glandular epithelium in the uterus is adenocarcinoma. A mixture of benign squamous epithelium with malignant glandular epithelium is called an adenoacanthoma. An adenoacanthoma has approximately the same prognosis as adenocarcinoma of the same grade and stage and should be treated similarly. If both adenomatous and squamous components were malignant, the tumor would be an adenosquamous carcinoma. Atypical adenomatous hyperplasia is a premalignant lesion in which there is crowding of glands and cytologic atypia. Endolymphatic stromal myosis is a low-grade stromal sarcoma.

3. **C,** Page 800; Figure 28-2 (from Droegemueller). The glands are dilated, but the cellular architecture is benign and there is no invasion. There is classic benign Swiss-cheese configuration; therefore, the diagnosis is cystic endometrial hyperplasia. Clear cell adenocarcinoma has many malignant cells with clear spaces. In this case, the spaces are not within the cells but are formed by groups of cells arranged in large dilated glands. Cellular leiomyoma would have whorls of connective tissue cells. A mixed müllerian tumor would have mitotic figures in connective tissue cells. Adenomatous hyperplasia has crowded glandular architecture with no invasion.

4. **D,** Page 807. Progression of adenomatous hyperplasia is slow and occurs in only a small number of cases. Usually the D&C will be therapeutic, but either progestin, if no pregnancy is wanted, or Clomid for ovulation induction, if pregnancy is desired, are proven treatments. Hysterectomy is not warranted for adenomatous hyperplasia alone. Repeat endometrial curettage should be done to assess completeness of cure.
5. **E,** Pages 806–807. A pap smear has a poor diagnostic rate probably not exceeding 50% for any endometrial pathology. Brushings or washings of the endometrium rely on cellular morphologic changes. Methods that deal with histologic specimens are easier to interpret. Therefore, the method that yields the most complete tissue specimen is the least likely to have errors of sampling or interpretation. A suction curettage, done carefully, is the best office sampling procedure.
6. **C,** Page 812. The involvement of the cervix by invasive carcinoma makes the endometrial carcinoma a stage II. Depth of the uterus does not influence the stage when the cervix is involved. The reason for doing a fractional D&C during the diagnostic process is to rule out cervical extension of endometrial invasive tumor and to rule out primary cervical carcinoma.
7. **E,** Pages 811–812. (Also see White A J et al: Primary squamous cell carcinoma of the endometrium, Obstet Gynecol 41:912. 1973.) Squamous cell carcinoma is a rare cancer of the endometrium with a poor prognosis that is usually associated with pyometra. White's study has documented no 5-year survival. The other tumors of the endometrium such as clear cell adenocarcinoma, papillary serous carcinoma, secretory carcinoma, and mucinous carcinoma are rare. Secretory and mucinous carcinoma have a relatively good prognosis, while clear cell and papillary serous carcinomas have a poor prognosis.
8. **E,** Page 815. As each factor increases in severity, the risk of nodal involvement increases. The risk of nodal involvement is even higher if more than one factor is brought into play. The grade of the tumor and the depth of myometrial invasion appear to be the most highly significant.
9. **A,** Page 828. Although the most common malignancy of the female genital tract is endometrial adenocarcinoma, fewer deaths occur from it than from either ovarian or cervical cancer. This is largely because it is detected and treated in an early stage. Early detection is possible because irregular uterine bleeding is an early and most common presenting symptom.
10. **C,** Pages 821–822. Progesterone is used in the management of both recurrences and metastasis of endometrial carcinoma. The tumor is more likely to respond if it is well differentiated. Response rates of 10% to 30% have been reported and seem to be higher in patients whose tumors have the largest number of progesterone receptors. Other forms of cytotoxic chemotherapy also have been used. Cytotoxic drugs seem to have a better response rate if the tumor is undifferentiated.
11. **D,** Page 820. Stage III adenocarcinoma of the endometrium has a 5-year survival rate of up to 40% with total abdominal hysterectomy and bilateral salpingo-oophorectomy and radiation if the patients have only subclinical spread of tumor. When there is a palpable mass, survival with radiation only is approximately 16%. The overall survival is approximately 30%.
12. **E,** Pages 821–822. The primary chemotherapeutic agent used in endometrial adenocarcinoma is a progestin. Endometrial carcinoma has a response rate of 10% to 30% to progestins and the highest response rates are in grade 1 tumors that have the greatest number of estrogen and progesterone receptors. Tamoxifen has also been used as it seems to increase the number of progesterone receptors in the tumor tissue. Neither of these are cytotoxic however. In the cytotoxic group, cyclophosphamide, duxorubicin, *cis*-platinum, and 5-FU are frequently used in combination for endometrial carcinoma. Mitomycin has been used primarily in gastric cancer.
13. **C,** Pages 823–824. The treatment for homologous uterine sarcoma is surgical. Metastases or recurrences are usually treated with multiple-agent chemotherapy. Radiation has not been shown to increase survival significantly, although it appears to decrease the risk of pelvic recurrence. Distant metastases are frequent and most often occur in the lungs or abdomen.
14. **C,** Page 821. Ninety percent of the adenocarcinomas of the endometrium that recur do so within 5 years, but as 10% recur later, prolonged follow-up is important. The most frequent site of recurrence is in the pelvis (approximately 50%), followed by lung (17%).
15. **E,** Page 823. Leiomyosarcomas comprise nearly 50% of all uterine sarcomas. They are diagnosed if the tumor contains over five mitoses per 10 high-power fields. The more mitoses present the worse the prognosis. Endolymphatic stroma myosis is a more be-

nign form of endometrial stromal sarcoma, both of which are rare. The heterologous rhabdomyosarcoma, liposarcoma, chondrosarcoma, and osteosarcoma are less common than the homologous types. In total, sarcomas comprise less than 5% of all uterine malignancies.

16. **E,** Pages 822–823. If a uterine sarcoma forms mesenchymal tissue normally found in the uterus, it is called a homologous sarcoma. If it forms mesenchymal tissue not normally found in the uterus, such as bone, fat, striated muscle, and cartilage, it is called heterologous. If the heterologous sarcoma is in combination with adenocarcinoma, it is called a malignant müllerian mixed tumor (MMMT). Prior pelvic radiation therapy is a predisposing factor, having been performed in approximately 12% of patients with MMMT. If an adenocarcinoma and a homologous sarcoma coexist, this tumor may be called a carcinosarcoma. Endolymphatic stromal myosis is a rare low-grade sarcoma made up of cells resembling the endometrial stroma. These are most often found in premenopausal females. Endometrial stromal sarcoma is a more malignant version of the same cell type.

17–19. **17, A; 18, E; 19, C;** Page 807. A young woman with benign endometrial hyperplasia symptoms may be given cyclic progestins (for example, Provera 10 mg for 10 to 14 days each month can be given). A postmenopausal woman with atypical endometrial hyperplasia (called CIS by some pathologists) should have definitive treatment with removal of the uterus unless medically contraindicated. A young anovulatory woman who desires pregnancy but who has atypical endometrial hyperplasia may be treated with clomiphene citrate to induce ovulation. If successful, this therapy will interrupt the continuous unopposed estrogen that had previously stimulated her endometrium.

20. **C,** Page 803. Adenomatous hyperplasia is identified by crowded irregular glands without significant cytologic atypia.

21. **A,** Page 800. Papillary serous carcinoma is a highly malignant form of endometrial carcinoma that has a papillary form resembling papillary serous adenocarcinoma of the ovary.

22. **E,** Page 803. Atypical adenomatous hyperplasia is a premalignant variant of endometrial hyperplasia. There is cytologic atypica but no invasion. On a lower power there would be crowding of the glands.

23. **B,** Page 800. Adenoacanthoma has malignant adenomatous cells and benign squamous cells.

24. **D,** Pages 802–803. This is an invasive carcinoma of the endometrium that has crowded glands and cellular atypia with stromal invasion. Figure 28-5 is moderately differentiated adenocarcinoma.

25. **C** (2, 4), Pages 806–807; Table 28-3 (from Droegemueller). Office aspiration, or suction curettage, can adequately sample the endometrium in most cases. If the patient continues to have bleeding or other symptoms, a repeat D&C may be indicated. The office procedure usually can be done under paracervical block and some patients benefit from an oral prostaglandin synthetase inhibitor taken 30 minutes before the procedure. A disadvantage of office curettage using a small suction curet is the possibility of missing other uterine pathology, such as polyps or small submucous fibroids.

26. **A** (1, 2, 3), Page 802; Table 28-1. The incidence of cancer of the endometrium is greatest between the ages of 55 and 65. Risk factors include unopposed estrogen from any source, such as estrogen-producing ovarian tumors, polycystic ovary disease, late menopause and obesity, or oral intake of estrogens. Unopposed estrogen, whether from exogenous or endogenous sources, provides prolonged estrogen effect on the endometrium. Progestins or Progesterone decreases estrogen receptor formation, stimulates the conversion of estradiol to estrone, and promotes sloughing of the endometrium when it is withdrawn. Hypertension, by itself and unrelated to obesity, is not a risk factor for endometrial carcinoma.

27. **E** (All), Page 814. Endometrial carcinoma spreads through round ligament lymphatics to the femoral nodes; through tubal and infundibular ligament lymphatics to the paraaortic nodes; and through the broad ligament lymphatics to the pelvic nodes. An endometrial tumor can also spread by direct extension through the uterine wall into the peritoneal cavity as well as through the fallopian tube lumen to the adnexa.

28. **A** (1, 2, 3), Page 813. Young women with endometrial carcinoma have a better prognosis than older women with this disease. White women fare better than black women. The stage of the disease is a well-recognized prognostic determinant. Fortunately, most endometrial carcinomas are diagnosed at stage I. Obesity per se does not affect survival independent of the other clinical factors. Pathologic prognostic factors are grade, type of tumor, depth of invasion, node involvement, and peritoneal spread.

29. **A** (1, 2, 3), Pages 819–820. The mainstay of therapy for stage II adenocarcinoma of the endometrium is surgery if the patient is able to tolerate it. Uterine and vaginal brachytherapy has been used before surgery in some cases and external irradiation to 40 Gray (Gy) has been given after surgery in others. Progesterone or progestins are generally used for stage III disease and in recurrences.

30. **A** (1, 2, 3), Page 817. The spread to nodes in Stage I, grade 1 adenocarcinoma is less than 2%, while with Stage I, grade 2 the risk is approximately 11%, and rises to 25% to 30% in Stage I, grade 3 adenocarcinoma. Stage II carries increased risk of pelvic node spread because there is cervical involvement. In Stage I, grade 1 carcinoma of the endometrium, the risk of nodal involvement is so low that routine sampling is not warranted.

CHAPTER 29
Neoplastic Diseases of the Ovary

DIRECTIONS: Select the one best answer or completion.

1. A 50-year-old woman has an asymptomatic ovarian carcinoma in one ovary. Although her peritoneal cavity is free of tumor, she has retroperitoneal nodes positive for the malignancy without other evidence of disease. At which stage is her ovarian tumor?
   A. Ia
   B. IIa
   C. IIb
   D. III
   E. IV

2. At what approximate age does the peak death rate from ovarian cancer occur?
   A. 40
   B. 50
   C. 60
   D. 70
   E. 80

3. The most common type of ovarian neoplasm originates in which cells?
   A. Germ cells
   B. Epithelial cells
   C. Stromal cells
   D. Lipoid cells
   E. Sex-cord cells

4. A rare virilizing tumor of the ovary is
   A. polyembryoma.
   B. mucinous cystadenocarcinoma.
   C. fibroma.
   D. dysgerminoma.
   E. Sertoli-Leydig.

5. A 61-year-old woman has a 3 cm right adnexal cyst found on routine exam. What is the appropriate management?
   A. Reassurance.
   B. Repeat the exam in 2 to 3 months.
   C. Suppress the ovary with cyclic estrogen and progesterone.
   D. Order CT or ultrasound.
   E. Laparotomy.

6. A 62-year-old woman has a breast mass and firm bilaterally-enlarged ovaries. Breast biopsy reveals a mucin-secreting carcinoma. What is the most likely diagnosis of the ovarian tumors?
   A. Dysgerminoma
   B. Clear cell carcinoma
   C. Fibroma
   D. Brenner tumor
   E. Krukenberg tumor

7. A 32-year-old woman comes to you for a routine gynecologic evaluation and renewal of her birth control pills containing 50 ug ethenylestradiol. On an otherwise normal pelvic exam you find a 5 cm left ovarian cyst. What would be the appropriate management?
   A. Yearly follow-up.
   B. Follow-up in 2 to 3 months.
   C. Double her dose of birth control pills.
   D. Order a CT scan.
   E. Laparotomy.

8. What is the most common type of epithelial tumor?
   A. Mucinous
   B. Endometroid
   C. Serous
   D. Clear cell
   E. Brenner

9. After complete resection of stage II ovarian carcinoma, chemotherapy using Alkeran is considered. A major long-term side effect is
   A. permanent destruction of lymphocytes.
   B. cardiac toxicity.
   C. increased risk of subsequent leukemia.
   D. stomatitis.
   E. pulmonary fibrosis.

10. A 62-year-old woman who is on no medications develops irregular uterine bleeding. On examination she has a pink rugated vagina and a 5 × 6 × 4 cm firm right ovarian mass. Office curettage reveals adenomatous endometrial hyperplasia without atypia. Which of the following ovarian tumors would best account for her symptoms?
    A. Serous cystadenoma
    B. Mucinous cystadenocarcinoma
    C. Teratoma
    D. Dysgerminoma
    E. Granulosa cell tumor

11. When discussing ovarian tumor management, a second-look procedure refers to
    A. a repeat thorough history and physical.
    B. a laparoscopy done after primary surgical treatment.
    C. a laparotomy done after 1 year of chemotherapy when no clinical evidence of disease exists.
    D. a laparotomy for staging after initial diagnosis but before definitive surgery.
    E. a laparotomy done to debulk tumor after the tumor has recurred.
12. What is the second most commonly found type of ovarian neoplasm?
    A. Epithelial
    B. Germ cell
    C. Stromal
    D. Lipoid
    E. Gonadoblastoma
13. Primary treatment of a pure 6 cm dysgerminoma confined to one ovary in a 22-year-old woman should include
    A. total abdominal hysterectomy, bilateral salpingo-oophorectomy, and omentectomy.
    B. unilateral salpingo-oophorectomy.
    C. chemotherapy.
    D. radiation therapy.
    E. radical hysterectomy and bilateral salpingo-oophorectomy.

DIRECTIONS: For each numbered item, select the one heading most closely associated with it. Each lettered heading may be used once, more than once, or not at all.

Match the following photomicrographs with the appropriate ovarian epithelial neoplasm.

(A) Serous
(B) Mucinous
(C) Endometriod
(D) Clear cell
(E) Brenner

14. Figure 29-1
15. Figure 29-2
16. Figure 29-3
    (A) Benign cystic teratoma
    (B) Dysgerminoma
    (C) Granulosa cell tumor
    (D) Krukenberg tumor
    (E) Endodermal sinus tumor
17. Figure 29-4
18. Figure 29-5
19. Figure 29-6
20. Figure 29-7

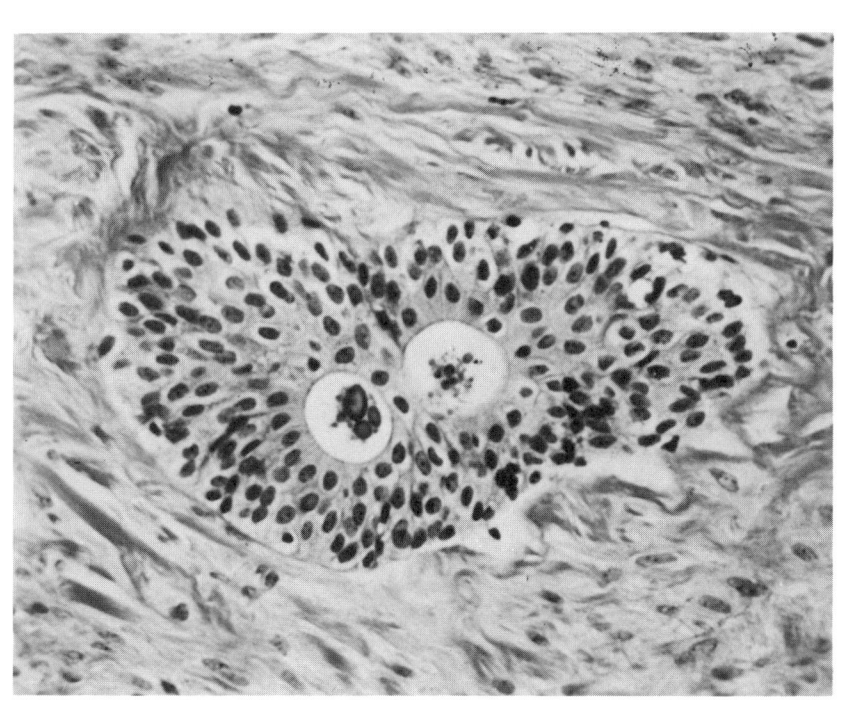

FIGURE 29-1.

(From Atlas of tumor pathology, Fascicle 16, 2nd series. Washington, DC, Armed Forces Institute of Pathology, 1979.)

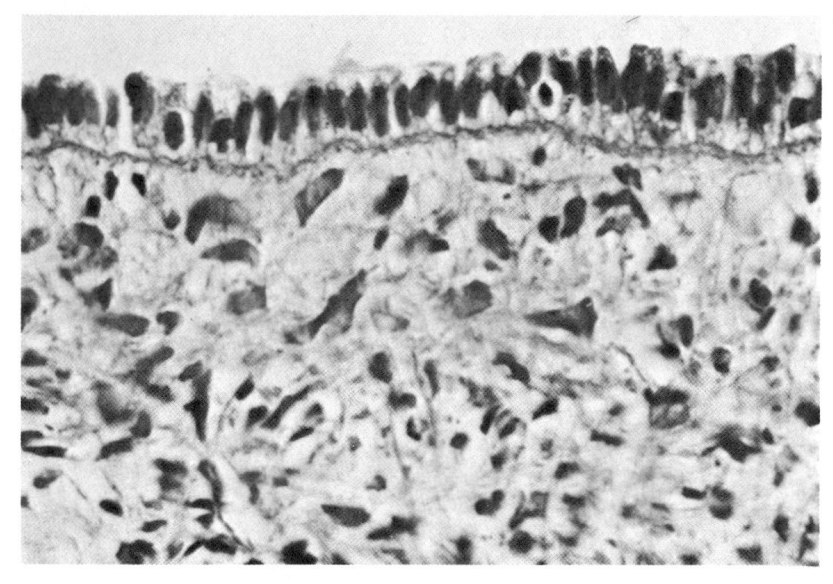

FIGURE 29-2.
(From Serov SF, Scully RE, Sobin LH: Histologic typing of ovarian tumors. Geneva, World Health Organization, 1973.)

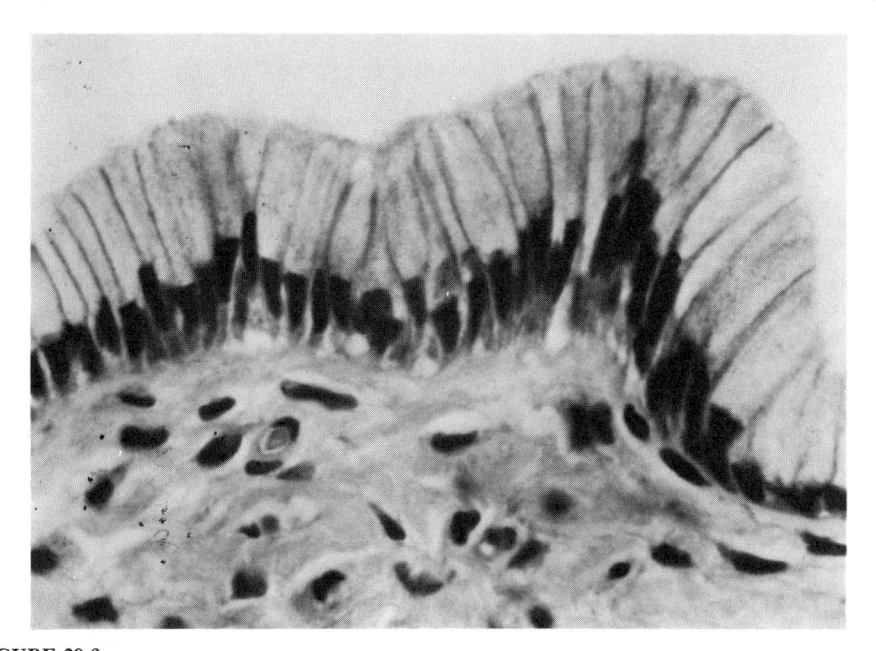

FIGURE 29-3.
(From Serov SF, Scully RE, Sobin LH: Histologic typing of ovarian tumors. Geneva, World Health Organization, 1973.)

DIRECTIONS: For each numbered item, indicate whether it is associated with
  A only (A)
  B only (B)
  C both (A) and (B)
  D neither (A) nor (B)

(A) Germ cell tumors of the ovary
(B) Epithelial tumors of the ovary
(C) Both
(D) Neither

21. Produce alpha-fetoprotein.
22. 80% produce CA-125.
23. Often contain tissue from more than one embryonic cell layer.

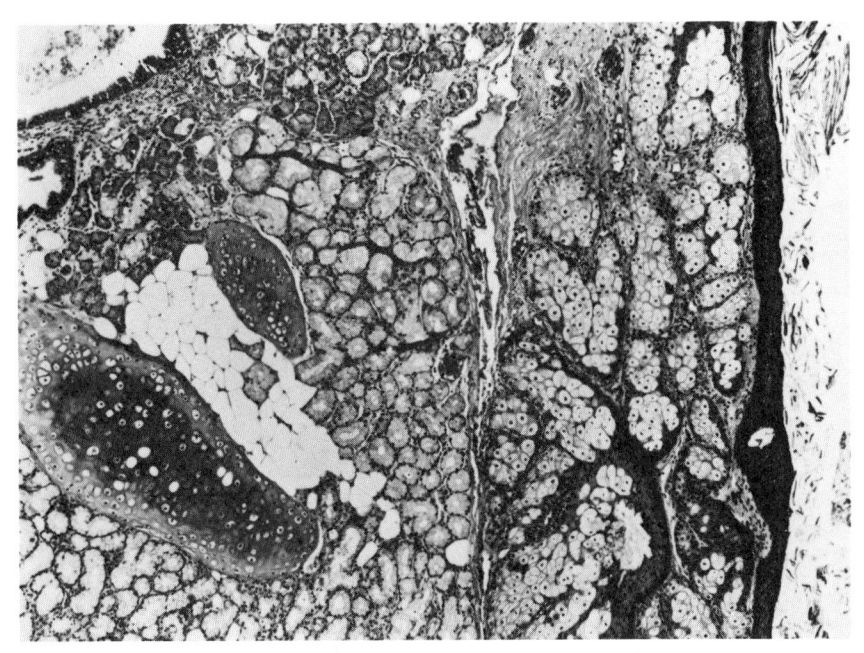

FIGURE 29-4.
(From Serov SF, Scully RE, Sobin LH: Histologic typing of ovarian tumors. Geneva, Switzerland, World Health Organization, 1973.)

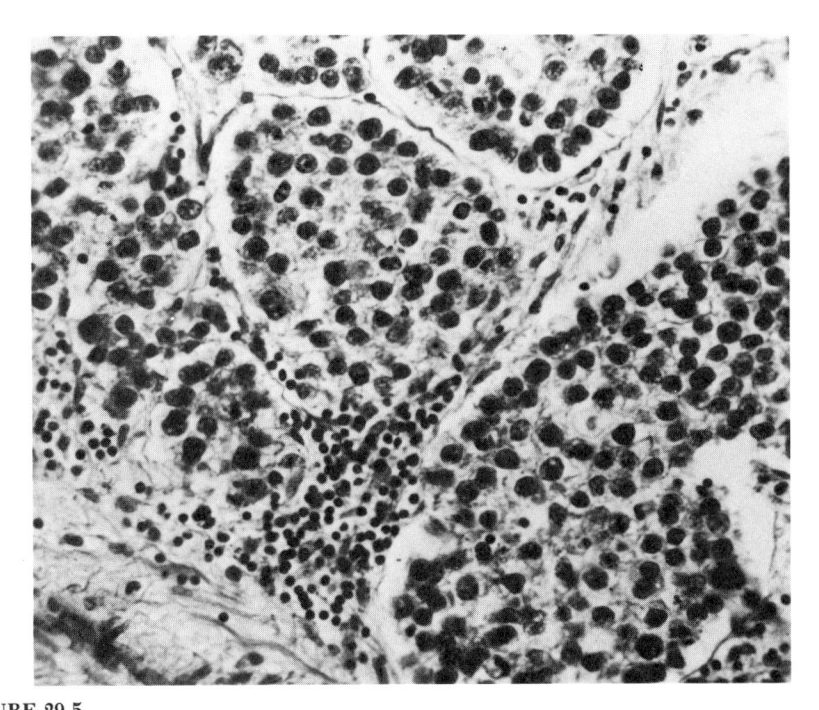

FIGURE 29-5.
(From Scully RE: Germ cell tumors of the ovary and fallopian tube. In Meigs JV, Sturgis SH, eds: Progress in gynecology, vol. 4. New York, Grune & Stratton, 1963.)

192 Gynecologic Oncology

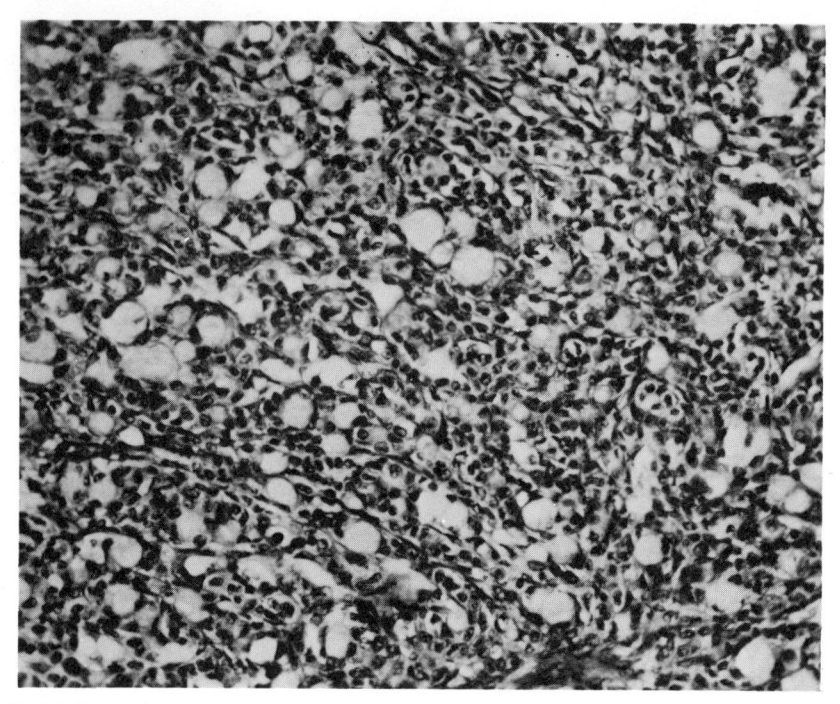

FIGURE 29-6
(From Droegemueller W, Herbst AL, Mishell DR, Stenchever MA: Comprehensive gynecology, St. Louis: The C.V. Mosby Co, 1987.)

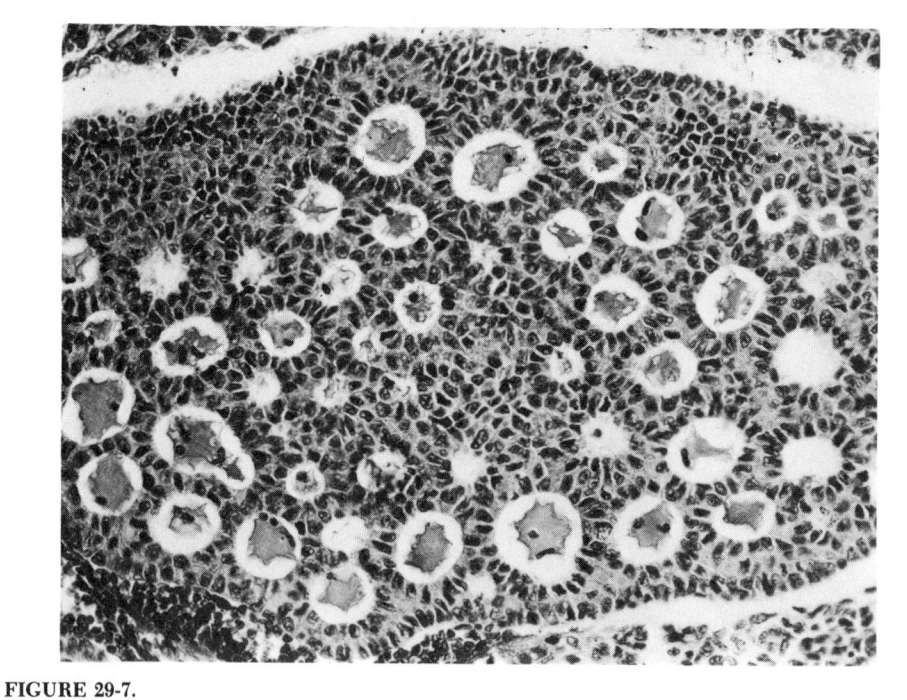

FIGURE 29-7.
(From Scully RE, Morris J: Functioning ovarian tumors. In Meigs JV, Sturgis SH, eds: Progress in gynecology, vol. 3. New York, Grune & Stratton, 1957.)

DIRECTIONS: Each question contains four suggested answers of which one or more is correct. Choose the answer
   A if 1, 2, and 3 are correct
   B if 1 and 3 are correct
   C if 2 and 4 are correct
   D if 4 only is correct
   E if all are correct

24. A 24-year-old woman had a large stage I mucinous cystadenocarcinoma of the ovary of low malignant potential which ruptured prior to surgery. This situation
   1. makes surgical removal easier.
   2. often leads to postoperative bowel obstruction.
   3. increases the subsequent risk of malignant change in residual tumor.
   4. is associated with pseudomyxoma peritonei.

25. Direct complications of ovarian carcinoma include
   1. hydrothorax.
   2. malnutrition.
   3. bowel obstruction.
   4. bone marrow suppression.

26. Which factors influence the occurrence of ovarian carcinoma?
   1. Frequency of ovulation.
   2. Eating a fatty diet.
   3. Living in an industrialized country.
   4. Family history.

27. You are performing surgery on a 39-year-old woman with 5–6 cm bilateral irregular adnexal masses on pelvic examination. What should you be prepared to do?
   1. A vertical incision.
   2. Peritoneal washings and/or ascitic fluid for cytology.
   3. Biopsy of the peritoneal surfaces and paraaortic nodes.
   4. Total abdominal hysterectomy and bilateral salpingo-oophorectomy.

28. Prognosis in cases of ovarian malignancy is related to
   1. stage.
   2. cell type.
   3. grade.
   4. amount of residual tumor.

29. True statements regarding borderline ovarian tumors are:
   1. They comprise approximately 20% of ovarian epithelial cancers.
   2. They have a very serious prognosis despite their benign appearance.
   3. They do not invade the ovarian stroma.
   4. They are more common in postmenopausal than in premenopausal women.

30. What should a work-up of a 58-year-old patient with a persistent left adnexal mass include?
   1. An IVP
   2. A chest x-ray
   3. Barium enema
   4. Cystoscopy

ANSWERS

1. **D**, Page 844, Table 29-4 (from Droegemueller). Staging of ovarian cancer is based on findings at the clinical examination and the surgical exploration, including the histology of the specimen and cytology of fluids. In this case the extension of the tumor to the retroperitoneal nodes placed the patient in stage III. About 10% to 20% of women with carcinoma apparently confined to one ovary have been found to have retroperitoneal lymph node involvement at the time of surgery. The 5-year survival rate for stage III ovarian carcinoma is approximately 15%.

2. **E**, Page 834; Figure 29-1 (from Droegemueller). Ovarian cancer causes more deaths than any other genital malignancy, although it is only the second most common genital cancer. This is due to lack of symptoms early in the disease. Until the tumor is widespread, patients are asymptomatic. Therefore, ovarian malignancies are detected late and treated late in the course of their progression. The highest death rate is in the late 70s and 80s.

3. **B**, Pages 835–836. Ovarian neoplasms are formed from tissues that constitute the ovary. These include the epithelial lining (the most common source of tumors), germ cells, sex cord cells, and stroma. Very rarely tumors will arise from lymphatics or blood vessels and nerves within the ovary. Occasionally carcinoma originating in other organs will metastasize to the ovary.

4. **E**, Pages 868–869. There have been only approximately 500 Sertoli-Leydig tumors reported. However, they are discussed frequently because they cause symptoms due to their hormone production. Sertoli-Leydig tumors are the male homolog of the granulosa theca cell tumors. They may produce androgens that cause virilization in young women. Most behave as low-grade malignancies with 5-year survivals of 70% to 90%. Higher survival rates occur when the tumor is better differentiated. Polyembryoma tumors and dysgerminomas are both rare malignancies of germ cell origin. A mucinous tumor is derived from the epithelium of the ovary and a fibroma from the nonfunctioning stroma.

5. **E**, Pages 836, 842. The ovary decreases in size in the postmenopausal years and should be no larger than 1.5 cm in the greatest diameter. At this age physiologic enlargement does not occur. Direct visualization should be accom-

plished to determine the origin of the cyst (for example, whether it is ovarian, tubal, parametrial, or bowel). If the cyst is ovarian, it should be removed as the probability of it being a neoplasm is extremely high. In that case, a total abdominal hysterectomy, bilateral salpingo-oophorectomy, and a careful exam of the peritoneal contents should be done. Retroperitoneal node sampling should be done if the neoplasm is malignant.

6. **E, Page 869.** Krukenberg tumors of the ovary contain mucin-producing signet-ring cells and are usually metastatic from the GI tract (most commonly) or the breast. In this case, with a known mucin-secreting tumor of the breast, bilateral ovarian metastases are most likely. Dysgerminomas may occur in the elderly but are most common in young women and are rarely bilateral. Fibromas and Brenner tumors are also rarely bilateral, and clear cell carcinomas are relatively rare malignant ovarian epithelial tumors.

7. **E, Page 842.** In a menstrual age woman not using birth control pills (BCP) or other ovarian suppressive treatment, the development of physiologic ovarian cysts is common and would require only observation for a short period of time. Most of them resolve within one cycle. However, as birth control pills containing 50 μg of ethinylestradiol suppress physiologic ovarian cysts, any cyst that occurs while on BCPs is much more likely to be a neoplasm. Therefore, they should be evaluated by an operative technique. A CT scan or ultrasound cannot reliably distinguish between physiologic or neoplastic lesions.

8. **C, Page 870.** Epithelial tumors are the most common neoplasms of the ovary and serous tumors are the most common of the epithelial tumors. Like most ovarian neoplasms, they can be either benign or malignant. The malignant serous tumors have the worst prognosis of all the epithelial tumors. They are bilateral in 33% to 66% of the cases.

9. **C, Pages 852–853.** Alkeran causes bone marrow depression within 2 weeks. It increases the risk of leukemia. This risk may range from 2% to as high as 10% within 8 years of therapy. It is therefore important to give Alkeran only if its benefits are significant. Stomatitis is more commonly seen as an acute side effect of the antimetabolites. Pulmonary fibrosis is a consequence of bleomycin and cardiac toxicity of adriamycin. Renal damage is of significant concern with *cis*-platinum.

10. **E, Pages 866–867.** Sex cord–stromal tumors account for about 6% of all ovarian neoplasms. Some of these produce hormones. This woman has signs of estrogen effect without being on any medications. Such symptoms together with a firm adnexal mass make the possibility of a granulosa or theca cell tumor quite likely. These tumors behave as low-grade carcinomas and are primarily treated surgically. A total abdominal hysterectomy and bilateral salpingo-oophorectomy should also be performed in a patient of this age with this tumor.

11. **C, Pages 855–856.** A second-look procedure is a laparotomy done after a year of chemotherapy when no clinical evidence of tumor exists. It is therefore done in a patient who is in clinical remission. This procedure includes extensive biopsy and cytologic sampling of the peritoneal cavity including the retroperitoneal nodes. It is done to determine the need to continue or discontinue chemotherapy. If the second-look surgery is negative, the 5-year survival in patients with epithelial ovarian cancer is approximately 80%.

12. **B, Pages 857–858.** Physiological cysts are the most common cause of ovarian enlargement. Of the neoplasms, epithelial tumors are the most common (approximately 65%) while germ cell derived tumors are the second most common (approximately 20% to 25%). The most frequent germ cell tumor is the benign cystic teratoma which, as its name implies, is benign and can be treated by simple removal. Only 2% to 3% of germ cell tumors are malignant. These include the very rare polyembryoma, embryonal carcinoma, and endodermal sinus tumors, as well as the relatively common dysgerminoma.

13. **B, Pages 863–864.** Unilateral salpingo-oophorectomy is the treatment of choice after careful evaluation to rule out spread to the other ovary or other pelvic or retroperitoneal structures. Approximately 20% will recur, but they can be treated by radiotherapy or additional surgery. Multiple-agent chemotherapy has also been utilized. It is important to carefully examine the tumor histologically for other malignant germ cell elements (mixed germ cell tumor). If other malignant germ cell elements are present, the prognosis is much poorer.

14–16. **14, E; 15, A; 16, B; Pages 836–838, 840.** Serous, mucinous, endometrioid, clear cell, and Brenner tumors are the five cell types that comprise the epithelial tumors of the ovary. They may form benign or malignant tumors. The clear cell tumor is always malignant. Serous tumors are the most common neoplasm and also are the most common of the malignancies. Their lining epithelium resembles tubal epithelium. Mucinous tumors resemble endocervical mucinous cells, and endometrioid tumors resemble the endometrium.

The Brenner tumor has islands of cells that resemble the Walthard cell nests of the ovary or the transitional epithelium of the bladder. Their nuclei are distinctive in that they look like coffee beans. Abundant ovarian stroma is found between these islands of epithelial cells. This is a rare tumor and almost always benign.

Clear cell tumors are malignant and are found in the endometrium, endocervix, and vagina as well as in the ovary. They have a clear cell and a hobnail cell pattern.

17. **A**, Page 858. Benign cystic teratomas (dermoids) contain cells derived from all germ layers. They can occur at any age but are most common during the reproductive years. There is histologic differentiation into different adult benign tissues, and they may even contain functional glands such as thyroid (struma ovarii). The rare malignant variants usually are associated with differentiation of the squamous components.

18. **B**, Page 863. The ovarian dysgerminoma consists of multiple germ cells with a stroma infiltrated by lymphocytes. It is analogous to the seminoma in the male. Dysgerminomas are most common in women under the age of 30 and are bilateral in about 10% of the cases.

19. **D**, Pages 869–870. The Krukenberg tumor contains mucin-filled signet-ring malignant cells. They are metastatic to the ovary, usually from the GI tract or breast. Therefore, if one is found in the ovaries, a careful search for the primary lesion should be undertaken.

20. **C**, Page 867. Granulosa cell tumors are made up of granulosa cells from the specialized stroma of the ovary. They contain some fibroblasts and theca cells in varying proportions. The histopathological section shown in the question also contains Call-Exner bodies. These are eosinophilic bodies surrounded by granulosa cells and are also found in normal follicles. This tumor is quite rare but is also discussed frequently because it can secrete hormones (primarily estrogen) and cause premature puberty or postmenopausal bleeding. They behave as low-grade malignancies and have a greater than 90% 10-year survival.

21–23. 21, **A**, Page 833; 22, **B**, Page 855; 23, **A**, Page 858. Approximately 80% of patients with epithelial ovarian cancer have increased amounts of the ovarian antibody designated CA-125, which can be used to monitor the development of recurrent disease. However, as this test has a high false negative rate, it cannot be used exclusively for such monitoring. Germ cell tumors are derived from the totipotential germ cell and therefore are capable of producing many of the proteins found during the development of the embryo such as alpha-fetoprotein, which is produced by endodermal sinus tumors. They may differentiate to mimic the three developmental layers of the embryo, namely, the ectoderm, endoderm, and mesoderm.

24. **C** (2, 4), Pages 849–850. The rupturing of a mucinous cystadenoma allows the spread of viable cells in the abdomen which produce a large amount of mucinous material. Their growth often leads to bowel obstruction, although it is not associated with bowel cancer. The intraabdominal accumulation of mucin is called pseudomyxoma peritonei and can cause disability and death, although it is not frankly malignant. The mucin is very difficult to remove surgically, although this attempt may be aided by a copious lavage with 5% dextrose in water. Residual cells may respond to cytoxan, adriamycin, and *cis*-platinum combination chemotherapy.

25. **A** (1, 2, 3), Pages 853, 856. Malignant or benign hydrothorax can occur with ovarian carcinoma. The fluid tends to reaccumulate, especially if the tumor is malignant. Bowel obstruction and malnutrition are common late sequelae of ovarian cancer. Bowel obstruction may be treated with resection and malnutrition may be treated by hyperalimentation. Bone marrow suppression is usually due to the treatment, either chemotherapy or radiation therapy, not the disease itself.

26. **E** (All), Pages 834–835. Women who ovulate less frequently, either because they took birth control pills or were often pregnant, appear to be less prone to develop ovarian carcinoma. Factors that increase the risk of ovarian carcinoma are living in an industrialized country and eating a diet high in animal fat. Familial occurrence of ovarian cancer has been reported. These genetically susceptible individuals are rare but may develop intraperitoneal carcinomatosis similar to ovarian cancer, even though their ovaries are removed prophylactically. Theoretically, these tumors arise from the multipotential coelomic epithelium.

27. **E** (All), Pages 851–852. In any case where invasive ovarian epithelial carcinoma is suspected, a vertical incision should be used, and peritoneal washings or ascitic fluid should be sent for cytology. Biopsy of peritoneal surface and sampling of paraaortic nodes would be indicated in stage I and II ovarian cancer. A total abdominal hysterectomy and bilateral salpingo-oophorectomy plus omentectomy should be done if ovarian cancer is found. An attempt should be made to reduce the tumor to the smallest residual mass, which may also require bowel or partial bladder resection.

28. **E** (All), Pages 846–848. The worse the stage and grade of the ovarian tumor, the worse the prognosis. Cell type is important. Undifferentiated and serous tumors have the worst prognosis. The amount of residual tumor after maximum removal is also a factor. The greater the amount of residual tumor, the less the patient responds to chemotherapy.

If total resection of a stage III tumor is accomplished, the 5-year survival is approximately 30%. It is only 10% if the resection is incomplete. The size of the residual tumor is also of prognostic value. Cases with greater than 1.5 cm residual tumor masses have a poorer outcome than cases with 1.5 to 0.5 cm masses of residual tumor, which in turn do have a poorer outcome than those with less than 0.5 cm residual tumor masses.

29. **B** (1, 3), Pages 848–849. By definition, borderline ovarian carcinoma (ovarian carcinoma of low malignant potential) does not invade ovarian stroma. Lack of invasion is one of the histologic requirements necessary to make the diagnosis of a borderline tumor. About 20% of ovarian epithelial carcinoma falls into the borderline category, and these tumors have a much better prognosis than frankly invasive ovarian cancer. Julian and Woodrull report that stage I borderline serous tumors have a 100% 5-year survival. These can be treated by unilateral salpingo-oophorectomy in young women who wish to retain their childbearing potential. As borderline tumors are more common in young women who desire to retain their childbearing potential, the relatively benign behavior is important to remember so that treatment can be modified accordingly.

30. **A** (1, 2, 3), Page 845. A patient with a suspected ovarian malignancy (which must be considered in any postmenopausal woman with an adnexal mass) should have a thorough history and physical, a chest x-ray, hematocrit, white blood count, and blood chemistry. They should also have an IVP to rule out renal or ureteral involvement. A barium enema is important to rule out bowel carcinoma and to establish a baseline of bowel integrity in the event of future radiation treatment. Cystoscopy is not necessary in patients with adnexal masses and no other finding.

CHAPTER 30

Premalignant and Malignant Diseases of the Vulva

DIRECTIONS: Select the one best answer or completion.

1. The histologic diagnosis is squamous carcinoma with penetration to 5 mm and capillary space/lymphatic involvement. Her clinical staging is T1NOMO. What is optimal treatment?
   A. Radical vulvectomy with bilateral inguinal-femoral node dissection.
   B. Radical vulvectomy with left inguinal-femoral node dissection.
   C. Radical vulvectomy alone.
   D. Laser excision of the visible lesion.
   E. Radiation therapy of the visible lesion.

2. During a lymphadenectomy of the inguinal-femoral nodes performed as part of the therapy of a stage II carcinoma of the vulva, the surgeon recognizes that several of the nodes contain tumor. Therapy now should include
   A. an ipsilateral deep pelvic lymphadenectomy.
   B. a bilateral deep pelvic lymphadenectomy.
   C. radiotherapy to ipsilateral deep pelvic nodes.
   D. radiotherapy to bilateral deep pelvic nodes.
   E. triple-agent chemotherapy.

3. A 28-year-old woman has biopsy-proven carcinoma in situ of a 2×3 cm acuminate lesion on the posterior fourchette. What is the best treatment for this patient?
   A. Total vulvectomy
   B. Skinning vulvectomy
   C. Topical 5-fluorouracil (5-FU)
   D. Multiple trichloroacetic acid applications
   E. Wide local excision

4. A diagnosis of Stage 1A carcinoma of the vulva is made in a 62-year-old woman based on International Society for the Study of Vulvar Disease (ISSVD) criteria of an excision biopsy of a lesion on the left labium majus. What is optimal treatment?
   A. Wide local excision
   B. Topical 5 fluorouracil
   C. Simple vulvectomy
   D. Radical vulvectomy
   E. Primary radiation therapy

5. What is the next step in your management of this patient?
   A. Oral conjugated estrogen
   B. Topical estrogen cream
   C. Vulval colposcopy
   D. Simple vulvectomy
   E. Topical testosterone cream

6. A 72-year-old woman presents with a 9-month history of progressive vulvar pruritus. Examination of the vulva reveals diffuse erythema with excoriations and a 1 1/2 cm, slightly raised lesion of the posterior left labium majus. What should be the next step in her management?
   A. Wide local excision of the raised lesion.
   B. Office biopsy of the raised lesion.
   C. Prescribe topical corticosteroid cream.
   D. Office laser vaporization of the raised lesion.
   E. Office cryocautery of the raised lesion.

7. A 71-year-old woman comes to your office with a "swelling" in her vagina for the past 4 months. Pelvic examination is unremarkable except for a 4 ×4 cm, slightly tender, moderately firm mass in the inferior medial portion of the right labium majus. What should she have next?
   A. Vulvar colposcopy (vulvoscopy)
   B. Treatment with topical fluorinated steroids
   C. Incision and drainage
   D. Biopsy of the mass
   E. Laser ablation of the mass

8. Biopsy of a 9 cm condylomatous mass on the left labium majus of a 48-year-old woman reveals verrucous carcinoma. What is the best treatment?
   A. Laser ablation
   B. Wide local excision
   C. Radical vulvectomy
   D. Radical vulvectomy with ipsilateral inguinal-femoral lymphadenectomy
   E. Radical vulvectomy with bilateral inguinal-femoral lymphadenectomy

9. A 71-year-old woman with a 2-year history of progessive vulvar itching presents for treatment. The vulva has a homogeneous "onion skin" appearance. The vulvar biopsy you obtain as part of your evaluation is shown in Figure 30-1. What is your diagnosis?
   A. Hyperplastic dystrophy without atypia
   B. Hyperplastic dystrophy with atypia (VIN 2)
   C. Paget's disease
   D. Carcinoma in situ
   E. Lichen sclerosus

DIRECTIONS: For each numbered item, indicate whether it is associated with
A only (A)
B only (B)
C both (A) and (B)
D neither (A) nor (B)

Stage IB Lesions
(A) Squamous cell carcinoma of the vulva
(B) Melanoma of the vulva
(C) Both
(D) Neither

10. This cancer often bypasses the inguinal-femoral nodes and spreads directly to deep pelvic nodes.
11. Treated by radical vulvectomy and bilateral inguinal-femoral lymphadenectomy.

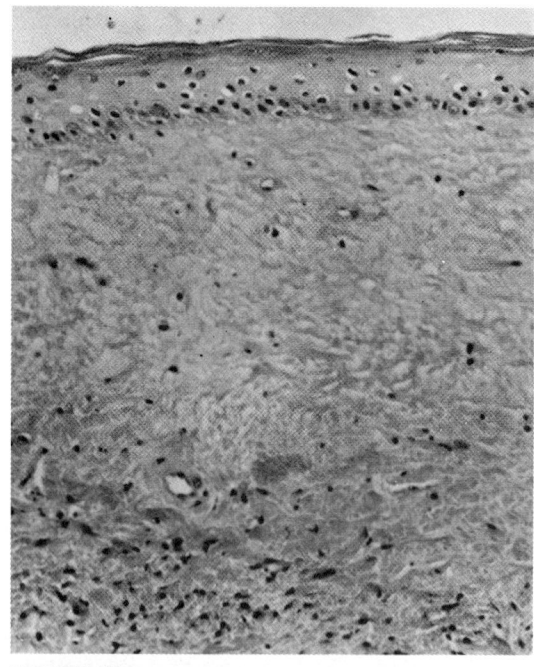

FIGURE 30-1.
(From Friedrich EG, Wilkinson EJ: The vulva. In Blaustein A, ed: Pathology of the female genital tract, 2nd ed. New York, Springer-Verlag, 1982.)

12. Depth of invasion most important prognostic factor
    (A) Pure lichen sclerosus
    (B) Pure hyperplastic dystrophy
    (C) Both
    (D) Neither
13. Best described as leukoplakia
14. Does not develop atypia or premalignant changes
15. May be classified using the vulvar intraepithelial neoplasia (VIN) rating
    (A) Femoral-inguinal lymph nodes
    (B) Deep pelvic nodes
    (C) Both
    (D) Neither
16. Primary sites of drainage for primary lesion of clitoris
17. Used in the TNM staging of vulvar carcinoma
18. Primary sites of drainage for primary lesion on labium majus
    (A) Figure 30-2
    (B) Figure 30-3
    (C) Both
    (D) Neither
19. Shows characteristics of hyperplastic vulvar dystrophy.
20. Consistent with changes of Paget's disease.
21. Topical fluorinated corticosteroids most efficacious.
    (A) Aneuploidy
    (B) Polyploidy
    (C) Both
    (D) Neither
22. Seen in DNA studies of vulvar biopsies showing vulvar atypia.
23. Requires total vulvectomy.
24. Associated with vulvar lesions that spontaneously regress.

DIRECTIONS: Each question contains four suggested answers of which one or more is correct. Choose the answer
A if 1, 2, and 3 are correct
B if 1 and 3 are correct
C if 2 and 4 are correct
D if 4 only is correct
E if all are correct

25. A 68-year-old woman has just had surgery for stage IB carcinoma of the vulva. She has positive inguinal-femoral nodes. Which factors are important in determining the next therapeutic step?
    1. Number of metastatic nodes
    2. Contiguity of metastatic nodes
    3. Size of metastatic nodes
    4. Proximity of metastatic nodes to the primary tumor

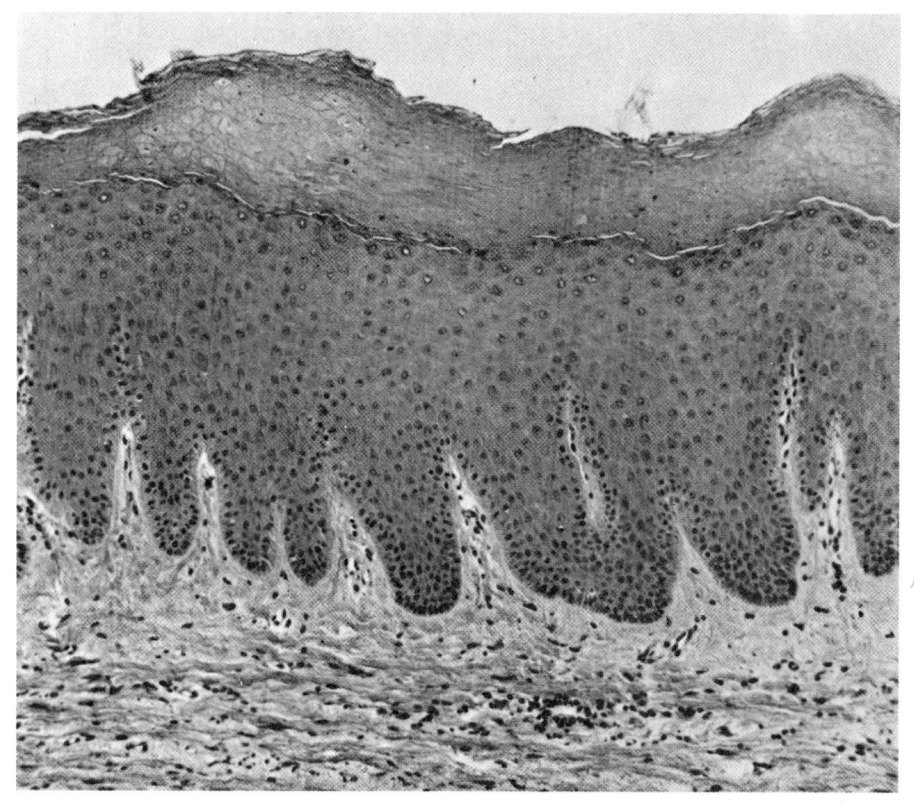

Premalignant and Malignant Diseases of the Vulva 199

FIGURE 30-2.
(From Friedrich EG, Wilkinson EJ: The vulva. In Blaustein A, ed: Pathology of the female genital tract, 2nd ed. New York, Springer-Verlag, 1982.)

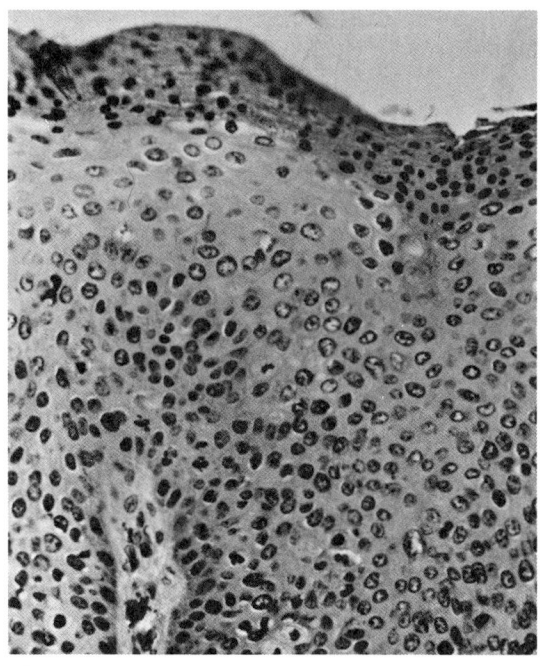

FIGURE 30-3.
(From Friedrich EG, Wilkinson EJ: The vulva. In Blaustein A, ed: Pathology of the female genital tract, 2nd ed. New York, Springer-Verlag, 1982.)

26. A 72-year-old woman presents with an 18-month history of progressive pruritus. The vulvar skin has a diffuse, reddened eczematoid appearance. The vulvar biopsy you obtained is reproduced in Figure 30-4. You advise the patient to
    1. have stool tested for blood.
    2. have mammography.
    3. have yearly cervical cytology.
    4. have total vulvectomy.
27. Which characteristics of stage I-A vulvar carcinoma are defined by the International Society for the Study of Vulvar Disease?
    1. A well-differentiated cellular architecture.
    2. A tumor less than 2 cm in diameter.
    3. Confluent tumor tongues penetrating stroma.
    4. Depth of invasion less than 1 mm from the basement membrane.

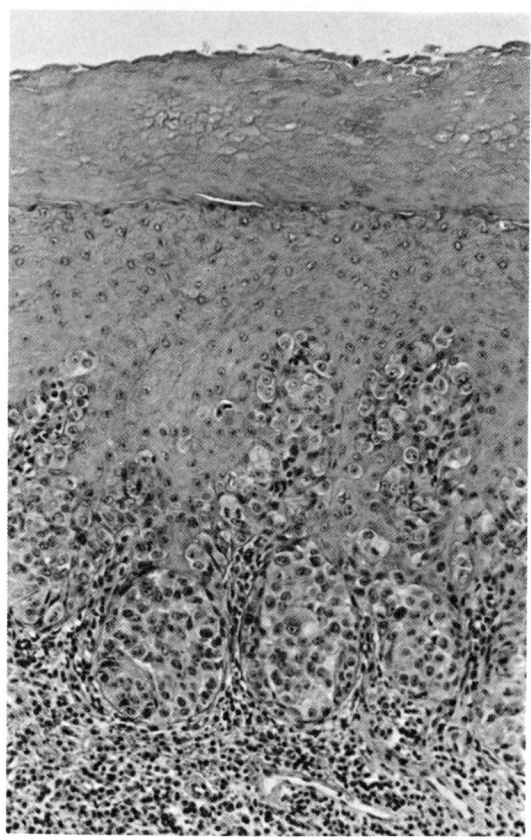

FIGURE 30-4.
(From Friedrich EG, Wilkinson EJ: The vulva. In Blaustein A, ed: Pathology of the female genital tract, 2nd ed. New York, Springer-Verlag, 1982.)

28. Excisional biopsy of a 4 mm pigmented, ulcerated lesion is performed on the left labium minus, near the clitoral hood of a 52-year-old woman. Histologic diagnosis confirms malignant melanoma. Correct observations regarding this lesion include:
    1. Melanoma is the most frequent nonsquamous malignancy of the vulva.
    2. Local excision is adequate treatment.
    3. Melanoma arises from compound nevi.
    4. Metastatic spread bypasses the inguinal-femoral node and progresses to the deep pelvic nodes.

ANSWERS

1. **A,** Pages 893–894. Effective therapy of Stage I or II and some early Stage III vulvar carcinomas can be accomplished with a radical vulvectomy and bilateral inguinal-femoral node dissection. Because of the patterns of lymphatic drainage, it is important with all invasive vulvar carcinomas to perform bilateral groin dissection. In view of recent evidence that suggests that deep pelvic nodes are virtually never involved unless the inguinal nodes are also involved, most oncologists now remove only the inguinal-femoral nodes at the time of primary surgery. Laser excision or primary radiation is unacceptable treatment.

    A deep pelvic node dissection can be done if, in the frozen or permanent section of histologic specimen, the inguinal-femoral nodes are found to be involved with tumor.

2. **D,** Page 894. A recent national cooperative randomized study suggests that radiation therapy to the deep pelvic nodes is superior to surgical therapy when it is known that the inguinal-femoral nodes contain tumor. This report shows improved survival for those who receive radiation of 4500 to 5000 rads.

    Although chemotherapy may be used for disseminated disease as a palliative measure, no chemotherapeutic regimen has been successful in treating this disease.

3. **E,** Page 887. Wide local excision is the best treatment for a patient with an isolated lesion of the posterior fourchette that proves to be carcinoma in situ.

    In the past, simple vulvectomy was widely practiced to treat carcinoma in situ of the vulva, but this disfiguring operation is now infrequently used and has been shown to be unnecessary. This is particularly true in younger women. Skinning vulvectomy has been advocated, followed by split-thickness vulvar skin grafting. In this case with a small lesion, such a procedure would constitute more treatment than is necessary. 5-Fluorouracil cream has also been used to treat carcinoma in situ of the vulva. It is successful in approximately 75% of cases. However, this treatment causes severe vulvar edema and pain over a prolonged period of time and usually is not prescribed for isolated lesions.

    Concentrated trichloroacetic acid applications are used to treat condyloma acuminata when they are *not* associated with severe vulvar intraepithelial neoplasia. This treatment is unacceptable for true cases of carcinoma in situ.

4. **D,** Page 893. For Stage IA lesions as defined by the ISSVD, therapy may be less extensive than is usually employed for invasive vulvar carcinoma. Based on currently available evidence, treatment for this lesion is controversial. Current tumor protocols are developed to evaluate the best therapy. It would appear that most patients with Stage IA carcinoma of the vulva would be treated with a modified radical or radical vulvectomy, according to this text. The lymph node dissection is omitted or deferred depending on the final pathologic evaluation of the primary tumor.

5. **E,** Page 884. The next step in managing a patient with lichen sclerosus would be topi-

cal testosterone cream. The efficacy of testosterone is excellent. It should be remembered that estrogen does not significantly affect changes in vulvar skin, although it promotes maturation and thickening of the vaginal epithelium. Vulvar colposcopy (vulvoscopy) is difficult since the colposcopic changes seen in the cervix are not present on the vulva. Simple vulvectomy is not warranted since the diagnosis has been established and the condition is benign.

6. **B**, Page 893. A typical invasive vulvar carcinoma usually appears as a slightly raised or polyploid mass. The patient frequently complains of a "sore" that has not healed. Prolonged vulvar pruritus is frequently associated with this disease. Delay in diagnosis is common because older patients frequently fail to seek prompt medical attention and often, when they do, a biopsy is not initially performed. In patients with this presentation, it is mandatory that office biopsy be performed immediately and certainly before initiating treatment. There is no need to perform wide local excision, as this well may be insufficient treatment. It is not an office procedure and will delay diagnosis. Topical treatment with corticosteroids is contraindicated before a tissue diagnosis is made. Both laser vaporization and office cryocautery of lesions such as this are contraindicated until a specific diagnosis is made.

7. **D**, Page 896. Bartholin's gland carcinoma is an adenocarcinoma and comprises 1% to 2% of vulvar cancers. An enlargement of the Bartholin's gland in a postmenopausal woman should raise the suspicion for this malignancy. Since this complaint is rarely associated with acute inflammation in a postmenopausal woman, one should biopsy all such masses in this age group. Empiric treatment with laser or topical agents is not warranted unless indicated by the biopsy results. Exam with a magnifying device such as a colposcope would not be useful in this patient since the lesion is below the epithelium. Simple incision and drainage is not appropriate unless representative samples of tissue are submitted for pathologic examination first.

These tumors are treated similarly to primary squamous cell carcinoma of the vulva, and radical vulvectomy with bilateral inguinal-femoral lymphadenectomy is the treatment of choice.

8. **B**, Page 896. Verrucous carcinoma is a rare tumor that may attain considerable size but is generally indolent in its behavior. Wide local excision is usually effective therapy. Radical vulvectomy, and radical vulvectomy with either ipsilateral or bilateral inguinal lymphadenectomy are not necessary. Laser ablation is insufficient to remove the deeper tissues. Radiation therapy is ineffective, can worsen the prognosis, and is therefore contraindicated for these tumors.

9. **E**, Pages 878–879. The changes shown in this photomicrograph are typical for lichen sclerosus. Usually the epithelium becomes markedly thinner with the loss or blunting of the rete ridges. The superficial portion of the dermis is hyalinized while the deep portion contains a lymphocytic infiltrate. This is not a premalignant condition, but it tends to be multifocal and usually reoccurs.

10–12. 10, **D**; 11, **C**; 12, **B**; Pages 897–898. It was previously believed that a melanoma of the vulva would metastasize to the deep pelvic nodes, bypassing the inguinal-femoral nodes. Recent studies have failed to demonstrate deep pelvic node involvement without inguinal node spread. This is similar to observations made with squamous cell carcinomas of the vulva.

The standard therapy for vulvar melanoma has been radical vulvectomy and bilateral inguinal-femoral node dissection for all lesions with the depth of penetration to level 3 or greater. This is the same therapy recommended for stage IB squamous cell carcinoma of the vulva.

Although melanomas are staged using the FIGO classification employed for squamous carcinomas, recent evidence indicates that staging is not as useful a prognostic indicator as depth of invasion. A system for vulvar melanoma classification is similar to that used by Clark for cutaneous melanomas. Five levels (I–V) have been defined (Figure 30-5). Regional node involvement is not likely to occur if the melanoma thickness measured from the surface epithelium to the deepest point is less than .76 mm. Most of these lesions correspond to level I or level II, according to the modified Clark system. Such melanomas can probably be successfully treated by wide local excision without inguinal-femoral node dissection. Although no long-term results are available, the 5-year survival has been reported to be excellent.

13–15. 13, **D**; 14, **A**; 15, **B**; Pages 878–879. The International Society for the Study of Vulvar Diseases (ISSVD) has provided a standard nomenclature to assist in minimizing the ambiguities previously used to describe premalignant vulvar disease.

Vulvar dystrophies are of two types: lichen sclerosus, a benign condition that does not develop atypia, and hyperplastic dystrophy, which may include atypia. Hyperplastic dystrophy with atypia may be classified as vulvar intraepithelial neoplasia (VIN), depending on the degree of cellular atypia on the biopsy specimen.

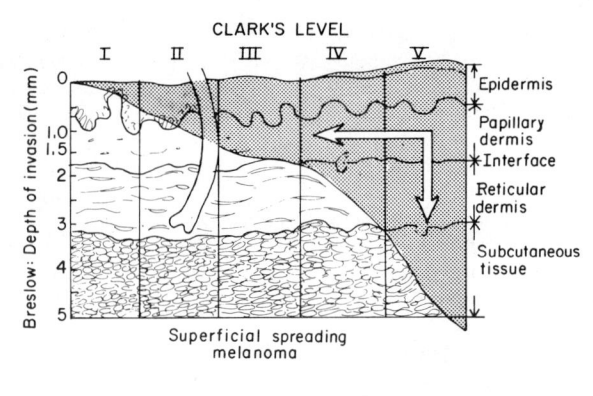

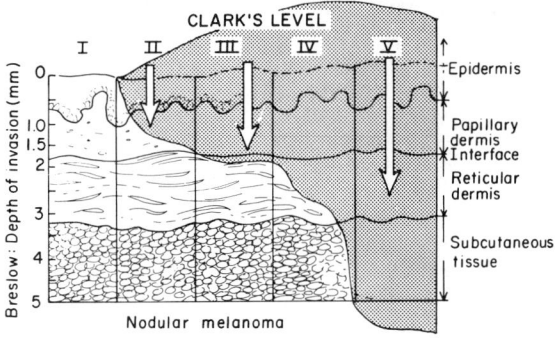

FIGURE 30-5.
Level of invasion for superficial spreading melanoma and nodular melanoma.
(From Podratz KC, Gaffey TA, Symmonds RE, et al: Gynecol Oncol 16:153, 1983.)

The term leukoplakia (white plaque) should not be used when describing vulvar changes.

These two types of dystrophies may be mixed, and if they are, the hyperplastic component may also be graded according to the VIN classification.

16–18. 16, **A**; 17, **C**; 18, **A**; Pages 889–890; Figure 30-15 (from Droegemueller). Knowledge of the lymphatic drainage of the vulva is important in order to stage vulvar carcinoma and plan surgical therapy. Recent studies have concluded that lesions in various quadrants of the vulva follow predictable patterns of spread. Radioactive dye studies confirm that over 90% of the lymphatic drainage of the labium majus or labium minus is to the ipsilateral femoral-inguinal lymph node complex. These same studies indicate that drainage from the clitoris and perineum follows a bilateral nodal distribution. No direct connection from the clitoris to the deep pelvic nodes has been demonstrated.

If the deep pelvic nodes are involved with the tumor, they are considered metastases and may be used in the TNM classification. It has been shown that when the deep pelvic nodes are involved, in almost every case the regional femoral-inguinal lymph nodes are involved first.

19–21. 19, **C**; 20, **D**; 21, **A**; Pages 879, 880, 884. Figure 30-2 depicts benign hyperplastic dystrophy and Figure 30-3 is a higher power view of vulvar intraepithelial neoplasia grade III. With hyperplastic dystrophy, there is a change in vulvar epithelial layers. Hystologically there is elongation and widening of the rete ridges, which may become confluent. The surface layer is hyperkeratotic and the tissue grossly is white or red. When atypical changes occur (Figure 30-3), there is a marked loss of the maturation process in the squamous epithelium as well as an increase in mitotic activity and in the nuclear-cytoplasmic ratio. Treatment for VIN III includes wide local excision or vaporization by laser. Treatment for hyperplastic dystrophy without atypia is best accomplished by topical corticosteroids.

Neither of these lesions are typical of Paget's disease. Paget cells are large pale cells that often occur in nests and infiltrate upward through the epithelium.

22–24. 22, **C**; 23, **D**; 24, **B**; Pages 886–887. Recent studies of nuclear DNA content of vulvar atypias suggest that not all lesions with this designation are premalignant. A polyploidy distribution of nuclear DNA is consistent with a benign process, while aneuploidy is consistent with true intraepithelial neoplasia with a potential chance of progressing to frank malignancy. Lesions containing polyploid DNA material have been noted to regress spontaneously.

Lesions associated with aneuploidy by DNA studies do not require total vulvectomy, even though they may be considered true intraepithelial neoplasia. This treatment is reserved for patients with extensive carcinoma in situ and, even here, the trend is to avoid total vulvectomy. Focal vulvar epithelial neoplasia may be treated by wide local excision or by laser vaporization.

25. **B** (1, 3), Pages 894–895. Survival of patients with vulvar carcinoma is directly related to the presence of metastatic disease in regional lymph nodes. After radical vulvectomy and bilateral node dissection, there is about 95% 5-year survival for patients with negative regional lymph nodes. As the number of metastatic nodes increase, the 5-year survival diminishes progressively. There is also a direct correlation between survival and metastatic nodal size. Those lesions associated with higher nodal tumor volume are generally associated with earlier recurrence and decreased survival rates.

The contiguity, that is, the number of nodes in sequence that contain metastatic disease, is not known to be related to recurrence or survival, and likewise the proximity of the first metastatic node to the primary tumor seems unimportant. These findings may relate to the diffuse drainage pattern from the primary tumor site to the regional nodes.

Information regarding the number and size of metastatic nodes is important in considering additional radiation therapy for patients with two or more positive lymph nodes.

26. **E** (All), Pages 880, 882–883, 888. This is a patient with Paget's disease. Paget's disease of the vulva is generally seen in postmenopausal women with a long history of vulvar pruritus and is frequently associated with other invasive carcinomas. The major importance of Paget's disease of the vulva is the frequent association with other invasive carcinomas. They may present as squamous carcinoma of the vulva or cervix, adenocarcinoma of the sweat glands of the vulva, or as Bartholin's gland carcinoma. Cases of adenocarcinoma of the GI tract accompanying Paget's disease have also been reported. Thus once a diagnosis of Paget's disease of the vulva is made, it is important for the gynecologist to rule out the presence of malignancy at other sites, including the breast.

If no primary malignancy is uncovered, a total vulvectomy is usually performed. It is important to remove the full thickness of the skin to the subcutaneous fat to be certain that all of the skin adnexal structures are excised, as they may have a subclinical malignancy. Those women who have been treated for Paget's disease of the vulva should have as part of the routine follow-up annual examination of the breast, cytologic evaluation of the cervix and vulva, and screening for gastrointestinal disease at least by testing for occult blood in the stool.

27. **C** (2, 4); Page 893. The International Society for the Study of Vulvar Disease has recommended that the term *microinvasion* be dropped and the designation *stage IA* be used for tumors less than 2 cm in diameter with depth of invasion less than 1 mm from the epidermal-stromal junction (basement membrane). This was instituted because the term *microinvasive carcinoma of the vulva* had no uniformly accepted definition. The purpose of identifying this group of tumors is to predict early tumors that are unlikely to spread to regional nodes and thus avoid the need for regional lymph node dissection. Cellular differentiation is not included in this classification, nor is the architecture of the tumor tongues important. Although there is almost no risk of metastases to regional nodes in stage IA lesions, late recurrence of these tumors can develop years after primary therapy.

28. **B** (1, 3), Pages 896–897. Melanoma is the most frequent nonsquamous cell malignancy of the vulva, comprising about 5% of primary cancers of this area. Although the diagnosis may be established by excisional biopsy, the treatment should be provided by radical vulvectomy and bilateral inguinal-femoral lymphadenectomy. Pelvic node dissection is reserved for those patients who have positive inguinal-femoral nodes. Melanomas may arise from either junctional or compound nevi. Although previously thought to bypass the inguinal femoral node complex and progress directly to the deep pelvic nodes, recent series have not demonstrated pelvic node involvement without inguinal node involvement.

CHAPTER 31
Premalignant and Malignant Diseases of the Vagina

DIRECTIONS: Select the one best answer or completion.

1. Recurrences of squamous cell carcinoma of the vagina are most likely to occur as
   A. local recurrence.
   B. bone metastases.
   C. liver metastases.
   D. lung metastases.
   E. brain metastases.

2. Which of the following treatment modalities is most frequently used in the treatment of squamous cell carcinoma of the vagina?
   A. Laser ablation
   B. Wide local excision
   C. Radical surgery
   D. Radiation therapy
   E. Chemotherapy

3. The current recommendation for the initial evaluation of girls exposed to DES in utero is to examine them
   A. following menarche.
   B. following menarche or by age 14, whichever is first.
   C. at age 18.
   D. when they are sexually active.
   E. under anesthesia.

4. The term *field defect* in gynecology denotes
   A. a blind spot in the visual field as a result of metastatic genital cancer.
   B. the propensity of the squamous epithelium of the lower genital tract to undergo premalignant change.
   C. herniation of fatty tissue through the inguinal canal.
   D. adenosis of the vagina as a result of in utero exposure to DES.
   E. in the treatment of vaginal carcinoma, an area not affected by radiation therapy.

5. Vaginal cancer stage II denotes
   A. ureteric involvement.
   B. the lesion extends to the pelvic wall.
   C. the lesion is limited to the vaginal wall.
   D. the lesion involves subvaginal tissue, but does not extend to the pelvic wall.
   E. the lesion involves the rectal mucosa.

6. An 80-year-old woman who is in good health has a routine gynecological examination. She had a total abdominal hysterectomy at age 45 for benign disease. The pap smear is reported as severe atrophy with inflammatory changes and a few atypical cells. Appropriate management consists of
   A. topical 5-FU.
   B. repeat pap smear in one year.
   C. a course of estrogen followed by repeat pap smear in 3 months.
   D. colposcopy.
   E. vaginectomy.

7. A patient with primary squamous cell carcinoma of the vagina is found to have hydronephrosis. The tumor seems to be filling the pelvis, but the bladder and rectum appear to be free of disease. The remainder of her evaluation fails to reveal distant disease. What is the appropriate stage to be assigned for this patient?
   A. 0
   B. I
   C. II
   D. III
   E. IV

8. A 60-year-old female presents to your office complaining of vaginal bleeding. Until this event she was healthy and was not receiving any medications. On examination, a fungating ulcerative lesion is found on the left lateral wall of the vagina near the fornix. What is the proper management?
   A. Pap smear
   B. Colposcopy
   C. Biopsy
   D. Vaginectomy
   E. Radiation therapy

9. A 41-year-old patient underwent total abdominal hysterectomy for moderate dysplasia of the cervix. This patient should be advised that she
   A. does not need to have a pap smear done anymore.
   B. needs a pap smear every 4 or 5 years.
   C. needs a pap smear every 2 or 3 years.
   D. needs a pap smear annually.
   E. should be followed with yearly colposcopic examinations only.

10. In carcinoma in situ (VAIN-III), abnormal cells are
    A. confined to the outer third of the epithelium.
    B. confined to the inner two thirds of the epithelium.
    C. throughout the entire thickness of the epithelium.
    D. invading the basement membrane.
    E. invading subepithelial tissues.
11. A 2-year-old girl is seen after passing a "grape-like" structure from the vagina. Otherwise, the girl is asymptomatic. One should
    A. obtain vaginal secretions for culture and sensitivity.
    B. admit the child for observation in the hospital.
    C. perform vaginoscopy under anesthesia.
    D. empirically treat the child with penicillin.
    E. warn the parents about the problem of the child's inserting foreign objects into the vagina.
12. A 72-year-old woman who is 10 years status posthysterectomy is referred for the evaluation of two abnormal pap smears. What is the next step in her management?
    A. Vaginectomy.
    B. Repeat pap smear in 3 months.
    C. Treat with cryotherapy.
    D. Perform colposcopy and biopsy suspicious areas.
    E. Treat with topical 5-FU.

DIRECTIONS: For each numbered item, indicate whether it is associated with
A only (A)
B only (B)
C both (A) and (B)
D neither (A) nor (B)

(A) Radical hysterectomy and vaginectomy
(B) Radiation therapy
(C) Both
(D) Neither
Appropriate treatment for:
13. VAIN-III
14. Stage II clear cell adenocarcinoma of the vagina
15. Stage III squamous cell carcinoma of the vagina
    (A) Clear cell carcinoma of the vagina
    (B) Squamous cell carcinoma of the vagina
    (C) Both
    (D) Neither
16. Histologically demonstrates hobnail cells
17. In utero exposure to DES
18. Chemotherapy is the first line of treatment
    (A) Endodermal sinus tumor of the vagina
    (B) Vaginal squamous cell carcinoma
    (C) Both
    (D) Neither
19. Affects mainly older women
20. Secretes α-feto-protein
    (A) VAIN-I
    (B) CIN I
    (C) Both
    (D) Neither
21. Associated with HPV infection
22. Requires radiation therapy
23. Can be detected on a pap smear
24. Characterized by abnormal maturation of the epithelium

DIRECTIONS: Each question contains four suggested answers of which one or more is correct. Choose the answer
A if 1, 2, and 3 are correct
B if 1 and 3 are correct
C if 2 and 4 are correct
D if 4 only is correct
E if all are correct

25. Malignant melanoma of the vagina
    1. is relatively common and therefore all pigmented lesions should be excised.
    2. affects older patients.
    3. rarely metastasizes.
    4. invades deeply into the tissues.
26. The diagnosis of sarcoma Botryoides is established in a 2-year-old. Proper management of the patient should include
    1. chemotherapy.
    2. surgery.
    3. radiation therapy.
    4. hormone therapy.
27. Which symptoms are most commonly associated with vaginal cancer?
    1. Vaginal discharge
    2. Urinary frequency
    3. Abnormal vaginal bleeding
    4. Tenesmus
28. The presence of an abnormal vaginal epithelium can be detected by using
    1. Lugol's stain.
    2. colposcopy.
    3. vaginal cytology.
    4. vaginogram.
29. True statements regarding vaginal carcinoma include:
    1. Most vaginal malignancies are metastatic from somewhere else.
    2. The most common histologic type of primary vaginal cancer is squamous cell carcinoma.
    3. HPV infection increases the risk of neoplastic changes in the vagina.
    4. Most vaginal malignancies occur in females exposed to DES in utero.

30. Appropriate modalities used in the treatment of Ca-in-situ of the vagina include
    1. vaginectomy.
    2. laser ablation.
    3. radiation therapy.
    4. 5-FU cream.
31. The interpretation of routine pap smears is adversely affected by
    1. vaginal infection.
    2. *Condylomata accuminata*.
    3. menopausal changes.
    4. menstruation.
32. Factors affecting the prognosis of patients with clear cell adenocarcinoma of the vagina include
    1. age of patient.
    2. size of tumor.
    3. depth of invasion.
    4. histologic pattern.
33. True statements concerning the treatment of vaginal cancer include:
    1. Vaginal cancer near the cervix is treated like cervical cancer.
    2. Squamous cell carcinoma Stage I of the vagina can be easily removed by carbon dioxide laser ablation.
    3. Vaginal cancer situated near the introitus is treated like vulvar cancer.
    4. Adjuvant radiation therapy is recommended in all cases of vaginal carcinoma.
34. Primary vaginal cancer
    1. accounts for 2% of all gynecologic malignancies.
    2. usually occurs as squamous cell carcinoma.
    3. Most commonly affects women over the age of 50.
    4. Often extends to the cervix to include the external os.
35. True statements regarding the use of laser in the treatment of vaginal intraepithelial neoplasia include:
    1. The depth of ablation is regulated in part by the wattage of the laser.
    2. Iodine staining of the vagina will outline areas requiring laser therapy.
    3. Follow-up every 4 months, including pap smear and colposcopy, is advised for the first year and every 6 to 12 months thereafter.
    4. The healing process requires only a few days.
36. Appropriate therapy for VAIN includes:
    1. cryotherapy.
    2. laser ablation.
    3. 5-fluorouracil cream.
    4. surgical excision.
37. A recognized or acceptable protocol for the initial treatment of a patient with malignant melanoma of the vagina may include
    1. radical surgery.
    2. radiation therapy.
    3. systemic chemotherapy.
    4. immunotherapy (Interleukin II).

ANSWERS

1. **A,** Page 909. Initially squamous cell carcinoma of the vagina recurs locally, just as squamous cell carcinoma of the cervix and vulva does. Although distant metastases do occur, most patients will present with local recurrences. Since an effective chemotherapy program for recurrent vaginal carcinoma has not been developed, in patients who have only localized recurrence, an exenterative procedure should be considered if the tumor was initially treated with radiation.
2. **D,** Pages 908–909. In recent years, radiation therapy has been the most frequent mode of treatment for squamous cell carcinoma of the vagina. External radiation therapy with megavoltage equipment is utilized initially to shrink the tumor. This is followed by a local cesium radium implant placed interstitially with needles or by intracavitary radiation using a tandem or ovoids similar to the delivery systems used for cervical carcinoma.
3. **B,** Pages 363, 910. The current recommendations for the initial evaluation of girls exposed to DES in utero are: 1. at any age when symptomatic 2. when a-symptomatic: at menarche, or at age 14, whichever comes first.
4. **B,** Page 901. Field defect describes the propensity of squamous epithelium of the lower genital tract (cervix, vagina, and vulva) to undergo premalignant changes. The epithelium of the lower genital tract is derived from a common embryonic origin. Since these structures are subjected to similar environmental stimulants, (for example, human papillomavirus and herpes simplex virus type II), similar premalignant changes might be anticipated. Areas of such neoplastic changes need not be contiguous and, in fact, may arise in multiple sites throughout the genital tract. The recognition of field defect is important since patients with CIN are more likely to also develop vaginal intraepithelial neoplasia (VAIN) or vulvar intraepithelial neoplasia (VIN).
5. **D,** Page 907. The staging of vaginal cancer according to FIGO is done following clinical evaluation. This includes EUA, cystoscopy, sigmoidoscopy, and imaging studies (that is, IVP, barium enema). Stage II involves subvaginal tissue, but does not extend to the pelvic wall.
6. **C,** Page 906. An abnormal pap smear requires further evaluation. Since estrogen deficient

state may adversely affect the interpretation of the pap smear, it should be repeated after the patient is given estrogen replacement therapy. Colposcopic evaluation of the atrophic vaginal epithelium may be difficult due to chronic inflammatory changes. If the repeat pap smear following ERT is abnormal, colposcopic evaluation and biopsies are necessary at that time.

7. **D**, Page 907. The lesion extends into the pelvis and obstructs a ureter, indicating that the lesion has extended to the pelvic wall. The appropriate stage to be assigned according to the FIGO classification is stage III.

8. **C**, Pages 906–911. A large fungating ulcerative lesion at this age group is likely to be a neoplasm. A biopsy of this or any significant lesion is a rapid and accurate mode of diagnosis and should be performed at the initial visit. Treatment should not be undertaken until a diagnosis is made. A diagnosis is based on biopsy, not on pap smear results.

9. **D**, Pages 758, 901. Considering what has been termed a field defect—the tendency to develop premalignant changes along the lower genital tract—this patient with premalignant changes of the cervix is more likely to develop premalignant changes of the vagina. If left undetected, this may progress to invasive cancer. A patient who has had moderate cervical dysplasia is at an increased risk to develop a vaginal or vulvar malignancy. As a screening tool vaginal cytology rather than colposcopy remains most cost effective.

10. **C**, Page 903. Carcinoma in situ (VAIN-III) denotes an intraepithelial neoplasm not invading the basement membrane or involving the subepithelial tissues but in which dysplastic cells extend throughout the entire epithelial layer.

11. **C**, Page 912. Although children sometimes insert foreign bodies into the vagina, passing a "grapelike" structure by a 2-year-old is extremely suspicious for the presence of a sarcoma botryoides. Since the prognosis for the child is directly related to the rapidity in which the diagnosis is established, one should perform vaginoscopy under anesthesia and biopsy all suspicious lesions as soon as possible.

12. **D**, Page 905. The patient presents with two abnormal pap smears and thus requires further evaluation. Once an abnormal smear from vaginal epithelium is identified, a biopsy is required for histologic identification. Some individuals might prefer to treat this woman for a few weeks with vaginal estrogen. Following this, they would perform colposcopy, biopsy suspicious areas, and perhaps repeat the pap smear. Since the patient already has had two abnormal pap smears, observation or repeat pap smears at regular intervals would delay detection of significant vaginal lesions. Neither cryotherapy nor vaginectomy is warranted until the disease and its extent are delineated.

13–15. 13, **D**; 14, **A**; 15, **B**; Pages 906–910. In a patient with vaginal intraepithelial neoplasia (VAIN), local excision or laser ablation of the epithelium is the procedure of choice.

Radiation therapy is most often utilized for treatment in patients with extensive vaginal carcinoma. Patients with stage III squamous cell carcinoma of the vagina would normally receive radiation therapy.

In young patients with clear cell adenocarcinoma, an attempt should be made to preserve ovarian function and coital function. Thus, radical hysterectomy with partial or complete vaginectomy, pelvic lymphadenectomy, and vaginal reconstruction is most often performed. When the tumor is extremely small, the use of local irradiation may be sufficient to ablate the tumor and preserve fertility. A stage II lesion would not fall into this category.

16–18. 16, **A**; 17, **A**; 18, **D**; Pages 907–911. Hobnail cells extruding into the lumina of tubular structures is characteristic appearance of the tubulocystic pattern of clear cell adenocarcinoma. Clear cell adenocarcinoma may have other patterns as well, such as solid or papillary. It affects young women, usually with a history of in utero exposure to DES. The tumor is rarely found in patients who do not have a history of DES exposure. Chemotherapy is reserved for patients with systemic disease or patients who failed other modalities of therapy.

19–20. 19, **B**; 20, **A**; Pages 901, 905. An endodermal sinus tumor (adenocarcinoma) is a rare vaginal tumor. It affects very young girls, usually under the age of 2. The tumor is aggressive, with an unfavorable prognosis since the tumor is usually fatal. It produces alpha-fetoprotein, which can be detected in the serum and can serve as a tumor marker. On the other hand, squamous cell carcinoma is the most common of the vaginal tumors, affecting mostly older women. It often occurs in a patient who has had or will develop other squamous cell tumors of the genital tract, particularly squamous cell carcinoma of the cervix.

21–24. 21, **C**; 22, **D**; 23, **C**; 24, **C**; Pages 901–902. VAIN is the abbreviation used to describe intraepithelial neoplasms of the vagina, while CIN is used to describe cervical intraepithelial neoplasms. Both conditions are a result of a faulty maturation process in the surface epithelium. Risk factors include previous venereal disease, herpes virus type II infection, human papilloma virus infection, and sexual activity at an early age with multiple sexual partners. Both lesions result in the exfoliation of abnormal cells into the vagina, which can be detected on a routine pap smear collected from the cervix and the posterior vaginal pool.

25. **C** (2, 4), Page 912. Malignant melanoma of the vagina is a rare neoplasm with only about 100 cases reported to date. It affects older patients (mean age 60). The lesion invades deeply into the subvaginal tissue and metastasizes extensively. Pigmented lesions of the lower genital tract are more likely than pigmented lesions elsewhere in the body to undergo malignant transformation and therefore, if there is any question regarding a pigmented lesion, it should be excised and submitted for histologic evaluation.

26. **A** (1, 2, 3), Page 913. Although exenterative procedures were performed in the past in the treatment of children with embryonal rhabdomyosarcoma (sarcoma Botryoides), effective control with less radical surgery appears to have been achieved with a multimodality approach consisting of chemotherapy (with vincristine, actinomycin D, and cyclophosphamide) and/or pelvic irradiation. When the tumor is reduced in size by this treatment, hysterectomy and vaginectomy often follow.

27. **B** (1 ,3), Page 907. The most common symptom of vaginal cancer is abnormal vaginal bleeding or discharge. Urinary frequency is sometimes noted in patients with a large anterior lesion, whereas tenesmus is noted in patients with a large posterior lesion. These symptoms appear only when the lesions are large and therefore quite late in the disease course. Similarly, pain is usually a symptom of an advanced tumor that has invaded deep into the tissues.

28. **A** (1, 2, 3), Pages 905–906. The presence of dysplastic vaginal epithelium is most frequently detected initially on pap smear. The abnormal area can be delineated by colposcopy or Lugol's stain. It should be biopsied for histologic evaluation. A vaginogram is a radiologic study of the vagina and would have no place in the evaluation of vaginal epithelial dysplasia.

29. **A** (1, 2, 3), Page 905. Primary vaginal cancer is rare. Most vaginal malignancies are metastatic, primarily from the cervix and endometrium. The most common histologic type of primary vaginal cancer is squamous cell carcinoma. As in cervical cancer, early sexual activity, multiple partners, previous herpes and human papillomavirus infection, and radiation increase a woman's risk for the later development of vaginal malignancy.

30. **C** (2, 4), Pages 905–906. While both vaginectomy and radiation therapy would ablate carcinoma in situ of the vagina, this would be considered overtreatment. The lesion is limited to the epithelial area only and thus removing the epithelial layer, either with laser therapy or the application of 5-FU cream, is sufficient. In both instances, follow-up is required to assure elimination of all abnormal areas. Like all patients with lower genital tract malignancies, the patient is at a higher risk of developing similar neoplasms along the lower genital tract. Close surveillance is necessary for the remainder of the patient's life.

31. **E** (All), Pages 743, 905–906. Inflammatory changes and estrogen deficiency affect the appearance of the exfoliating cells and thus make interpretation of cytologic smears more difficult. HPV infection results in cellular changes which can be mistakenly thought to be neoplastic. It is recommended that an infection be treated and cleared and that patients with severe atrophic changes be given hormonal replacement treatment. The cytologic smears should be repeated following completion of therapy. Menstrual blood obscures the sample, creating technical difficulties.

32. **E** (All), Page 910. Favorable factors in survival of patients with clear cell adenocarcinoma of the vagina include:
    1. Low stage
    2. Older age
    3. Tubulocystic pattern
    4. Small tumor diameter
    5. Reduced depth of invasion
    6. No lymph node involvement

33. **B** (1, 3), Pages 907–909. The lymphatic drainage of the upper vagina is similar to the lymphatic drainage of the cervix, while drainage of the lower vagina is similar to the lymphatics of the vulva. This fact has important therapeutic implications. Tumors of the upper vagina are treated as cervical cancer, whereas tumors of the lower vagina are treated as vulvar cancer. Stage I vaginal carcinoma denotes invasive cancer limited to the vaginal wall that cannot be removed by local ablation. The most common treatment for vaginal cancer is radiation. Since early cancer of the cervix and the vulva are treated surgically, vaginal carcinomas near these areas are often treated surgically. Adjuvant radiation therapy should be given to patients in whom the margins are not clear or lymph node involvement is detected.

34. **A** (1, 2, 3), Page 907. Primary vaginal cancers account for only 2% of all gynecologic malignancies. The most common type is squamous cell carcinoma, which predominantly affects women over the age of 50. To be considered a primary vaginal neoplasm, the tumor must arise in the vagina and not involve the external os of the cervix superiorly or the vulva inferiorly. If the tumor does involve either of these organs, it is considered to be a primary cervical or vulvar lesion, respectively, unless it is of the clear cell variety.

35. **A** (1, 2, 3), Pages 905–906. Laser therapy is useful in the management of vaginal intraepithelial neoplasia. Abnormal epithelium can be removed by adjusting the wattage to 15 or 20 watts and allowing the laser to vaporize to a depth of 2 to 4 mm. The healing usually requires a few weeks. Regular follow-up every 4 months, including a pap smear and colposcopy, is advised during the first year and every 6 to 12 months thereafter. These patients are more prone to develop intraepithelial neoplasms throughout the lower genital tract and must be monitored appropriately for these changes.
36. **E** (All), Pages 905–906. The premalignant changes of VAIN are localized to that epithelial layer alone. Ablation of the epithelium results in eradication of the disease. Cryotherapy, laser ablation, 5-fluorouracil cream application, and surgical excision of small lesions are all accepted methods of removing these lesions. Patients needs to be followed closely over the next year to insure that the lesions have been eradicated. These patients are more prone to develop premalignant changes in other organs (field defect); thus, long-term follow-up is required.
37. **E** (All), Page 912. Treatment of patients with malignant melanoma of the vagina consists of radical surgery with wide excision of the vagina, uterus, and dissection of the retroperitoneal nodes (pelvic and/or inguinal). Lower vaginal lesions require treatment similar to vulvar carcinoma, whereas upper vaginal lesions require treatment similar to cervical carcinoma. Adjunctive radiation therapy and chemotherapy also have been used. Despite all this, the 5-year survival is dismal. Local recurrence is common and the disease is usually fatal. Recently, introduction of immunotherapy with autotransfusion with white blood cells treated with Interleukin II have shown some response, and malignant melanoma is considered one of the diseases to be approved for such treatment.

CHAPTER 32

Malignant Disease of the Fallopian Tube

DIRECTIONS: Select the one best answer or completion.

1. At the time of exploratory laparotomy for a right adnexal mass in a 60-year-old patient, a dilated right fallopian tube is discovered. When opened it is found to be filled with tumor. No other tumors are noted, but the peritoneal fluid is found to be positive for malignant cells. What is the "unofficial stage" of the tubal carcinoma?
   A. Ia
   B. Ib
   C. Ic
   D. II
   E. III

2. A 57-year-old patient complains of vaginal bleeding, a profuse, intermittent watery discharge, and lower abdominal pain. On pelvic examination, a 5 cm right adnexal mass is palpated. These findings are most typical of
   A. functional ovarian cyst.
   B. ovarian carcinoma.
   C. endometrial carcinoma.
   D. fallopian tube carcinoma.
   E. leiomyosarcoma.

3. What percentage of patients with fallopian tube carcinoma have positive vaginal cytology?
   A. 10%
   B. 30%
   C. 50%
   D. 70%
   E. 90%

4. Where does the least common primary female genital tract malignancy originate?
   A. Ovary
   B. Fallopian tube
   C. Uterus
   D. Vagina
   E. Vulva

5. The family of a patient with tubal carcinoma confined to the tube (stage I) asks about the prognosis. You would tell them that 5-year survival is
   A. less than 5%.
   B. 10% to 20%.
   C. 30% to 40%.
   D. 50% to 60%.
   E. 70% to 80%.

6. In performing an exploratory laparotomy for a suspected tubal carcinoma, what should be the first step upon entering the abdominal cavity?
   A. Ligation of the distal and proximal ends of the affected tube.
   B. Palpation of the liver.
   C. Palpation of the paraaortic nodes.
   D. Obtaining peritoneal cytology.
   E. Removal of the adnexa.

7. A 62-year-old patient has persistent uterine bleeding despite two D&Cs and two trials of conjugated equine estrogens–progestin therapy. No endometrial pathology has been found and the pelvic examination is unremarkable. What should be the next step?
   A. Vaginal hysterectomy
   B. Abdominal hysterectomy
   C. Laparoscopy
   D. Irradiation of the pelvis
   E. Hysteroscopy with laser ablation of the endometrium

8. At the time of exploratory laparotomy, a 30-year-old gravida 1, para 1 is found to have a primary tubal carcinoma confined to the right tube. What is the appropriate operation?
   A. Right salpingectomy.
   B. Right salpingo-oophorectomy.
   C. Bilateral salpingectomy.
   D. Bilateral salpingo-oophorectomy.
   E. Total abdominal hysterectomy with bilateral salpingo-oophorectomy.

9. Where is the most frequent site of metastatic spread of tubal carcinoma?
   A. Liver
   B. Lung
   C. Bone
   D. Peritoneum
   E. Retroperitoneal nodes

10. Adenocarcinoma of the fallopian tube occurs most commonly in patients who are
    A. 40–49 years old
    B. 50–59 years old
    C. 60–69 years old
    D. 70–79 years old
    E. 80–89 years old

11. How is the diagnosis of primary tubal carcinoma most commonly made?
    A. History
    B. Physical examination
    C. Ultrasound
    D. CT scan
    E. Surgical exploration
12. The classic symptoms in a postmenopausal woman suggestive of tubal carcinoma are included in which triad?
    A. Pain, watery discharge, anorexia.
    B. Bleeding, watery discharge, adnexal mass.
    C. Bleeding, pain, adnexal mass.
    D. Anorexia, watery discharge, bleeding.
    E. Anorexia, pain, adnexal mass.
13. In which cancer is pain the most frequent presenting symptom?
    A. Ovary
    B. Fallopian tube
    C. Endometrium
    D. Cervix
    E. None of the above

DIRECTIONS: For each numbered item, indicate whether it is associated with
A only (A)
B only (B)
C both (A) and (B)
D neither (A) nor (B)

(A) Primary tubal carcinoma
(B) Primary ovarian carcinoma
(C) Both
(D) Neither

14. Commonly spreads to paraaortic nodes
15. Overall 5-year survival exceeds 50%
16. Less common than metastatic disease

DIRECTIONS: Each question contains four suggested answers of which one or more is correct. Choose the answer
A if 1, 2, and 3 are correct
B if 1 and 3 are correct
C if 2 and 4 are correct
D if 4 only is correct
E if all are correct

17. Which criteria are used to diagnose primary tubal carcinoma?
    1. The tumor is primarily within the lumen of the tube.
    2. The mucosa of the tube is involved with the tumor.
    3. A transition can be demonstrated between the malignant and nonmalignant tubal epithelium.
    4. The serosal surface of the tube is tumor-free.
18. Staging tubal carcinoma
    1. was officially adopted by FIGO in 1986.
    2. may not be altered by the findings encountered during surgery.
    3. is partially based on clinical findings, histologic grade, and depth of invasion.
    4. is based on the system used for primary ovarian carcinoma.
19. A 52-year-old patient is found to have stage I carcinoma of the fallopian tube, confined to the tubal lumen with negative peritoneal cytology. What is the proper therapy?
    1. Whole abdominal radiation.
    2. Intraperitoneal ^{32}P.
    3. Cyclophosphamide (Cytoxan) and Megestrol acetate (megace).
    4. Total abdominal hysterectomy, bilateral salpingo-oophorectomy, paraaortic node biopsy, omentectomy.
20. A 58-year-old asymptomatic patient is seen in your office for a routine office visit. A pap smear is performed. It is reported as "cells consistent with adenocarcinoma." The differential diagnoses should include adenocarcinoma of the
    1. endometrium.
    2. ovary.
    3. endocervix.
    4. fallopian tube.
21. A 48-year-old patient undergoes surgery for a left adnexal mass. While exploring the pelvis, you note a tumor of the left fallopian tube. If you suspect metastatic cancer to the tube, you should pay particular attention to the
    1. ovaries.
    2. intestines.
    3. uterus.
    4. breasts.
22. Abnormal uterine bleeding is the most common complaint associated with malignancies of the
    1. cervix.
    2. uterus.
    3. fallopian tube.
    4. ovary.
23. The term "hydrops tubae profluens" is associated with
    1. vaginal discharge.
    2. pelvic pain.
    3. a disappearing pelvic mass.
    4. vaginal bleeding.

ANSWERS

1. **C**, Page 919. Although there is no official FIGO staging system for primary tubal carcinoma, the commonly suggested system places a tumor confined to one tube with positive washings at Ic. Had the washings been negative, the stage would be Ia. If confined to both tubes with negative washings, the stage would be Ib.

2. **D**, Page 916. The triad of bleeding, watery discharge, and adnexal mass (hydrops tubae profluens) in a postmenopausal woman is considered highly suggestive of tubal carcinoma. These findings, however, only rarely occur together. The diagnosis is usually made postoperatively as the physician's index of suspicion is low.

   An adnexal mass in a menopausal patient must not be considered functional. The diagnosis of ovarian carcinoma is less likely because of the watery vaginal discharge. Postmenopausal bleeding should be considered endometrial carcinoma until proven otherwise, but the watery discharge and adnexal mass suggest a different primary process. Leiomyosarcoma would present as a uterine mass without the watery discharge rather than as an adnexal mass.

3. **A**, Page 917. Only 10% of the patients with tubal carcinoma have positive vaginal cytology. Therefore, the pap smear is not a reliable screening tool, and a negative smear does not rule out the possibility of tubal carcinoma.

4. **B**, Page 916. Fallopian tube carcinoma comprises approximately 0.3% to 1.1% of gynecologic malignancies. Up to 90% are metastatic from other sites, usually arising in the ovary or uterus. Metastatic tumors are 10 times more frequent than primary cancers of the fallopian tube.

5. **E**, Page 920. The overall 5-year survival for all stages of tubal carcinoma combined is 38%. Patients with disease confined to the tube have the best prognosis, expecting a 70% to 80% 5-year survival.

6. **D**, Page 920. In carrying out operative staging for presumed tubal or ovarian cancer, the first surgical procedure performed once in the peritoneal cavity should be the obtaining of peritoneal cytology using 200 to 300 ml of normal saline mixed with 5000 units of heparin. If any other manipulations are carried out prior to obtaining appropriate cytology, one runs the risk of shedding tumor cells into the peritoneal cavity, thus altering the staging evaluation.

7. **C**, Page 917. In a patient with postmenopausal uterine bleeding for whom D&C fails to reveal the cause of the bleeding, the possibility of tubal carcinoma must be considered. Laparoscopy can aid in establishing this diagnosis. Hysterectomy would not necessarily address the possibility of adnexal pathology, although an abdominal approach would allow thorough inspection of tubes and ovaries. Irradiation of the pelvis for bleeding of unknown etiology is inappropriate. Hysteroscopy with laser ablation of the endometrium would not rule out an adnexal etiology for the bleeding.

8. **E**, Page 920. Although the patient described is young and of low gravidity and parity, the appropriate operation is total abdominal hysterectomy with bilateral salpingo-oophorectomy. If no intraperitoneal spread is apparent, paraaortic node biopsy should be performed. An omentectomy should also be done.

9. **D**, Page 919. The peritoneum is the most frequent site of metastatic spread of tubal carcinoma. Retroperitoneal nodes are also a common site. Hepatic and pleural fluid metastases are less common and denote stage IV disease when they occur.

10. **B**, Pages 916–917 and Fig. 32-1 (from Droegemueller). The average age of women with adenocarcinoma of the fallopian tube is 54.9 years. As indicated in Figure 32-1, the decade in which most cases occur is 50–59 years.

11. **E**, Page 916. Although tubal carcinomas may present with excessive bleeding or discharge, and although an adnexal mass is occasionally found, history and physical examination do not usually lead one to the correct diagnosis. Similarly, imaging studies are not pathognomonic. The diagnosis is most frequently made after surgical exploration for other diagnoses.

12. **B**, Page 916. The classic description of tubal carcinoma is the triad of abnormal uterine bleeding, adnexal mass, and watery discharge in a postmenopausal woman. Pain is reported but less frequently. Anorexia is not typically associated with tubal carcinoma.

13. **E**, Pages 776, 809, 845, 916. Pain does not represent the most frequent presenting symptom in any of the malignancies of the female genital tract. In the case of tubal carcinoma, pain may occur, but it is less frequent than abnormal or excessive vaginal bleeding or discharge.

14–16. 14, **C**; 15, **D**; 16, **A**; Pages 846, 916, 920. (Also see Richardson GS, Scully RE, Nikrui, N et al: Common epithelial cancer of the ovary, NEJM 312:415, 1985.) Both ovarian and tubal carcinoma commonly spread to the paraaortic nodes. This is of particular importance when the primary tumor appears to be confined to the ovary or tube. Paraaortic nodes should be palpated and sampled. The overall 5-year survival for both malignancies is below 50%. In cases of tubal carcinoma, survival is approximately 38%. Whereas metastatic tumors to the ovary comprise only a small portion of tumors in the ovary, 90% of tubal cancers are metastatic, mostly from ovary, uterus, or the gastrointestinal tract.

17. **A** (1, 2, 3), Pages 917–918. (Also see Hu, Taymor, and Hertig: Primary carcinoma of the fallopian tube, Am J Obstet Gynecol 59:58, 1950.) The criteria used in the diagnosis of primary tubal carcinoma were suggested by Hu et al. They include:
    1. The primary tumor is grossly within the lumen of the tube.
    2. The mucosa of the tube is involved with the tumor, which displays a papillary or medullary pattern.
    3. A transition can be demonstrated between the malignant and nonmalignant tubal epithelium if the tubal wall is involved to a great extent.

18. **D** (4), Pages 812–813, 844, 919. A staging system for primary tubal carcinoma has not been officially adopted by FIGO. Since the spread of the disease is similar to that of epithelial carcinoma of the ovary, many authors have suggested a staging system similar to the one for ovarian cancer. As described in the text, the suggested staging system is accomplished clinically, at the time of surgery. The histologic grade and depth of invasion are considerations in determining the prognosis of endometrial, not tubal, adenocarcinoma.

19. **D** (4), Page 920. Therapy for stage I tubal carcinoma confined to the lumen with negative cytology usually consists of primary surgery only (total abdominal hysterectomy, bilateral salpingo-oophorectomy, paraaortic node biopsy, and omentectomy). If peritoneal cytology is positive, intraperitoneal ^{32}P or whole abdominal radiation is also used. Chemotherapy is reserved for widespread intraperitoneal disease or for recurrent metastatic carcinoma.

20. **E** (All), Page 917. Vaginal cytology has been reported to be positive in approximately 10% of fallopian tube carcinomas. Ruling out endometrial carcinoma must be the primary consideration; however, the diagnoses of tubal carcinoma, as well as endocervical or ovarian carcinoma, should be considered in patients with vaginal cytology positive for adenocarcinoma in whom endometrial carcinoma has been excluded.

21. **A** (1, 2, 3), Page 916. Since 90% of tubal cancers are metastatic, it behooves the clinician to know that the likely primary sites are in the ovary, uterus, and gastrointestinal tract.

22. **A** (1, 2, 3), Pages 776, 809, 845, 916. Abnormal or excessive vaginal bleeding is the most commonly associated sign of cancers of the cervix, uterus, and fallopian tube. Ovarian cancer tends to present as a vague swelling of the abdomen caused by ascites unless the ovarian neoplasm is the relatively rare granulosa cell tumor.

23. **A** (1, 2, 3), Page 916. Hydrops tubae profluens, sometimes associated with tubal carcinoma, refers to a symptom complex of abnormal vaginal discharge and pelvic pain associated with a pelvic mass. This mass may disappear after the discharge is noted. This symptomatology is presumably explained by blockage of the distal part of the tube, peristalsis of the tube resulting in vaginal discharge, and disappearance of the mass as the dilated tube is emptied.

CHAPTER 33
Gestational Trophoblastic Disease

DIRECTIONS for questions 1–7: Select the one best answer or completion.

1. A 37-year-old gravida 5, para 4 is referred with a confirmed diagnosis of a hydatidiform mole. This was not a planned pregnancy; the patient felt that she had completed her childbearing. During the evaluation of this patient, it is noted that the uterus is greater than expected by dates and that she has bilateral ovarian cysts approximately 10 cm in diameter. What would you recommend?
   A. Sharp curettage
   B. Chemotherapy
   C. Hysterotomy
   D. Hysterectomy
   E. Hysterectomy with bilateral oophorectomy

2. Which is the most common site of metastasis for gestation trophoblastic neoplasia (GTN)?
   A. Brain
   B. Lung
   C. Liver
   D. Ovary
   E. Vagina

3. A 30-year-old gravida 3, para 2 delivered a normal 3000g male infant 4 weeks ago. On the first postpartum day she had a bilateral tubal ligation. She has continued to have what is considered excessive bleeding. A D&C has been performed. The tissue is pictured in Figure 33-1. What is this?
   1. A hydatidiform mole
   2. A partial mole
   3. A choriocarcinoma
   4. Evidence of retained secudines
   5. A normal finding

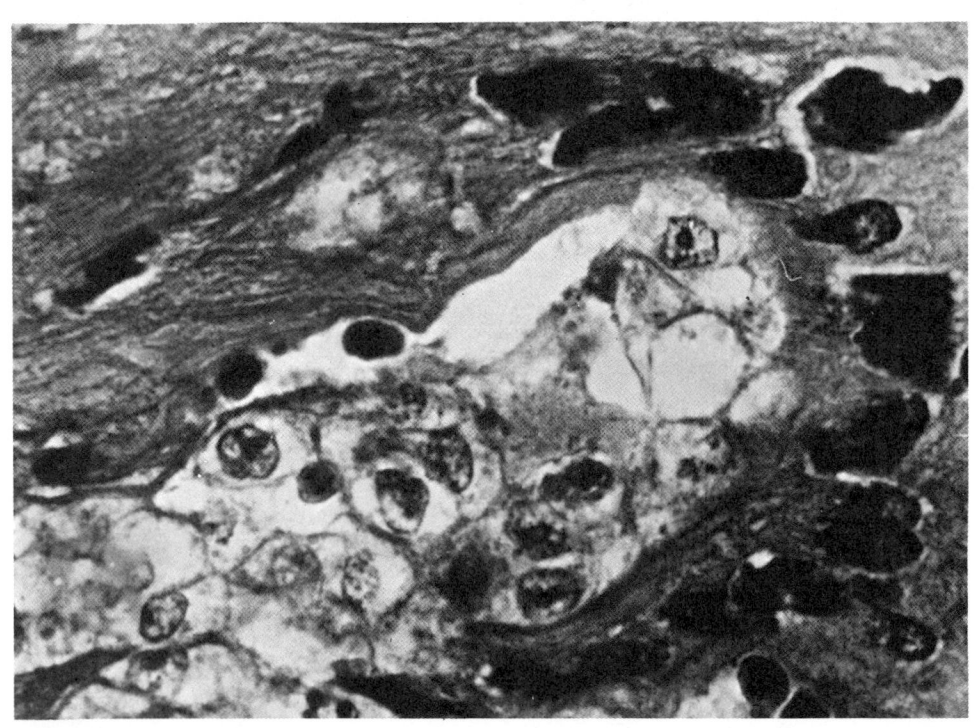

FIGURE 33-1.

4. A 25-year-old gravida 4, para 3 has a hydatidiform mole. Her last menstrual period was 14 weeks ago. The uterus is consistent with a 14-week pregnancy. The ovaries are not palpable. Appropriate follow-up after evacuation should include all of the following **EXCEPT**
   A. an initial chest x-ray.
   B. a chest x-ray if the β-HCG plateaus.
   C. oral contraception.
   D. a pelvic examination every 2 weeks until normal.
   E. a sensitive test, specific for β-HCG every 2 weeks for 1 year.
5. All of the following are indications of high risk gestational trophoblastic neoplasia **EXCEPT**
   A. disease present for more than 4 months.
   B. pretreatment serum β-HCG greater than 40,000 mIU/ml.
   C. GTN following a term pregnancy.
   D. brain metastasis.
   E. liver metastasis.
6. Choriocarcinoma is most likely to develop after
   A. a normal pregnancy.
   B. a partial mole.
   C. a hydatidiform mole.
   D. an ectopic pregnancy.
   E. an incomplete abortion.
7. The risk of developing a hydatidiform mole is highest if pregnancy occurs in women who are
   A. less than 20 years of age.
   B. 20 to 29.
   C. 30 to 39.
   D. 40 to 49.
   E. over 50 years of age.

DIRECTIONS for questions 8–9: For each numbered item, select the one heading most closely associated with it. Each lettered heading may be used once, more than once, or not at all.

    Blood Types
   Wife   Husband
(A) A   A
(B) A   0
(C) B   A
(D) AB   0
(E) The couple's blood type has not been shown to be a risk factor

8. A woman at a higher risk for developing a hydatidiform mole
9. A woman at a higher risk for developing a choriocarcinoma

DIRECTIONS for questions 10–12: For each numbered item, select the one heading most closely associated with it. Each lettered heading may be used **only once**.

(A) Partial mole
(B) Androgenesis
(C) Complete mole
(D) Gestational trophoblastic neoplasia

10. A condition with some normal and some swollen villi plus some fetal or cord or amniotic membrane elements associated with polyploidy.
11. A placental abnormality involving swollen placental villi and trophoblastic hyperplasia with loss of fetal blood vessels.
12. Malignant gestational trophoblastic disease or gestational trophoblastic tumor. It can be either metastatic or nonmetastatic.

DIRECTIONS for questions 13–20: For each numbered item, indicate whether it is associated with
  A only (A)
  B only (B)
  C both (A) and (B)
  D neither (A) nor (B)

(A) Partial Mole
(B) Complete Mole
(C) Both
(D) Neither

13. Hyperplasia of the syncytiotrophoblast
14. Hyperplasia of the cytotrophoblast
15. Usually a 47, XY karyotype
16. Both maternal and paternal origin
17. Immediate evacuation of a 32-week–sized uterus
   (A) Current terminology
   (B) Previous terminology
   (C) Both
   (D) Neither
18. Chorioadenoma destruens
19. Moderate risk, gestational trophoblastic malignancy
20. Incomplete hydatidiform mole

DIRECTIONS for questions 21–33: Each question contains four suggested answers of which one or more is correct. Choose the answer
  A if 1, 2, and 3 are correct
  B if 1 and 3 are correct
  C if 2 and 4 are correct
  D if 4 only is correct
  E if all are correct

21. Each of four patients has had a hydatidiform mole evacuated from her uterus. After consulting the graph in Figure 33-2, indicate those patient(s) who should be treated for gestational trophoblastic neoplasia.
    1. Patient 1
    2. Patient 2
    3. Patient 3
    4. Patient 4

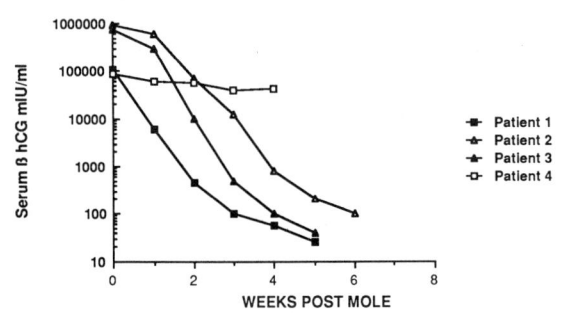

FIGURE 33-2.

22. A 20-year-old gravida 1, para 0 is seen at 21 weeks of pregnancy by menstrual dates. The uterus is the size of a 25-week gestation. Having made the diagnosis of a hydatidiform mole, you would
    1. start oxytocin immediately.
    2. follow the initial therapy with a hysterotomy.
    3. give prophylactic chemotherapy.
    4. perform a suction curettage.
23. Appropriate treatment regimens for low risk (metastatic) gestational trophoblastic neoplasia (GTN) include
    1. one additional course of chemotherapy after a negative β-HCG has been obtained.
    2. Actinomycin D.
    3. VP-16 (etoposide).
    4. Methotrexate.
24. Malignant sequelae following a hydatidiform mole are more common when the signs and symptoms include
    1. a uterus large for dates.
    2. preeclampsia before the 24th week of gestation.
    3. ovarian enlargement.
    4. hyperemesis gravidarum.
25. Signs and symptoms of a hydatidiform mole include
    1. abdominal pain.
    2. ovarian enlargement.
    3. hyperemesis gravidarum.
    4. uterus small for dates.
26. A 32-year-old gravida 5, para 4 is now 20 weeks pregnant by her menstrual dates. The uterus is felt to be the size of a 16-week gestation. An ultrasound is obtained and is pictured in Figure 33-3. The β-HCG is markedly elevated for 20 weeks. In discussing the possible outcomes, you would tell this patient that
    1. the fetus has a life expectancy of less than 1 month.
    2. she has an increased likelihood of developing preeclampsia.
    3. she will need to have serial β-HCG levels obtained postpartum.
    4. there is a 20% risk of malignant sequelae.
27. It is well established that individuals more likely to develop a hydatidiform mole include a woman
    1. with a history of a prior hydatidiform mole.
    2. in her twenties.
    3. who is Mexican.
    4. who is black.
28. True statements about the *recurrence* of gestational trophoblastic neoplasia (GTN) include:
    1. metastatic low risk usually occurs within 1 year following treatment.
    2. metastatic low risk is 10%.
    3. nonmetastatic is 1% to 2%.
    4. metastatic high risk is 50%.
29. True statements about gestational trophoblastic neoplasia (GTN) include:
    1. one third arise after a molar pregnancy.
    2. one third arise after a normal pregnancy.
    3. one third arise after an abortion or ectopic pregnancy.
    4. Given a complete mole, approximately 20% will develop into GTN.
30. Normal trophoblastic tissue
    1. divides rapidly.
    2. invades locally.
    3. contains multinucleated cells.
    4. metastasizes.
31. Which tests currently are used in the diagnosis and management of a complete or partial mole?
    1. An amniogram
    2. A serum β-HCG
    3. An arteriogram
    4. Ultrasound

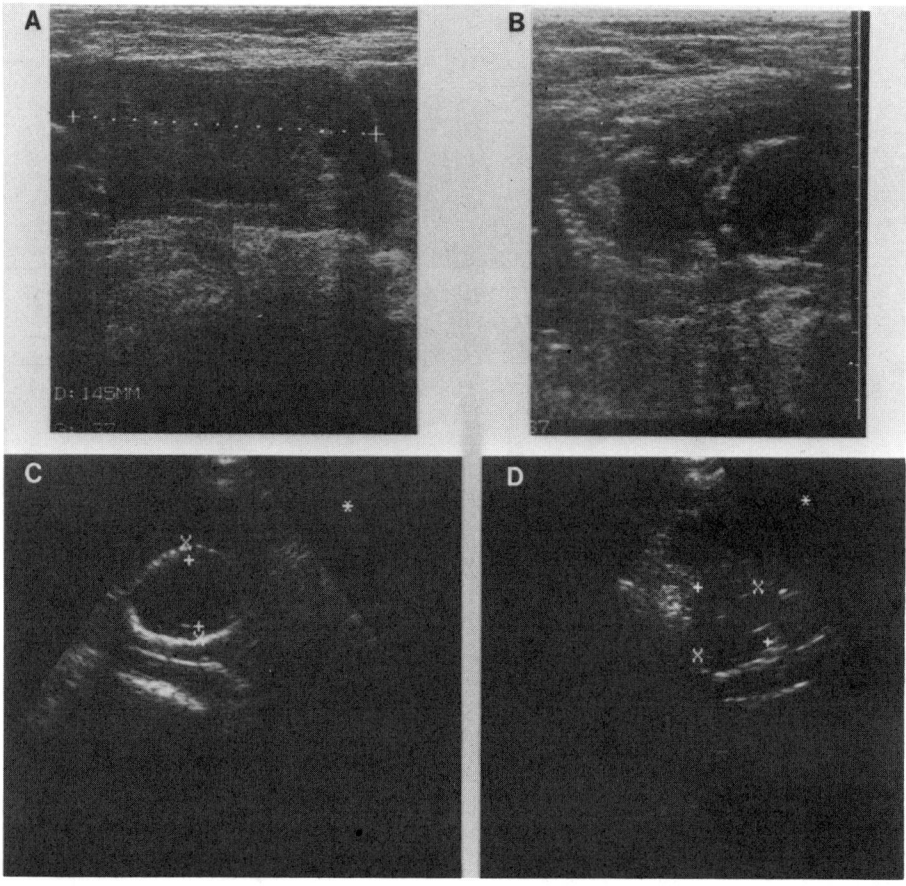

FIGURE 33-3.

32. A patient's uterus is symmetrically large for dates. The referring physician ordered a β-HCG. The result is charted on the laboratory's report shown in Figure 33-4. Your differential diagnosis includes
   1. twins.
   2. a complete mole.
   3. incorrect dates.
   4. leiomyomata.

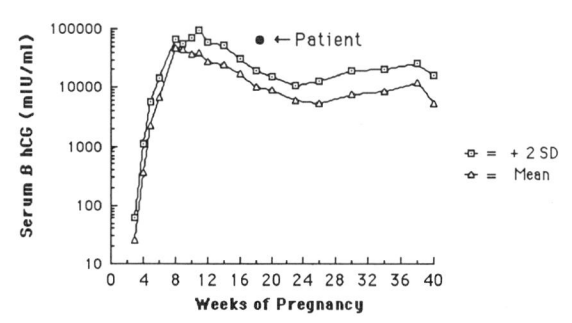

FIGURE 33-4.

33. Having established the differential diagnosis in question 32, you order an ultrasound. The image is reproduced in Figure 33-5. Given the most likely diagnosis, abnormal laboratory tests sometimes reported with this problem include
   1. elevated serum thyroxine.
   2. decreased serum fibrinogen.
   3. x-ray evidence of a pulmonary lesion.
   4. polycythemia.

ANSWERS

1. **D,** Page 931. If the patient has completed childbearing, hysterectomy should strongly be considered if the patient is older with an enlarged uterus or theca lutein cysts. The ovarian lutein cysts regress after termination of the pregnancy, and oophorectomy should not be performed unless there is other ovarian pathology.
2. **B,** Page 933. The most frequent site of metastatic GTN is the lungs (80% to 90% of cases), and less frequently the liver, brain, ovary, and vagina. However, metastatic disease can occur at any site. Given the diagnosis of GTN, a careful survey for metastatic disease should be initiated using CT examination of the brain and the abdomen. Tests of

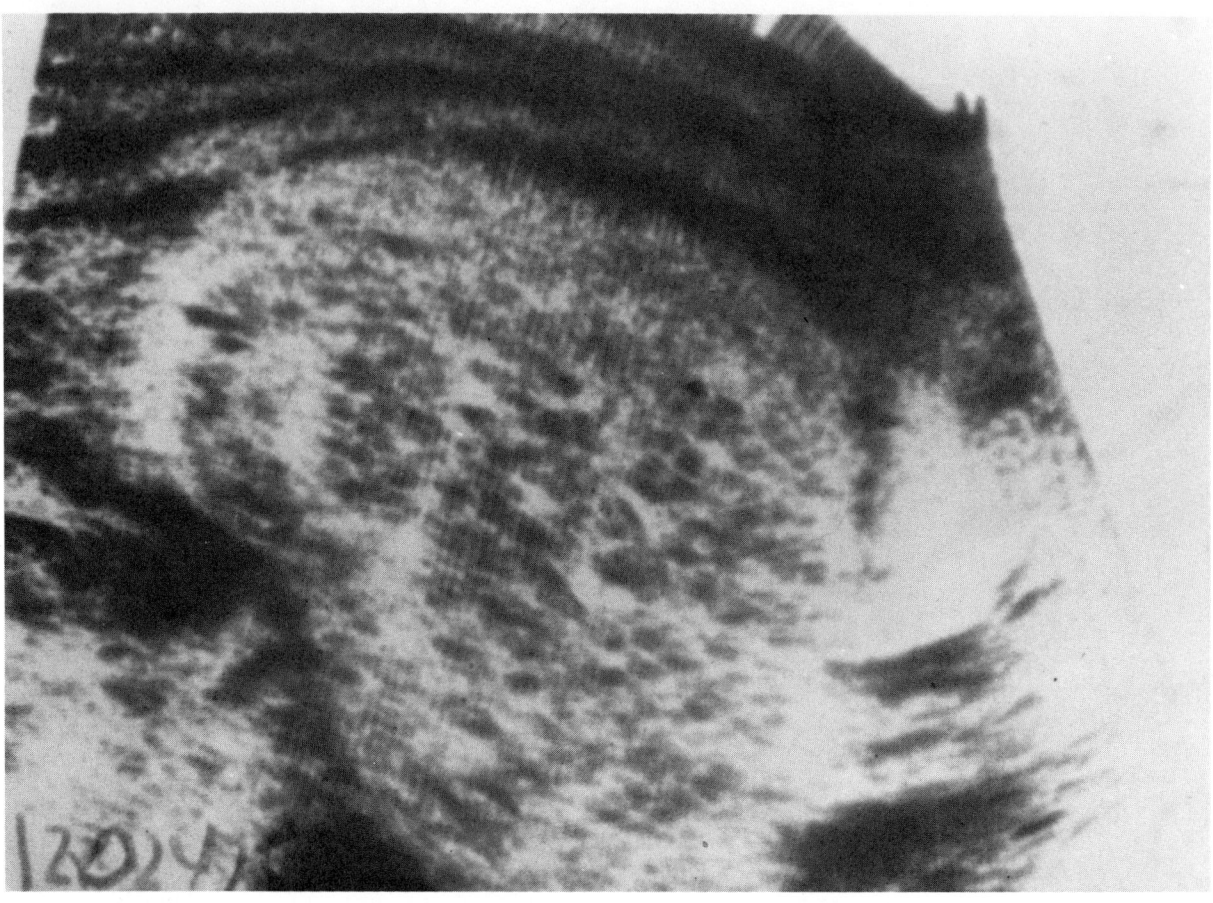

FIGURE 33-5.

renal and liver chemistries should also be performed in addition to a hematologic profile.

3. **C**, Pages 926, 928. The photomicrograph depicted in Figure 33–1 (from Bigelow B: Gestational trophoblast diease. In Blaustein A, ed: Pathology of the female genital tract, 2nd ed. New York, Springer-Verlag, 1982) is a high-power view of a choriocarcinoma. Central pale cytotrophoblasts are surrounded by syncytiotrophoblasts. These tumors tend to be hemorrhagic and necrotic. No villi are seen. With a complete or partial hydatidiform mole, the villi are edematous and lack fetal blood cells. One would expect to see villi rather than hemorrhage or necrosis with retained secundines. Choriocarcinoma may develop after a normal pregnancy. Trophoblastic tissue regresses within 2 to 3 weeks after normal delivery. The finding of trophoblastic cells in the uterus more than 3 weeks after delivery should lead one to consider the possibility of choriocarcinoma. This scenario is indeed rare as the incidence of choriocarcinoma following a normal term pregnancy is 1 in 40,000 in the United States.

4. **E**, Page 933. Management of a patient with a hydatidiform mole includes
   1. A chest x-ray initially and repeated if abnormal or if the β-HCG plateaus or rises.
   2. Contraception for 1 year.
   3. A pelvic examination every 2 weeks until normal, then every 3 months
   4. Weekly serum determinations of β-HCG until normal for two values, then monthly for 1 year.

5. **C**, Pages 934, 937. Recent evidence indicates that GTN after term pregnancy may be considered as low risk unless one of the poor prognosis factors is also present. High risk GTN is gestational trophoblastic neoplasia in which one or more of the following are present: The initial serum titer is >40,000 mIU/ml; the disease has been present more

than 4 months; brain or liver metastases are present; prior chemotherapy has failed.

6. **C**, Page 928. Although most choriocarcinomas occur after complete molar pregnancies, occurrences have been reported after incomplete moles and rare choriocarcinomas have developed after normal pregnancy (1 per 40,000 term pregnancies). The disease also follows incomplete abortion and ectopic pregnancy.

7. **E**, Page 928. The risk of developing a hydatidiform mole in women who are pregnant is lowest in the 25–29 year age bracket. If the risk assigned to this group is 1, the risk in a woman under 20 years of age is 1.53 and in women over 50 it is 80.76, this being the highest risk group. Since not many women who are 50 years of age become pregnant, numerically few hydatidiform moles are seen in this age group.

8–9. 8, **E**; 9, **B**; Page 928. Studies have shown that women with type A blood married to men with type O and vice versa are at higher risk for choriocarcinoma in comparison to matings of other blood groups. No differential in the risk for hydatidiform mole for ABO blood groups has been demonstrated.

10–12. 10, **A**; 11, **C**; 12, **D**; Pages 923, 927. A partial mole is a molar pregnancy with some normal and some swollen villi plus some fetal or cord or amniotic membrane elements associated with polyploidy.

A hydatidiform mole is a placental abnormality involving swollen placental villi and trophoblastic hyperplasia with loss of fetal blood vessels. There are two types, partial and complete. A complete mole is the most common type of gestational trophoblastic disease (GTD), occurring in the United States in 0.75 per 1000 pregnancies.

Gestational trophoblastic neoplasia is malignant gestational trophoblastic disease or gestational trophoblastic tumor. It can be either metastatic or nonmetastatic.

13–17. 13, **C**; 14, **B**; 15, **D**; 16, **A**; 17, **B**; Pages 924–925, 931. The three morphologic characteristics of a complete mole are: (1) a mass of distended villi that appear as large grapelike dilations, (2) a loss of fetal blood vessels in the villi, and (3) hyperplasia of the syncytiotrophoblast and cytotrophoblast. With a partial mole, in addition to the presence of a fetus, there is hyperplasia of the syncytiotrophoblast only.

With complete mole, only paternal chromosomes are present; there are 46 chromosomes and they are nearly always 46, XX, although a few moles with 46, XY karyotype have been reported. This is the result of a process known as androgenesis, which is the impregnation of an inactive egg by a paternal haploid sperm that duplicates its chromosomes to provide a diploid complement (See Figure 33-2, page 925).

Incomplete or partial moles are triploid and have 69 chromosomes of both maternal and paternal origin (See Figure 33-3, page 926).

Immediate evacuation of a 32-week-sized uterus may be an ethical, legal problem. If the size of the fetus corresponds to uterine size, theoretically, the fetus is viable so that it would be illegal to terminate the pregnancy. The malignant potential of a partial mole is lower than that for a complete mole. These fetuses are markedly abnormal and do not survive. The abnormalities are usually evident by ultrasound evaluation. Thus, if you chose answer C, you should not consider this response entirely incorrect.

18–20. 18, **B**; 19, **D**; 20, **A**; Pages 928–929. Previously the term *hydatidiform mole* referred to a molar pregnancy; *invasive mole* or *chorioadenoma destruens* referred to a molar pregnancy that had invaded the uterus away from the implantation site; and *choriocarcinoma* referred to the malignant variation that metastasized and was often fatal. The current classification of gestational trophoblastic disease is:

Hydatidiform Mole
1. Complete
2. Incomplete

Gestational trophoblastic neoplasia
1. Nonmetastatic
2. Metastatic
   a. Low risk
   b. High risk

21. **D** (4), Page 933. Usually, there is a gradual decline of BHCG after evacuation of a hydatidiform mole, reaching a normal range of 3 to 5 mIU/ml by the 14th week after evacuation. There may be an abnormal regression curve after evacuation of a mole, such as that shown in patient 4, and in such instances the patient requires therapy for gestational trophoblastic neoplasia. A rise in titer or a plateau in titer (failure to decrease over a 3-week interval) indicates the presence of postmolar trophoblastic neoplasia.

22. **D** (4), Pages 931, 937. Intravenous oxytocic agents are used during the evacuation and immediately postoperatively to aid in uterine contraction and to help reduce blood loss. However, it is not advisable to use oxytocic drugs before evacuation of the molar pregnancy because of the risk of disseminating abnormal trophoblastic cells. Suction curettage has proven to be safe and effective even with a larger uterus. After evacuation by suction curettage is complete, a gentle sharp curettage should be performed to ensure completion of the procedure. There is no need

to do a hysterotomy. Prophylactic chemotherapy has not gained widespread acceptance because giving chemotherapy at the time of evacuation of the mole exposes the patient to toxic and dangerous drugs, even though 80% of patients with a complete mole do not require further treatment.

23. **E** (All), Page 934. There are several different regimens that employ either methotrexate or actinomycin D for low risk GTN therapy. VP-16 (etoposide) has also been effectively used as single-agent therapy. One additional course of the agent being used should be given after a negative β-HCG has been obtained.

24. **A** (1, 2, 3), Page 929. Malignant sequelae following a hydatidiform mole appear to be more common among those with an enlarged uterus and preeclampsia. Enlargement of the ovaries is associated with a higher frequency of future malignant change (approximately 50%) as compared to less than 15% for those without ovarian enlargement.

25. **E** (All), Page 929. Signs and symptoms associated with a hydatidiform mole include abnormal bleeding in early pregnancy, lower abdominal pain, preeclampsia before 24 weeks of gestation, hyperemesis gravidarum, a uterus large for dates, a uterus small for dates, enlargement of the ovaries, absent fetal heart tones and fetal parts, expulsion of swollen villi, and rarely hyperthyroidism.

26. **A** (1, 2, 3), Pages 925, 930, 936. Also see Szulman AE, Surti U: The syndromes of partial and complete molar gestation. *Clin Obstet Gynecol* 27:172, 1984. The ultrasound depicted in Figure 33-3 reveals placenta tissue suggestive of a hydatidiform mole (A), oligohydramnios (B), hydrocephaly (C), and a cystic structure (D) which in this patient is a theca lutein cyst. This is a case of a partial mole associated with an abnormal fetus. Survival beyond the early neonatal period has not been reported. An increase in the incidence of preeclampsia has been observed with hydatidiform moles. Comparing 200 patients, Szulman and Surti found the incidence of preeclampsia in patients with complete moles to be 6% and those with partial moles 8%. Although partial moles are rarely followed by GTN, the patient should be followed with serially β-HCG determinations.

27. **B** (1, 3), Page 928. A history of prior hydatidiform mole increases the risk of a subsequent mole by 20 to 40 times. The lowest incidence of hydatidiform mole in women who are pregnant is in the 20 to 40 age group. Mexicans have a relatively high incidence of molar pregnancies. The increased frequency of moles in lower socioeconomic groups and in underdeveloped areas has led to the suggestion that poor nutrition is a factor in the development of the disease. The evidence is conflicting, and a dietary etiology is not supported by current data. A decreased rate has been reported among blacks in the United States in comparison to whites.

28. **B** (1, 3), Pages 934–935, 937. Recurrence of metastatic low-risk GTN seldom occurs more than 1 year after treatment. The recurrence rate for low-risk metastatic GTN is approximately 5%. The recurrence rate for non-metastatic GTN is 1% to 2%. Nonmetastatic GTN and metastatic low-risk GTN are almost 100% curable by chemotherapy. As many as 20% of patients with metastatic high-risk GTN who attain a negative β-HCG titer have a recurrence. Patients with metastatic high-risk GTN are successfully treated with chemotherapy in more than 70% of cases.

29. **D** (4 only), Page 933. GTN develops after approximately 20% of complete hydatidiform moles. Conversely, about half the cases of GTN arise after molar pregnancy while one fourth occur after normal pregnancy and one fourth after abortion or ectopic pregnancy.

30. **E** (All), Page 923. Trophoblastic tissue is unusual insofar as it shares certain characteristics with malignancies, such as the ability to divide rapidly, to invade locally, and occasionally to metastasize to distant sites such as the lung. The syncytiotrophoblast is a multinucleated cell layer.

31. **C** (2, 4), Page 930. The most valuable aid in the diagnosis of a hydatidiform mole is ultrasound. Other diagnostic tests, such as amniograms and arteriograms, were previously used. HCG is important in the diagnosis and follow-up of a molar pregnancy, but you should use a sensitive RIA, receptor assay, or ELIZA **specific** for the β subunit. Always know the specificity and sensitivity of the test you are using. A *single* elevated β-HCG is not diagnostic because the patient may have twins or her dates may be in error. One should have a baseline β-HCG before beginning treatment.

32. **A** (1, 2, 3), Pages 930–931. Levels of β-HCG can appear elevated in a twin pregnancy. This patient's value would fall into an acceptable range if she were really 12, not 18 weeks.

Patients with a complete mole have an elevated β-HCG. A single β-HCG is often not diagnostic, especially if the level is not elevated. In 30% to 50% of cases, the uterus will be large for dates.

Patients with an incomplete mole tend to have lower levels of β-HCG. Although a patient with leiomyomata will have a uterus large for dates, this alone will not explain the elevated β-HCG. The myomata would have to coexist with incorrect dates.

33. **A** (1, 2, 3), Page 931. Occasionally a patient with a mole will manifest hyperthyroidism, disseminated intravascular coagulation, or trophoblastic disease in the lungs. These patients can develop pulmonary insufficiency. They may be anemic due to blood loss.

PART FIVE: ENDOCRINOLOGY AND INFERTILITY

CHAPTER 34: Dysmenorrhea and Premenstrual Syndrome

DIRECTIONS for questions 1–3: Select the one best answer or completion.

1. A 20-year-old woman has been arrested and charged with the murder of her husband. In her defense she has entered a plea of temporary insanity by virtue of premenstrual syndrome. You have been subpoenaed to testify as a gynecologist regarding her premenstrual syndrome. On the witness stand the prosecuting attorney asks you to define PMS. Your testimony should indicate that it is a syndrome characterized by symptoms which
   A. occur no more than 14 days prior to menstruation.
   B. occur no more than 5 days prior to menstruation.
   C. occur in severe form in more than 10 per cent of patients.
   D. are sometimes absent immediately after menstruation.
   E. may be present one month and absent another.

2. The defense attorney of the woman in question 1 has entered into evidence a graph of the defendant's "symptoms" over the past 2 months. You are asked to review Defendant's Exhibit A (Figure 34-1). Based on this graph you might reasonably testify that the accused
   A. has PMS.
   B. is a manic-depressive.
   C. was insane at the time of the murder.
   D. has severe dysmenorrhea.
   E. none of the above.

3. A 20-year-old nulligravid patient presents with a history of severe lower abdominal cramping pain, nausea, vomiting, and diarrhea occurring approximately 8 hours after the onset of menstruation and lasting 1 to 2 days. The patient's periods occur regularly every 26 to 28 days and last 5 days. She is not sexually active, uses no birth control, and normally takes extra strength Tylenol™ (Acetaminophen) with little relief. Her physical examination including pelvic is unremarkable.

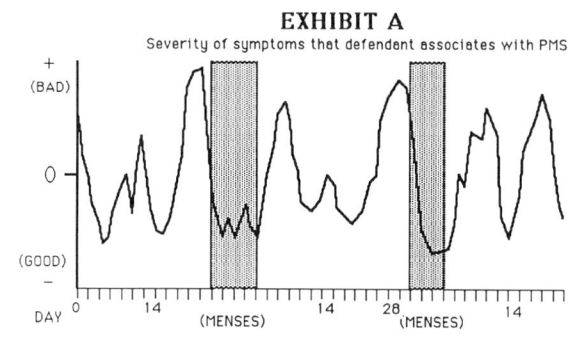

EXHIBIT A
Severity of symptoms that defendant associates with PMS

FIGURE 34-1.

The cause of these symptoms is most likely
   A. adenomyosis.
   B. endometriosis.
   C. cervical stenosis.
   D. excess prostaglandins.
   E. leiomyomata.

DIRECTIONS for questions 4–15: For each numbered item, indicate whether it is associated with

A only (A)
B only (B)
C both (A) and (B)
D neither (A) nor (B)

(A) Premenstrual syndrome
(B) Dysmenorrhea (primary or secondary)
(C) Both
(D) Neither

4. Lower abdominal pain just prior to menstruation.
5. Pelvic heaviness and bloating.
6. Prostaglandin mediated.
7. May respond to nonsteroidal anti-inflammatory drug (NSAID) therapy.
8. Approximately 15% of sufferers have severe symptoms.

(A) Primary dysmenorrhea
(B) Secondary dysmenorrhea
(C) Both
(D) Neither

9. Likely to improve with mild to moderate strength analgesics.
10. Likely cause of menstrual discomfort in a 42-year-old multiparous woman.
11. Generally associated with a normal pelvic examination.
12. Likely to have a familial pattern.
13. Is a major cause of school absences.
14. Associated with throbbing abdominal pain and a sense of pelvic heaviness.
15. Symptoms start 2 to 3 days prior to menses.

DIRECTIONS for questions 16–28: Each question contains four suggested answers of which one or more is correct. Choose the answer
A if 1, 2, and 3 are correct
B if 1 and 3 are correct
C if 2 and 4 are correct
D if 4 only is correct
E if all are correct

16. Primary dysmenorrhea is
    1. most common in the late teens or early twenties.
    2. associated with ovulatory menstrual cycles.
    3. likely to improve during oral contraceptive therapy.
    4. likely to improve after insertion of an intrauterine contraceptive device (IUD).
17. True statements about PMS include:
    1. PMS is caused by an excess of estrogen just prior to menstruation.
    2. Endorphins appear to play a pivotal role in the development of symptoms.
    3. Many of the symptoms associated with PMS are caused by fluid storage causing weight gain, abdominal swelling, and breast tenderness.
    4. PMS is a multifactorial psychoendocrine disorder.
18. Which are contraindications to the use of nonsteroidal anti-inflammatory agents for the treatment of primary dysmenorrhea?
    1. Aspirin sensitive asthma
    2. a history of diarrhea with menstruation
    3. gastric ulcer
    4. premenstrual syndrome
19. Which of the following would be useful in making the diagnosis of premenstrual syndrome?
    1. A clinical trial of 200 mg/day of Vitamin B_6
    2. Endometrial biopsy to assess corpus luteal function
    3. Serum estrogen level
    4. A diary of symptoms over a 2 to 3 month period
20. Treating PMS patients with bromocriptine
    1. causes a greater improvement in mood than does placebo treatment.
    2. reduces the elevated levels of prolactin found in these patients.
    3. relieves breast tenderness in doses as small as 1 mg/day.
    4. is only appropriate when breast tenderness is the major symptom.
21. Why has prostaglandin $F_{2\alpha}$ been implicated as a possible cause of primary dysmenorrhea?
    1. It is found in higher amounts in women with dysmenorrhea.
    2. It is capable of stimulating the smooth muscle of the gastrointestinal tract.
    3. It is capable of stimulating the smooth muscle of the uterus.
    4. Inhibition of its production through the use of nonsteroidal anti-inflammatory drug gives clinical relief of symptoms.
22. The role of progesterone in the treatment of PMS is based on
    1. the observation that PMS symptoms are absent during pregnancy.
    2. small controlled trials that show statistical superiority over other therapies.
    3. large, open, uncontrolled trials.
    4. evidence of reduced levels of progesterone in patients with PMS.
23. What is appropriate initial therapy for premenstrual symptoms in a 29-year-old gravida 3, para 2, abortus 1 white female who has had her "tubes tied"?
    1. Reassurance
    2. A balanced diet emphasizing increased protein
    3. Vitamin B_6 100 mg p.o. b.i.d.
    4. A combination oral contraceptive
24. In a 19-year-old nulligravid patient with the clinical diagnosis of primary dysmenorrhea, appropriate therapy consists of two tablets of the following at the onset of pain and then 1 t.i.d. prn.
    1. Anaprox™ 275 mg.
    2. Ponstel™ 250 mg.
    3. Motrin™ 800 mg.
    4. Indomethacin 25 mg.

25. Why has fluid retention been implicated in PMS?
    1. An increase in total body weight.
    2. An increase in abdominal girth.
    3. Presence of cerebral edema.
    4. A perception of swelling.
26. A 35-year-old gravida 3, para 3 health food store owner asks your opinion about using vitamin B_6 in a dosage of 650 mg twice a day for the treatment of PMS. Your response should state that this regimen
    1. will help to slow the metabolism of estrogen.
    2. is potentially dangerous.
    3. is based on evidence of B_6 deficiencies.
    4. has not been conclusively proven effective.
27. A 34-year-old woman gravida 2, para 2 wearing an IUD presents with a history of heavy, crampy periods since the birth of her child 1 year ago. She had experienced menstrual pain during most of her periods prior to her pregnancy. This discomfort had responded to therapy with Motrin™ (ibuprofen), and her current discomfort is somewhat worse than she remembers prior to pregnancy. She has recently tried an over-the-counter ibuprofen medication without success. This patient's physical examination including pelvic examination is normal and her IUD string is visible. Which are possible diagnoses?
    1. Primary dysmenorrhea
    2. Premenstrual syndrome
    3. Secondary dysmenorrhea
    4. Pelvic inflammatory disease
28. To help this patient's complaints (Question 27) you might reasonably recommend
    1. an additional pregnancy.
    2. a nonsteroidal anti-inflammatory agent.
    3. monthly doses of a broad-spectrum antibiotic.
    4. removal of the IUD with the use of an alternative birth control method if desired.

ANSWERS

1. **A**, Page 945. (Also see Premenstrual Syndrome and Dysmenorrhea, Dawood MY, McGuire JL and Demers LM (eds.), Urban & Schwarzenberg, Baltimore, 1985.) Probably the best working definition of premenstrual syndrome is one that restricts the recurrence of significant, distressing symptoms to no more than 14 days before menses. These symptoms must recur episodically and predictably over no less than 3 consecutive cycles. In addition, the symptoms must spontaneously and completely disappear with, or soon after, the onset of menstrual flow. While PMS is though to affect anywhere from 5% to 95% of women, only about 2% to 3% have severe symptoms.

2. **E**, Pages 945, 949. The pattern of symptoms illustrated is typical of patients who have complaints that become linked or entrained with the recurrent rhythm of the period, not true PMS. No mention of menstrual pain has been made to support the diagnosis of dysmenorrhea. As a gynecologist you are not in a position to diagnose what that disorder is nor to make legal assessments regarding her guilt or accountability.

3. **D**, Pages 941–944. Primary dysmenorrhea is caused by an excess of prostaglandin $F_{2\alpha}$. This prostaglandin excess also contributes to the frequent presence of nausea, vomiting, and diarrhea not seen with adenomyosis or cervical stenosis. The pain associated with endometriosis generally precedes the onset of menstrual flow and improves after flow is established.

4–8. 4, **A**; 5, **C**; 6, **B**; 7, **C**; 8, **B**; Pages 942, 945. While the most commonly recognized symptoms of premenstrual syndromes are emotional, many somatic pre-period symptoms may be present. When these symptoms exist solely in the premenstrual period, they may correctly be termed a part of premenstrual syndrome. These same somatic symptoms may also be present in primary or secondary dysmenorrhea and the differentiation between these and PMS is based on the timing of the complaints. By definition, dysmenorrhea is pain appreciated **during** menses. Even though both PMS and dysmenorrhea may respond to NSAID therapy, there is no evidence currently available that prostaglandins play a significant role in the development of PMS. Severe symptoms are found in 2% to 3% of PMS patients and 10% to 15% of women with dysmenorrhea.

9–15. 9, **C**; 10, **B**; 11, **A**; 12, **A**; 13, **A**; 14, **B**; 15, **D**; Pages 941–944. The best therapy for secondary dysmenorrhea is ultimately directed toward the cause, but both primary and secondary dysmenorrhea may be successfully treated with analgesics. The distinction between primary and secondary is most often made on the basis of a normal pelvic examination in primary dysmenorrhea. The peak age of incidence for primary and secondary dysmenorrhea is very different. Primary dysmenorrhea is much more likely in younger women and thus accounts for a significant number of school absences. In older women secondary dysmenorrhea is much more likely even though primary dysmenorrhea is still possible. While causes of secondary dysmenorrhea such as fibroids may have a familial pattern, it is primary dysmenorrhea that is most closely associated with a familial tendency. The symptoms of pelvic heaviness and throbbing pain are more common with secondary dysmenorrhea. The pain of primary dysmenorrhea is usually described as sharp or "laborlike" in character. In neither primary nor secondary dysmenorrhea do the symptoms start appreciably before the onset of menstrual flow.

16. **A** (1, 2, 3), Page 942. Almost 40% of dysmenorrheic women report the onset of symptoms during the first years of menstruation. The peak incidence occurs in the late teens to early twenties and then declines with advancing age. Because primary dysmenorrhea is associated with ovulatory cycles, suppression of ovulation with oral contraceptives will often provide at least some measure of relief. While some studies indicate no effect of IUD use on the incidence of dysmenorrhea, many authors feel that it may contribute to menstrual pain and classify it as a cause of secondary dysmenorrhea. Progesterone releasing IUDs are less likely to be associated with dysmenorrhea.

17. **C** (2, 4), Pages 945–948. While many possible causes for PMS have been advanced over the years, most remain unproven. Currently the best that can be said is that PMS is a multifactorial psychoendocrine disorder. There is growing evidence that the endorphins have a central role in most symptoms of PMS. Both estrogen excess and fluid storage have been postulated as causes for PMS, but controlled studies have not supported their importance in the etiology of this syndrome.

18. **B** (1, 3), Page 943. Aspirin sensitive asthma, inflammatory bowel disease, and ulcer disease are contraindications for most NSAIDs. While there is an incidence of from 3% to 10% of diarrhea with the use of NSAIDs, many studies have indicated that there is a reduction in the incidence of period-related diarrhea with these drugs. PMS is not a contraindication to the use of these drugs and, indeed, patients may respond favorably to their use.

19. **D** (4), Page 949. The most useful tool for making the diagnosis of premenstrual syndrome is a diary of symptoms. There is no evidence of corpus luteal dysfunction and no support for changes in estrogen levels that would be helpful in making the diagnosis. Since the value of B_6 therapy is debatable, any response noted would be nondiagnostic because of the possibility of a placebo effect.

20. **D** (4), Page 947. Studies have been unable to demonstrate an abnormal level of prolactin in women with PMS. In controlled studies of bromocriptine use in PMS, only breast tenderness responded and only in doses above 5 mg/day.

21. **E** (All). (See Ylikorkala O, Dawood MY, New concepts in dysmenorrhea, Amer J Obstet Gynecol 130:833847, 1978.) Prostaglandin $F_{2\alpha}$ has been found in levels of 5 to 10 times the usual amount in women with primary dysmenorrhea. This is a potent stimulator of smooth muscle both in the uterus and in the gastrointestinal tract. In the uterus, this prostaglandin $F_{2\alpha}$ action may be responsible for intrauterine pressures in excess of 400 mmHg. (During contraction of the uterus in a menstruating woman, the intrauterine pressure is 60–80 mmHg.) In the gastrointestinal tract, the increased motility caused by the stimulatory effects of prostaglandin $F_{2\alpha}$ may account for the frequent observation of nausea, vomiting, and diarrhea in patients with primary dysmenorrhea. While the success of NSAID therapy supports the role of prostaglandins in primary dysmenorrhea, it does not by itself conclusively establish the cause and effect relationship.

22. **B** (1, 3). (See Dalton K., Diagnosis and clinical features of premenstrual syndrome. In Premenstrual Syndrome and Dysmenorrhea, Dawood MY, McGuire JL, Demers LM (eds.), Urban & Schwarzenberg, Baltimore, 1985.) The use of progesterone therapy in PMS has been most vocally championed by Dr. Katharina Dalton of England. She observed that PMS symptoms were absent in her own pregnancy and in her patients during pregnancy. This has led to the use of progesterone in uncontrolled open trials of more than 30,000 patients worldwide. Despite this experience, to date no controlled blind study has been able to confirm a superiority over placebo. No study has been able to confirm any consistent alteration in progesterone levels.

23. **A** (1, 2, 3), Page 949. Though unproven by double blind trials, reassurance, a good diet, and an exercise program are always appropriate. Supplementation with small doses of vitamin B_6 is probably very reasonable therapy in almost any patient with PMS. A substantial number of patients will benefit from just undergoing the process of investigation and the identification of a diagnostic condition. Many patients with true PMS will show intolerance to oral contraceptive pills. This intolerance, combined with a lack of benefit, make them a poor choice for therapy.

24. **A** (1, 2, 3), Pages 942–943. Anaprox™ (naproxen sodium), Ponstel™ (mefenamic acid), and Motrin™ (ibuprofen) are all approved for the treatment of dysmenorrhea and would be appropriate in the absence of contraindications. Because of evidence of receptor site activity by the fenamates (Ponstel™ and Meclomen™), there may be some theoretical advantage favoring these agents. In practice this may be reflected in a

slightly faster onset of action. For most patients, however, these differences are probably of little consequence. Indomethacin has been shown to be effective in treating dysmenorrhea, but its higher incidence of side effects and lack of official approval make it a second line drug.

25. **D** (4), Page 947–948. Controlled studies have been unable to demonstrate any change in abdominal measurements or in total body weight, even in those patients who complain of swelling and bloating. Cerebral edema has not been proven. These patients do believe that during the period of symptomatology they are bloated and swollen.

26. **C** (2, 4), Pages 946–947. (Also see Hagen I, Neshem B-I, Tamtland T: Acta Obstet Gynecol Scand 64:667–670, 1985.) The rationale for using B_6 as therapy for PMS comes from the fact that B_6 is consumed in the metabolism of estrogen. Vitamin B_6 is also involved in the production of serotonin in the brain. Because reduced levels of serotonin have been found in patients with depression, some authors have postulated that replacing B_6 may favorably affect the emotional symptoms of PMS. Vitamin B_6 therapy for PMS has not been adequately studied to make any case for efficacy. While some patients may experience improvement, there are no blind studies to suggest a response greater than seen with placebo. Indeed, one recent double-blind, placebo-controlled trial shows a 4.2% median response for B_6 therapy (100 mg/day) versus a 21% median response for placebo (Hagen et al.). Peripheral nerve damage has been reported in dosages above 200 mg/day. Dosage in the magnitude suggested for this patient should not be used. There is no evidence that additional B_6 will have any effect on the rate of estrogen metabolism, even though it is a coenzyme in the process.

27–28. 27, **B** (1, 3); 28, **C** (2, 4); Pages 941–944. (Also see (2) Dawood MY (ed.): Dysmenorrhea, Williams and Wilkins, Baltimore, 1981; (3) Chan WY, Dawood MY, Fuchs F: Relief of dysmenorrhea with the prostaglandin synthetase inhibitor ibuprofen: Effect on prostaglandin levels in menstrual fluid, Am J Obstet Gynecol 135:102, 1979; (4) Dawood MY, McGuire JL and Demers LM (eds.): Premenstrual Syndrome and Dysmenorrhea, Urban & Schwarzenberg, Baltimore, 1985.) While the most likely diagnosis for this patient is dysmenorrhea secondary to an IUD, continuing primary dysmenorrhea is still a possibility. There is no historic or physical evidence for either PMS or PID. The patient's history suggests that she may have had primary dysmenorrhea before her pregnancy. Studies reported by Dawood indicate that pregnancy and delivery may not relieve dysmenorrhea (2). As many as 20% of women with dysmenorrhea will experience a return of symptoms with the return of ovulation (3). The lack of response of the patient's symptoms to over-the-counter strengths of ibuprofen most likely reflects inadequate dosage rather than an indication of nonprostaglandin-mediated etiology.

When IUD use was more common, they represented a not uncommon cause for secondary, though iatrogenic, dysmenorrhea. It has been postulated that the increased prostaglandins found with IUD use not only may have been partially responsible for the contraceptive effect, but also may have been the reason for the associated menstrual pain. This association is supported by studies that indicate moderate success in treating these women with therapeutic doses of prostaglandin inhibitors (4). To attempt to differentiate between secondary dysmenorrhea from her IUD and primary dysmenorrhea, it may be necessary to advise the removal of the IUD. For a discussion of other considerations in the use of IUDs see Chapter 11.

CHAPTER 35

Abnormal Uterine Bleeding

DIRECTIONS: Select the one best answer or completion.

1. The rationale for the therapeutic use of conjugated estrogen (CE) for the immediate treatment of dysfunctional uterine bleeding is based on the fact that it
   A. stabilizes endogenous serum clotting factors.
   B. causes a decrease in platelet adhesiveness.
   C. causes decidualization of the endometrium.
   D. leads to rapid proliferation of the endometrium.
   E. is followed by a uniform endometrial slough upon withdrawal.

2. An 18-year-old patient presents with a 2 month history of intermittent, irregular bleeding. Her last normal menstrual period was 3 months ago. Prior to that, her cycle was regular at 28 days. A pelvic examination is normal. What would you do next?
   A. An endometrial aspiration
   B. Pelvic ultrasound
   C. A pregnancy test
   D. Laparoscopy
   E. Hysteroscopy

3. A 45-year-old patient who had menorrhagia for 6 months underwent a dilation and curettage. The uterus was normal in size. The cavity felt smooth, and the pathologist noted this was a secretory endometrium. What is the best subsequent management option?
   A. Cyclic medroxyprogesterone acetate
   B. Continuous medroxyprogesterone acetate
   C. Continuous conjugated estrogens
   D. Cyclic danazol
   E. Combination oral contraceptives

4. A 22-year-old woman presents with "heavy menstruation," which is now in its seventh day. Pelvic examination is normal except for the presence of clotted blood filling the posterior fornix. A BHCG screen is negative and an office hematocrit is 35%. One recognized approach would be
   A. high dose conjugated estrogen (CE) therapy (10 mg/day in divided doses) until bleeding stops.
   B. medroxyprogesterone acetate (MPA) (10 mg/day for 10 days).
   C. combination oral contraceptives with 35 mcg of estrogen (2 tablets/day) until bleeding stops.
   D. office endometrial aspiration.

5. Assuming that the bleeding is markedly diminished within 24 hours, the next step in the treatment of the patient described in question 4 should include
   A. continuing conjugated estrogen (CE) at its present dose and adding medroxyprogesterone acetate 10 mg/day for 2 weeks.
   B. doubling the CE and continuing this dose for 2 weeks.
   C. a cycle of oral contraceptives.
   D. stopping the CE and beginning a cycle of oral contraceptives.
   E. office endometrial aspiration.

6. What is the mean volume of blood lost during normal menstruation?
   A. 15 ml
   B. 35 ml
   C. 55 ml
   D. 75 ml
   E. 95 ml

7. A 38-year-old woman presents with heavy vaginal bleeding of 9 days duration. Her pulse is 110, blood pressure 80/60, and pelvic examination is normal. The most efficacious treatment is
   A. parenteral high dose conjugated estrogen for 10 days.
   B. dilation and curettage.
   C. medroxyprogesterone acetate 20 mg/day for 10 days.
   D. danazol 400 mg/day for 10 days.
   E. four oral contraceptive tablets daily for 10 days.

8. A 14-year-old girl presents to the emergency room with a 3 day history of excessive menstrual flow. Her hemoglobin is 8.2 and her hematocrit is 23. A pregnancy test is negative. The blood pressure is 80/40 and the pulse 120. What is the most likely diagnosis?
   A. Von Willebrand's disease
   B. Factor VIII deficiency
   C. Leukemia
   D. Anovulation
   E. Endometrial polyps

9. A 28-year-old woman presents with complaints of missed menses for 7 days followed by spotting and then "late flow." These delayed cycles have occurred approximately 3 or 4 times per year for the past 2 years. A sensitive urine pregnancy test is negative at the time of her office visit. Endometrial biopsy done on the fourth day of her "late flow" reveals mixed proliferative and secretory endometrium. What is the diagnosis?
   A. Inadequate corpus luteum
   B. Anovulation
   C. Repetitive subclinical abortions
   D. Chronic ectopic pregnancy
   E. Halban's syndrome

10. A 38-year-old, 5 feet 4 inch, 135 pound gravida 2, para 2 woman presents with a 4 month history of progressively heavier, irregular menstruation. A BHCG test is negative. The pelvic examination is normal. What is the best choice for further investigation?
    A. Office hysteroscopy
    B. Office endometrial aspiration
    C. Serum clotting studies
    D. Hysterosalpingogram
    E. Pelvic ultrasound

11. After successful treatment of an acute episode of anovulatory bleeding in a 13-year-old, long-term treatment is best accomplished by which of the following?
    A. Dilation and curettage
    B. Cyclic oral contraceptives
    C. Cyclic conjugated estrogens
    D. Cyclic medroxyprogesterone acetate
    E. Cyclic danazol

12. A 42-year-old woman with Class III valvular heart disease has a history of progressive menorrhagia over the past 8 months. Previous attempts at using M.P.A. have failed. Endometrial aspiration shows proliferative endometrium without inflammation. The hemoglobin is 10.8. What is the treatment of choice?
    A. Cyclic oral contraceptives
    B. Nonsteroidal anti-inflammatory drugs
    C. Antibiotic therapy
    D. Endometrial laser vaporization
    E. Dilation and curettage

DIRECTIONS: For each numbered item, select the one heading most closely associated with it. Each lettered heading may be used once, more than once, or not at all.

(A) Danazol
(B) Ergot alkaloid
(C) Epsilon aminocaproic acid
(D) Medroxyprogesterone acetate

13. Inhibitor of fibrinolysis and is associated with a 50% reduction in menstrual blood loss in patients with menorrhagia.
14. Does not reduce menstrual blood loss in patients treated for menorrhagia.
15. Enhances activity of 17-α-dehydrogenase to favor conversion of estradiol to estrone.

DIRECTIONS: For each numbered item, indicate whether it is associated with
   A only (A)
   B only (B)
   C both (A) and (B)
   D neither (A) nor (B)

(A) Hysteroscopic laser photovaporization
(B) Hysteroscopic cryotherapy
(C) Both
(D) Neither

16. Recurrence of menorrhagia same as the recurrence after D&C.
17. An alternative to hysterectomy.
18. Used to treat early endometrial carcinoma.

(A) Organic uterine bleeding
(B) Dysfunctional uterine bleeding
(C) Both
(D) Neither

19. Considered endocrinologic in origin.
20. May present as menorrhagia.
21. Bleeding from marked atrophic vaginitis.

(A) High dose conjugated estrogen therapy
(B) High dose oral contraceptive therapy
(C) Both
(D) Neither

22. Effective for control of severe anovulatory bleeding.
23. Affords rapid endometrial cell growth and proliferation.
24. Decreases estrogen receptors in the endometrial cells.

DIRECTIONS: Each question contains four suggested answers of which one or more is correct. Choose the answer

A if 1, 2, and 3 are correct
B if 1 and 3 are correct
C if 2 and 4 are correct
D if 4 only is correct
E if all are correct

25. The histologic appearance of the endometrium of a patient who is anovulatory reveals
    1. proliferation of the endometrium.
    2. an acute inflammatory cell infiltrate.
    3. areas of necrosis of the endometrium.
    4. an eosinophilic infiltrate.
26. True statements regarding characteristics of normal menstruation include:
    1. The mean cycle interval is 28 days.
    2. Menstrual discomfort requires therapy.
    3. The mean duration of menstrual flow is 4 days.
    4. Blood flow requires no more than 20 sanitary pads or regular tampons per month.
27. Which pharmacologic actions of nonsteroidal anti-inflammatory drugs (NSAIDs) are used in treating menorrhagia?
    1. Inhibiting platelet aggregation
    2. Blocking conversion of arachidonic acid into prostaglandins
    3. Blocking formation of prostacyclin
    4. Increasing thromboxane formation
28. Which are characteristics of the hematologic profile of women who have greater than 80 ml blood loss per menstrual cycle?
    1. Reduced serum iron level
    2. Lower mean hemoglobin
    3. Lower mean hematocrit
    4. Decreased platelet aggregation
29. Medroxyprogesterone acetate (MPA)
    1. Long-term use stimulates secretory activity in the endometrial cell.
    2. Inhibits estrogen receptor replenishment in the cytosol.
    3. Reduces vascularity in the basalis layer of the endometrium.
    4. Activates 17-hydroxysteroid dehydrogenase.

ANSWERS

1. **D**, Page 956. The rationale for the therapeutic use of estrogen for the immediate treatment of DUB is based on the fact that estrogen in pharmacologic doses causes rapid growth of the endometrium. Thus bleeding that results from most causes of dysfunctional bleeding will respond to such therapy because a rapid growth of endometrial tissue occurs over the denuded and raw epithelial surface. Acute bleeding from most causes is usually controlled by this method. Appreciable changes in either systemic or local clotting factors or changes in platelet adhesiveness have not been well documented. Decidualization of the endometrium does not occur in the absence of progestin therapy and likewise uniform endometrial slough after estrogen withdrawal does not occur unless the estrogen treatment has been followed by adequate doses of progestins.

2. **C**, Page 955. The most common causes of intrauterine bleeding during the reproductive age are accidents of pregnancy such as a threatened, incomplete, or missed abortion or an ectopic pregnancy. This warrants performance of a sensitive β-HCG test, either by serum or urine, as part of the immediate diagnostic evaluation. Endometrial aspiration and hysteroscopy are contraindicated in this patient until a diagnosis of pregnancy is ruled out.

   After results of the pregnancy test are available, one might perform pelvic ultrasound and/or laparoscopy in this patient with normal pelvic exam findings, if one were concerned about a pregnancy abnormality.

3. **A**, Pages 956–957, 960–961. After dilation and curettage is used to treat acute bleeding in a women in her late reproductive years, further therapy is indicated if the histology shows secretory endometrium. This is best accomplished by using cyclic medroxyprogesterone acetate to effect an orderly withdrawal bleeding each month. Continuous MPA will be associated with degrees of endometrial atrophy from which the patient is likely to bleed again. Both cyclic and continuous conjugated estrogens are contraindicated since they will cause excessive endometrial proliferation which may cause further irregular, heavy bleeding. Cyclic danazol is not indicated and is a less cost effective measure to control bleeding in the patient. Since this woman is 45 and thus in a perimenopausal age group, she could be treated even though the endometrium is secretory. At this time it is possible that she is not ovulating each month. Oral contraceptives are contraindicated in this patient.

4. **A**, Pages 956–957. There are several approaches to the treatment of acute "endocrinologic" uterine bleeding. Each has its advocates. In this 22-year-old patient, acute bleeding is usually controlled adequately by administration of oral conjugated estrogens (CE) in a dose of 10 mg/day in divided doses until the bleeding markedly slows or stops. In this age group, it is important to have ruled out pregnancy. Judging from the amount of bleeding and the age of the patient, the bleeding is likely to be sec-

ondary to anovulation. Endometrial aspiration is not indicated in this patient with a low risk for neoplastic disease. This procedure will not remove the underlying cause for her bleeding. Likewise, dilation and curettage is not necessary unless there is a poor clinical response to estrogen therapy.

Medroxyprogesterone acetate (MPA) is less effective in providing immediate relief from the bleeding. Oral contraceptive agents containing 50 mcg of estrogen have been used in the immediate treatment of this problem.

5. **A, Pages 956–957.** When high dose conjugated estrogen therapy has been successful in reducing the amount of uterine bleeding within the first 24 hours, immediate progestin support of the endometrium is also required. Therefore conjugated estrogen therapy is continued at the same dosage and a progestin, usually medroxyprogesterone acetate (MPA), 10 mg/day is added. Both hormones are continued for 2 weeks, after which treatment is stopped to allow withdrawal bleeding.

Doubling the CE dose for 2 weeks is likely to cause abnormal hyperplasia of the endometrium and more bleeding. Initiation of oral contraceptives at this point is unnecessary in this patient who already has responded to conjugated estrogens. Stopping the conjugated estrogens after the initial high dose treatment is likely to be associated with further endometrial bleeding, which would render the response to the initiation of oral contraceptives ineffective. Since this patient has responded to high dose CE therapy, office endometrial aspiration is unnecessary at this point. If the patient were not to respond to the above outlined therapy, endometrial sampling or D&C would be indicated.

6. **B, Page 954.** There are two reliable objective methods that can be used to quantify menstrual blood loss. One involves radioisotope tagging of a patient's red cells; the other involves photometric measurement to quantify the amount of hematin collected on sanitary napkins. Using these techniques, it has been found in several studies that the mean amount of menstrual blood loss in normal women (women with normal hemoglobin, hematocrit, and plasma iron) is about 35 ml.

7. **B, Pages 960–961.** A dilation and curettage should be used to stop the acute bleeding episode in patients over the age of 35, since the incidence of anatomical problems and pathologic findings is increased in this age group. The performance of the D&C can be both diagnostic and therapeutic. The D&C is the quickest way to stop acute bleeding and is indicated for patients with severe menorrhagia who may be hypovolemic. It should be remembered that, although the D&C is effective for the treatment for acute bleeding, long-term cures are unusual since the underlying pathophysiology is unchanged.

8. **D. Pages 954–955.** Certain systemic diseases, especially disorders of blood coagulation such as Von Willebrand's disease and prothrombin (Factor VIII) deficiency, may often present as abnormal uterine bleeding. Other disorders that produce platelet deficiencies, such as leukemia, occasionally present in this fashion. Coagulation disorders are found in about 20% of adolescent females who require hospitalization for abnormal uterine bleeding.

Although routine screening for coagulation defects is indicated in an adolescent with dysfunctional uterine bleeding, the most common causes are anovulation and pregnancy.

9. **E, Page 955.** Certain disorders that may cause dysfunctional uterine bleeding relate to the life span of the corpus luteum. Prolonged life of the corpus luteum has been reported as a cause for abnormal bleeding similar to that presented by this patient (Halban's syndrome or a persistent corpus luteum). The etiology is uncertain and the treatment is expectant. This entity must be differentiated from early pregnancy loss by obtaining a sensitive serum or urine pregnancy test. Since this disorder is associated with a normal appearing secretory endometrium, the diagnosis is made if a biopsy is obtained on the fourth day of the patient's flow is both proliferative and secretory and the β-HCG assay is negative.

10. **B, Page 956.** In this age group, having ruled out pregnancy and given a normal pelvic examination, one must rule out malignancy even though it is unlikely. A cost effective method is to perform an office endometrial aspiration. An endometrial biopsy is ideally obtained at the onset of the bleeding episode to help determine whether or not ovulation has occurred. This knowledge will help determine therapy.

Office hysteroscopy is not indicated until the endometrial histology is known. Hysterosalpingogram and pelvic ultrasound are unnecessary tests in this patient. Serum clotting studies are largely unrevealing in a patient in this age group with a relatively short history of a bleeding abnormality.

11. **D, Page 957.** Adolescent anovulatory patients represent an ideal model for the use of progestins in the treatment of dysfunctional uterine bleeding. Because these patients are likely to have immaturity of the hypothalamic-pituitary axis, progestin therapy for 10 days each month is a reasonable mode of treatment to produce regular cyclic bleeding until maturity of the positive feedback system is achieved. Although controversial, it is probably best that oral contraceptives not be used in these patients since this therapy prolongs hypothalamic-pituitary

inhibition. Dilation and curettage is not indicated in this patient, whose acute bleeding episode has been controlled. Cyclic conjugated estrogens and cyclic danazol therapy are not indicated. Danazol is expensive and carries with it the risk of undesirable side effects.

12. **D**, Pages 961–962. (Also see Goldrath MH, Fuller TA, Segal S: Laser Photo Vaporization of Endometrium for the Treatment of Menorrhagia, Am J Obstet Gynecol 140:14, 1981.) Laser photovaporization of the endometrium for treatment of menorrhagia has been recently advocated by some investigators. This procedure for endometrial ablation may be used as an alternative to hysterectomy in patients where other modalities have failed or are *contraindicated*. This technique has been reported by Goldrath et al., who showed that it was curative in 160 of 180 patients.

Cyclic oral contraceptives are contraindicated in this patient and the efficacy of nonsteroidal anti-inflammatory drugs and antifibrinolytics in patients with systemic disease is poor. Dilation and curettage may only afford temporary relief.

13–15. 13, **C**; 14, **B**; 15, **D**; Pages 959–960. (Also see Nilsson L and Rybo G: Treatment for Menorrhagia, Am J Obstet Gynecol 110:713, 1971.) Episolon-aminocaproic acid is one of a number of potent inhibitors of fibrinolysis and therefore has been used in the treatment of various hemorrhagic conditions including menorrhagia. It is associated with a significant reduction of blood loss in these patients, resulting in about a 50% reduction in menstrual blood loss. The blood loss reduction was greatest in those patients who originally exhibited the greatest menstrual blood loss.

Ergot derivatives are not recommended. They are rarely effective and have a high incidence of side effects including nausea, vertigo, and abdominal cramps. One study demonstrated no reduction of blood loss among 82 women with menorrhagia who were treated with Ergot alkaloid preparations. This preparation is not effective at the cellular level. It is effective postpartum because myometrial contraction is important in reducing blood loss.

One mechanism of action of medroxyprogesterone acetate is to enhance the conversion of a potent estrogen, estradiol, to the less potent estrogen, estrone. This effectively reduces the cellular proliferation of the endometrium and thus reduces blood loss in patients with menorrhagia.

16–18. 16, **B**; 17, **A**; 18, **D**; Pages 961–962. Both cryotherapy and laser vaporization have been advocated for use in women with menorrhagia when other treatment modalities have failed. In both cases the procedure is done through an operating hysteroscope. Currently, evidence suggests that cryocautery is not effective. It has a recurrence rate of menorrhagia similar to that of dilation and curettage.

Laser photovaporization shows more promise with recent reports indicating high cure rates. There is minimal endometrial regeneration and the side effects seem to be minimal. Long-term data are not yet available. If these results continue to be favorable and are confirmed by others, this procedure may be used as an alternative to a hysterectomy in patients who fail other medical treatment regimens, or as an alternative to hysterectomy in patients who are poor surgical risks. Neither of these modalities is currently indicated for the treatment of endometrial cancer.

19–21. 19, **B**; 20, **C**; 21, **A**; Page 954. The etiology of abnormal uterine bleeding is usually divided into two major categories, organic and dysfunctional (or endocrinologic). The organic causes can be subdivided into systemic disease and reproductive tract disease. This implies an abnormal metabolic or anatomic etiology.

Dysfunctional uterine bleeding or endocrinologic bleeding usually refers to an aberration in the ovulatory mechanism or dysfunction of the hormonal milieu of the menstrual cycle. Heavy menstruation (menorrhagia) can be either dysfunctional or organic in origin.

22–24. 22, **C**; 23, **A**; 24, **B**; Page 957. Both high dose conjugated estrogen therapy and high dose combination oral contraception therapy are effective in controlling uterine blood loss from anovulation. Some gynecologists feel that high dose oral contraceptive therapy, such as four tablets of oral contraceptives containing 50 mcg of estrogen taken in 24 hours, provides a more efficient therapy for this problem. One controlled study suggests that the efficacy of conjugated estrogens is greater. A reason for this is that the combined use of estrogen and progestin as found in oral contraceptives does not afford as rapid endometrial cellular growth as estrogen alone, since the progestin component of the oral contraceptives decreases the estrogen receptors and increases the estradiol dehydrogenase in the endometrial cell, thus inhibiting the growth-promoting action of estrogen.

If conjugated estrogens are used alone in the immediate treatment of this entity, it is important to remember to add a potent progestin such as medroxyprogesterone acetate once the bleeding has diminished to afford endometrial stabilization and effect orderly withdrawal bleeding after 2 weeks.

25. **B** (1, 3), Pages 955–956. In most patients with dysfunctional uterine bleeding, ovula-

tion fails to occur. There is continuous estradiol production without corpus luteum formation and progesterone secretion. This leads to a continually proliferating endometrium and the formation of areas of necrosis which occur as the endometrium outgrows its blood supply. In contrast to normal menstruation, uniform slough of the endometrium to the basalis layer does not occur and thus there is excessive uterine blood flow. Acute inflammation or eosinophilic infiltration typically is not part of the histology of the endometrium of patients with dysfunctional uterine bleeding. Chronic endometrial inflammation may contribute to irregular bleeding patterns. It is discussed in Chapter 22.

26. **B** (1, 3), Page 953. To define abnormal uterine bleeding, it is necessary to first recognize the characteristics of normal menstrual flow. The mean cycle interval is 28 days plus or minus 7 days and the mean duration of flow is 4 days. Bleeding for more than 7 days is abnormally prolonged and termed menorrhagia. Subjective assessments of menstrual blood loss (MBL) are poorly correlated with objective measurements of MBL. One study suggests that 40% of women with blood loss greater than 80 ml considered their menstrual flow to be small or moderate in amount. Determining the number of sanitary pads used is an unreliable indication of MBL. There is a great variability of absorption among different types of sanitary pads as well as marked variations in the fastidiousness among patients in their need to change sanitary products. Although considered a part of normal menstruation, the discomfort experienced usually does not require specific therapy.

27. **A** (1, 2, 3), Page 958. Nonsteroidal antiinflammatory drugs have been shown to significantly reduce menstrual blood loss, primarily in patients who ovulate. The exact details of their mechanism of action is unclear. They block fatty acid cyclooxygenase which catalyzes the conversion of arachidonic acid into prostaglandins. These drugs also block the formation of prostacyclin and decrease the formation of thromboxane. Thromboxane increases platelet aggregation.

28. **A** (1, 2, 3), Page 954. (Also see Hallberg L and Nilsson L: Determination of Menstrual Blood Loss, Scan J Clin Lab Invest 16:244, 1964.) Using quantitative methods, Hallberg et al. found that individuals with a monthly menstrual blood loss of greater than 80 ml have a significant lower mean hemoglobin, hematocrit, and serum iron levels. Therefore, a menstrual blood loss greater than 80 ml should be regarded as hypermenorrhea. The anemia demonstrated in these patients is secondary to blood loss and is not related to abnormal clotting factors or platelet aggregation abnormalities. Abnormalities of these factors may contribute to excessive blood loss in a smaller select group of patients (see question 35.7).

29. **C** (2, 4), Page 957. Medroxyprogesterone acetate, given to patients with adequate amounts of endogenous estrogen, produces regular withdrawal bleeding. When used as maintenance therapy over longer periods of time, MPA is usually prescribed in a dose of 10 mg daily for 10 to 13 days each month.

Unlike natural progesterone, progestins act as antiestrogens. They diminish the effect of estrogen on the target cells by inhibiting estrogen receptor replenishment in the cytosol and induce the activation of 17-hydroxysteroid dehydrogenase, which converts estradiol to the less active estrone. These findings account for the antimitotic, antigrowth effect of progestins. Natural progesterone stimulates secretory activity which does not occur with long term use of MPA. There is no evidence suggesting that endometrial vascularity is reduced by the use of MPA.

CHAPTER 36

Amenorrhea

DIRECTIONS: Select the one best answer or completion.

1. Normal pubertal development is the result of
   A. ovarian maturation.
   B. increased sensitivity of the hypothalamic-pituitary-gonadal axis to circulating estrogen.
   C. decreased REM sleep.
   D. maturation of the hypothalamic-pituitary-gonadal axis.
   E. weight loss.

2. A 17-year-old states she has never had a period. On examination, the findings are as shown in Figure 36-1. What is the most likely diagnosis?
   A. Pregnancy
   B. Androgen insensitivity
   C. Gonadal dysgenesis
   D. Imperforate hymen
   E. Rokitansky-Küster-Hauser syndrome

3. Given the probable diagnosis in Question 2, what would be the most useful initial diagnostic test?
   A. Buccal smear
   B. FSH
   C. Serum estrogen
   D. GnRH (LH-RH) stimulation test
   E. Bone age

4. Eight months after the delivery of her second child, a patient complains of still not having a period. The patient did not breastfeed because she could not produce milk. Pregnancy test and progestin withdrawal test are negative. What is the most likely diagnosis?
   A. Sheehan's syndrome
   B. Hyperprolactinemia
   C. Polycystic ovarian disease
   D. Androgen insensitivity
   E. Rokitansky syndrome

5. Anorexia nervosa is characterized by all the following **except**
   A. dry skin.
   B. hypotension.
   C. tachycardia.
   D. hypothermia.
   E. constipation.

6. A 14-year-old with normal secondary sexual development is seen in the emergency department complaining of abdominal pain. Her history reveals that this patient has never menstruated. On examination, you palpate a large central abdominopelvic mass which extends to the umbilicus and feels like an enlarged uterus. Fetal heart tones are not heard. What is the most likely diagnosis?
   A. Rokitansky syndrome
   B. Androgen insensitivity
   C. Complete transverse vaginal septum
   D. Pregnancy
   E. Gonadal dysgenesis

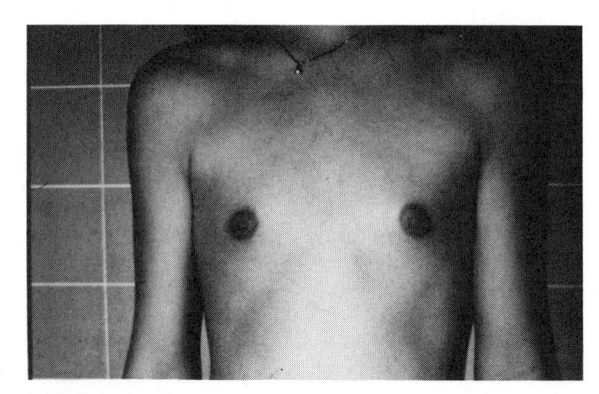

FIGURE 36-1.

7. Of the following conditions, which is the most common cause of secondary amenorrhea in adolescent girls?
   A. Polycystic ovarian disease
   B. Anorexia nervosa
   C. Hyperprolactinemia
   D. Rokitansky syndrome
   E. Gonadal dysgenesis

8. A 27-year-old marathon athlete asks for your advice regarding her menstrual cycles. In the past 4½ years she has menstruated only once. The examination is within normal limits. Appropriate advice would be to ask the woman to
   A. reduce physical activity to a minimum.
   B. increase caloric intake and gain weight.
   C. take oral contraceptive pills.
   D. await the results of a progestin withdrawal test.
   E. obtain a psychiatric evaluation.

9. A 17-year-old who has had regular periods every 28 to 30 days since she was 12 is now 2 weeks late for her period. Past medical history is negative, and the physical exam is within normal limits. Which of the following tests is indicated?
   A. Serum prolactin
   B. FSH
   C. β-HCG
   D. Serum estradiol
   E. Karyotype

10. A 16-year-old white female presents to her doctor's office complaining that she is 4 weeks late for her period. She is sexually active. Past medical history is negative, and the physical exam is within normal limits. The pregnancy test is negative. What is the most likely diagnosis?
    A. Ectopic pregnancy
    B. Anovulation
    C. Gonadal failure
    D. Hypothyroidism
    E. Anorexia nervosa

11. Which is an appropriate management of the anovulatory adolescent patient?
    A. Clomiphene citrate
    B. Progestin withdrawal
    C. Pergonal
    D. GnRH agonist
    E. Premarin

12. A 14-year-old high school student is referred for evaluation of primary amenorrhea. She is an excellent athlete and runs almost 5 miles daily. On examination it is noted that her breasts are Tanner stage 1, and pubic development is graded as Tanner stage 2. The remainder of the examination is within normal limits. Appropriate evaluation should include
    A. pregnancy test.
    B. serum estrogen levels.
    C. serum FSH levels.
    D. karyotype.
    E. serum testosterone levels.

DIRECTIONS: For each numbered item, select the one heading most closely associated with it. Each lettered heading may be used once, more than once, or not at all.

(A) Low levels of FSH
(B) Normal FSH
(C) High FSH
(D) High ACTH levels

13. Turner's syndrome
14. Positive progestin withdrawal test
15. Kallman's syndrome
16. Resistant ovary syndrome (Savage syndrome)

DIRECTIONS: Each question contains four suggested answers of which one or more is correct. Choose the answer
   A if 1, 2, and 3 are correct
   B if 1 and 3 are correct
   C if 2 and 4 are correct
   D if 4 only is correct
   E if all are correct

17. Typically patients with Rokitansky syndrome are differentiated from patients with androgen insensitivity by
    1. a history of primary amenorrhea.
    2. progesterone withdrawal test results.
    3. the presence of a short blind vagina.
    4. karyotype.

18. What would one expect a patient with anorexia nervosa to have?
    1. Low FSH
    2. Low T_4
    3. Low T_3
    4. Normal estrogen

19. Which of the following karyotypes may be obtained from individuals with gonadal dysgenesis?
    1. 45,X
    2. 46,XX or 46,XY
    3. 45,X/46,XX
    4. 45,X/46,XY

20. Which procedures are appropriate in the management of patients with androgen insensitivity syndrome?
    1. Gonadectomy
    2. Breast augmentation
    3. Vaginal dilation
    4. Hysterectomy

21. Asherman's syndrome is associated with
    1. secondary amenorrhea.
    2. dilation and curettage.
    3. tuberculous endometritis.
    4. elevated FSH levels.
22. Gonadectomy should be performed on patients with
    1. androgen insensitivity.
    2. Turner syndrome.
    3. pure gonadal dysgenesis.
    4. Rokitansky syndrome.
23. The somatic features of Turner's syndrome include
    1. short stature.
    2. normal breast development.
    3. web neck.
    4. cubitus varus.
24. Ovarian failure may be caused by
    1. autoimmune disorder.
    2. X-chromosome deletion.
    3. autosomal recessive disorder in 46,XX individuals.
    4. X-linked recessive disorder in 46,XY individuals.
25. In a 15-year-old presenting with primary amenorrhea and a large uterine mass, which diagnoses should be considered?
    1. Rokitansky syndrome
    2. Imperforate hymen
    3. Longitudinal vaginal septum
    4. Pregnancy
26. When Asherman's syndrome is suspected, which procedures are useful in establishing the diagnosis?
    1. Hysterogram
    2. Hysterotomy
    3. Hysteroscopy
    4. Laparoscopy
27. Findings associated with anorexia nervosa include
    1. weight loss of at least 25% of original body weight.
    2. onset before age 25.
    3. a distorted attitude towards food.
    4. absence of other medical or psychiatric disorders.
28. True statements regarding female athletes with exercise-induced amenorrhea include:
    1. Prolactin levels are extremely low.
    2. β-endorphin levels are elevated during exercise.
    3. Exercise-induced amenorrhea causes high FSH levels.
    4. The amenorrhea associated with exercise is stress related.

ANSWERS

1. **D,** Pages 966–968. Prior to puberty, gonadotrophin levels are low because the hypothalamic-pituitary-gonadal axis is extremely sensitive to the negative feedback of the low level of circulating estrogen. As the axis matures, this sensitivity diminishes and an *episodic* nocturnal rise in LH is observed. Next, pulses of FSH and LH are noted both at night and during the daytime. FSH and LH stimulate the gonad to produce estrogen which, in turn, affects secondary sexual development.
2. **C,** Pages 972–973. The combination of primary amenorrhea and absent breast development suggests failure of the gonads to produce estrogen. The only condition listed characterized by absent estrogen production is gonadal dysgenesis. In all other conditions, the amenorrhea is associated with adequate and appropriate breast development. The Rokitansky syndrome, also known as the Meyer-Rokitansky-Küster-Hauser syndrome, is characterized by an incomplete to atretic vagina and a rudimentary to bicornuate uterus. The tubes and ovaries are normal, and hence pubertal development is normal except for a lack of menstruation. The lower vagina usually consists of a short blind pouch. On rare occasions, a patient may have a functional endometrium and thus develop hematometra. Renal (50%) and skeletal malformations (10–15%) are moderately common.
3. **B,** Pages 972–973. Although all the tests listed have a place in the workup of a patient with delayed puberty, a determination of the FSH serum concentration would be most valuable in this patient. A high FSH level will confirm gonadal failure, while a low FSH level will suggest constitutional delay or pituitary failure. A karyotype is important after the diagnosis of gonadal failure is established, since some of these patients will have a mosaic containing a Y chromosome. Because it contains a great deal more information, a karyotype is preferred over a buccal smear.
4. **A,** Pages 985–986. This postpartum patient was unable to produce milk which is the typical presentation of a patient whose pituitary gland was destroyed during pregnancy and delivery due to hemorrhage or thrombosis. This constellation of events is called Sheehan's syndrome. It is important to evaluate the function of other endocrine organs, particularly the thyroid and the adrenal glands, because "multigland" hormonal replacement therapy may be indicated. Androgen insensitivity is found in a genetic male while Rokitansky syndrome includes an absent vagina. The clinical presentation is not typical of

polycystic ovarian disease since a withdrawal bleed is expected in response to progestin therapy.
5. **C,** Page 982. Patients with anorexia nervosa have bradycardia, not tachycardia. These patients may also have dry skin, hypotension, hypothermia, and constipation.
6. **C,** Pages 966, 970–971. The large central mass is probably an enlarged uterus. The association of primary amenorrhea, an enlarged uterus, and pain suggest an obstruction of the outflow tract and retention of menstrual flow. The patient has normal sexual development indicating an active hypothalamic-pituitary-ovarian axis and adequate estrogen production, excluding the possibility of gonadal dysgenesis. If, in fact, the large abdominopelvic mass is a uterus, androgen insensitivity syndrome is excluded since a uterus is absent in these individuals. The absence of fetal heart tones makes pregnancy an unlikely possibility. Rokitansky syndrome with a uterus is very rare and is therefore far less likely than a complete transverse vaginal septum.
7. **B,** Pages 981–983. Any patient who presents with postpubertal amenorrhea should be considered to be pregnant until proven otherwise since pregnancy is the most common cause of amenorrhea in young females. Adolescents with anorexia nervosa, excessive stress, hyperprolactinemia, Rokitansky syndrome, and gonadal dysgenesis can all present with primary amenorrhea, but eating disorders are probably the most common cause of secondary amenorrhea in adolescents who are not pregnant.
8. **D,** Pages 979–981. It is now believed that amenorrhea associated with strenuous exercise is also related to stress. While reducing physical activity to a minimum or increasing caloric intake to gain weight may alleviate the problem, most athletes refuse to do so. Amenorrhea by itself does the patient no harm. However, it reflects a hypoestrogenic state, which makes the patient susceptible to developing osteoporosis. Prior to the initiation of estrogen replacement therapy (ERT), a progestin withdrawal test is done. If positive (bleeding occurs), the patient is presumed to produce adequate amounts of estrogen, and ERT is not required. If negative, ERT is suggested to prevent the deleterious effects of estrogen deficiency on the bones.
9. **C,** Page 987. The most common cause of secondary amenorrhea in young women is pregnancy. Although hyperprolactinemia, gonadal failure, and chromosome abnormalities may cause secondary amenorrhea, these are relatively rare. This patient has not met the criteria for secondary amenorrhea. Nevertheless, a pregnancy test should be performed. If the pregnancy test is negative, the patient can be reassured. It is most likely that she will resume normal menstruation. If she has 6 months of amenorrhea, a workup should be initiated.
10. **B,** Pages 987–990. Anovulation is relatively common at both ends of the reproductive age group, that is, the young adolescent girls in the first 2 years after puberty and the perimenopausal women. Thus, anovulation is the most likely diagnosis in this patient whose hormonal and chromosomal studies are probably normal. If there is doubt, other laboratory tests such as FSH, TSH, prolactin, estrogen, and karyotype can be performed.
11. **B,** Pages 987, 990. Patients who suffer from chronic anovulation have unopposed estrogen production. Overgrowth of endometrium follows, and abnormal uterine bleeding occurs following a period of amenorrhea. Although the patient can be followed without treatment, progestin withdrawal would reassure the patient that there is no significant pathology as well as counteract the action of unopposed estrogen. Although clomiphene citrate induces ovulation, and therefore can be used to treat chronic anovulation, the use of this medication should be reserved for patients who wish to become pregnant.
12. **C,** Pages 972–974, 979–981. Although exercise-induced amenorrhea is relatively common in this age group, this young woman has not begun her secondary sexual development. Therefore, as with all girls her age who have not commenced developing breasts, complete evaluation is required. The absence of breast development signifies lack of estrogen production, and serum FSH levels at this point would be most helpful in determining whether estrogen deficiency is on the basis of gonadal dysgenesis or on the basis of hypothalamic-pituitary disorder. Elevated FSH levels would indicate gonadal failure, and low FSH levels would suggest a hypothalamic disorder. Pregnancy test and a karyotype are not indicated at the present time. Estrogen levels are difficult to interpret and testosterone is helpful when the patient is hirsute. In patients with low FSH levels, consideration should be given to performing the GnRH stimulation test to determine the level of maturation of the hypothalamic-pituitary ovarian axis.
13–16. 13, **C;** 14, **B;** 15, **A;** 16, **C;** Pages 970–977. Normal levels of FSH suggest adequate estrogen production, and thus following progestin administration, withdrawal bleeding is expected. High levels of FSH indicate a hypoestrogenic state on the basis of gonadal failure or resistance (gonadal dysgenesis, Turner's syndrome, resistant ovary syndrome). Withdrawal bleeding following progestin administration is not expected. Kallman's

syndrome denotes individuals with hypogonadotrophic hypogonadism and anosmia. FSH levels are low as a result of inadequate production.

17. D (4), Page 965. Patients with the typical Rokitansky syndrome and patients with androgen insensitivity have a short blind vagina and no uterus. Usually, they present to the physician complaining of primary amenorrhea. Because they have no outflow tract and Rokitansky syndrome often has no functioning uterus, a progestin withdrawal test is negative in both groups. The difference between these two groups of patients is the mechanism by which the müllerian duct fails to develop. In patients with androgen insensitivity, müllerian inhibiting factor produced by the testes causes regression of the müllerian duct.

Except for the karyotype, the findings are similar in both conditions. Patients with Rokitansky syndrome have a normal female karyotype (46,XX), while patients with androgen insensitivity syndrome possess a normal male karyotype (46,XY).

18. B (1, 3), Page 982. Patients with anorexia nervosa have a hypothalamic disorder interfering with normal GnRH release. Thus FSH and estrogen levels are extremely low. In addition, the peripheral conversion of T_4 to T_3 is impaired, resulting in low levels of T_3 but T_4 levels within the normal range.

19. E, Pages 972–973. Gonadal failure is usually the result of X chromosome deletion in all cells (45,X) or in some of the cells (mosaic). A number of karyotypes have been found including, but not limited to, 45,X; 45,X/46,XX; and 45,X/46,XY. Some individuals may have a single gene defect resulting in gonadal dysgenesis (pure gonadal dysgenesis). These conditions are transmitted either as an autosomal recessive disorder in genetic females (46,XX) or as an X-linked recessive disorder in genetic males (46,XY).

20. B (1, 3), Pages 974, 977. Patients with androgen insensitivity have normal testes located in the abdominal cavity or the inguinal canal. These gonads, if left in situ, are at increased risk of developing a malignancy, and thus should be removed when pubertal development is complete. Estrogen replacement therapy should be given following castration. The vagina of these individuals is short and requires dilation and elongation. This can be achieved either by graduated dilation (Frank's method) or surgically (McIndoe-Reed Procedure). These patients have no uterus and therefore hysterectomy is not performed. Breast development is adequate, requiring no augmentation.

21. A (1, 2, 3), Pages 977–978. Asherman's syndrome is characterized by intrauterine adhesions obliterating the endometrial cavity. The most frequent cause of Asherman's syndrome is a vigorous endometrial curettage, usually postpartum or postabortal. Tuberculous endometritis is a rare cause of Asherman's syndrome. As a result of Asherman's syndrome, patients have secondary amenorrhea, despite normal FSH and estrogen levels.

22. B (1,3), Pages 976–977. Prophylactic gonadectomy should be performed on all patients with a Y chromosome complement. Thus, patients with androgen insensitivity and patients with pure gonadal dysgenesis, who have 46,XY chromosome complement, require gonadectomy to eliminate the risk of developing a neoplasm (gonadoblastoma) in the gonad. Patients with Turner syndrome, whose karyotype is 45,X, and patients with Rokitansky syndrome, who have a normal 46,XX karyotype, do not require gonadectomy. A word of caution—some patients with gonadal dysgenesis who seemingly have a 45,X karyotype may have mosaicism in which the 45,X cell line is mixed with a 46, XY cell line. These patients would also need gonadectomy.

23. B (1,3), Pages 972–973. Patients with Turner's syndrome have gonadal dysgenesis and a karyotype of 45,X. In addition to primary amenorrhea and absent breast development, these individuals have other somatic abnormalities, the most prevalent being stature under five feet (the gene for stature being located on the short arm of the X chromosome). In addition, web neck, short fourth metacarpal, shield chest, widely spaced nipples, and cubitus valgus are some of the more prevalent somatic anomalies observed. Because of the short stature and these morphometric features, the diagnosis is usually made prior to puberty.

24. E (All), Page 986. Ovarian failure may result from deletion of genetic material on the X chromosome. When one X chromosome is missing in its entirety, the typical Turner's syndrome results. However, various degrees of deletion have been described. If X chromosome material is missing, ovarian failure can occur. Individuals with premature ovarian failure may have antibodies to endocrine organs, suggesting an autoimmune etiology. An infectious etiology such as mumps oophoritis has also been observed. Patients with a normal karyotype 46,XX may suffer from ovarian failure on the basis of an autosomal recessive disorder. Genetic males with 46,XY karyotype may present with "ovarian" failure on the basis of an X-linked recessive disorder. Because gonadal function is lost in utero, the external genitalia are not stimulated by androgens. As a result, the external genitalia develop to appear female. These individuals

are raised as girls and there is no secondary sexual development at the time of expected puberty.

25. **C** (2, 4), Page 966. A 15-year-old presenting with primary amenorrhea and a large abdominal mass may suffer from an outflow tract obstruction with the subsequent accumulation of menstrual flow behind the obstructing membrane. Thus, an imperforate hymen is a likely diagnosis. Although pregnancy is uncommon in patients who have not had a menstrual period, ovulation may occur in the first cycle, so pregnancy should always be considered. Patients with Rokitansky syndrome usually have no uterus and would not likely have a uterine mass. Primary amenorrhea is not a manifestation of a longitudinal vaginal septum.

26. **A** (1, 3), Pages 977–978. Asherman's syndrome denotes intrauterine synechiae. These can be diagnosed by hysterogram or during hysteroscopy. On hysterogram, synechiae can be seen as filling defects, or there may be complete obliteration of the uterine cavity. During hysteroscopy intrauterine adhesions are seen directly and can be interrupted through an operating hysteroscope. Laparoscopy and hysterotomy have no place in the diagnosis and management of intrauterine adhesions.

27. **E** (All), Page 982. All the findings listed are helpful in making the diagnosis of anorexia nervosa. In addition, at least two of the following manifestations are usually seen: 1) amenorrhea, 2) lanugo hair, 3) bradycardia, 4) periods of overactivity, 5) episodes of spontaneous or self-induced vomiting after meals.

28. **C** (2, 4), Pages 979–982. It is believed that amenorrhea associated with strenuous exercise is related to stress as well as to weight loss. Prolactin, β-endorphin, and catecholestrogen levels are significantly higher and LH and FSH significantly lower in women who exercise strenuously.

Chapter 37: Hyperprolactinemia, Galactorrhea, and Pituitary Adenomas

DIRECTIONS for questions 1–14: Select the one best answer or completion.

1. A 37-year-old with galactorrhea has a prolactin of 40 ng/ml on two occasions. Her thyroid function studies are normal. Twenty minutes after a 500 μg IV bolus of thyrotropin-releasing hormone (TRH) the prolactin is 90 ng/ml. The next step would be to
   A. observe for 3 months.
   B. obtain an anteroposterior and lateral coned-down views of the sella turcica.
   C. obtain a CT (computerized tomography) scan.
   D. start bromoergocryptine.
   E. refer for surgical resection.

2. A patient who has been treated for a prolactin-secreting microadenoma has just delivered and wishes to breast feed. You would advise her
   A. not to breast feed.
   B. to take bromoergocryptine while breast feeding.
   C. to take bromoergocryptine for 2 to 3 weeks after breast feeding.
   D. to have a serum prolactin determination before you decide what to advise.
   E. to have a CT (computerized tomography) scan before you decide what to advise.

3. All of the following can cause galactorrhea and hyperprolactinemia EXCEPT
   A. Cushing's disease.
   B. low dose oral contraceptives.
   C. chronic renal disease.
   D. hypothyroidism.
   E. chest trauma.

4. A 20-year-old gravida 0 complains of galactorrhea. She has no other complaints. Her periods are regular, occurring every 28 days. Her physical examination is normal. A serum prolactin is reported to be 18 ng/ml. At this point you would order
   A. a computerized tomography (CT) scan.
   B. a hypocycloidal tomography.
   C. a pneumoencephalography.
   D. all of the above.
   E. none of the above.

5. "Big-big" prolactin
   A. is the principle form of prolactin measured in bioassays.
   B. is the principal form of prolactin measured in immunoassays.
   C. is a dimer of the small monomeric form.
   D. has reduced binding to mammary tissue membranes in comparison to the monomeric form.
   E. constitutes 50% of the secreted form.

6. Select the patient in Figure 37-1 whose serum prolactin is most typical of the normal patient.
   A. Patient A
   B. Patient B
   C. Patient C
   D. Patient D
   E. Patient E

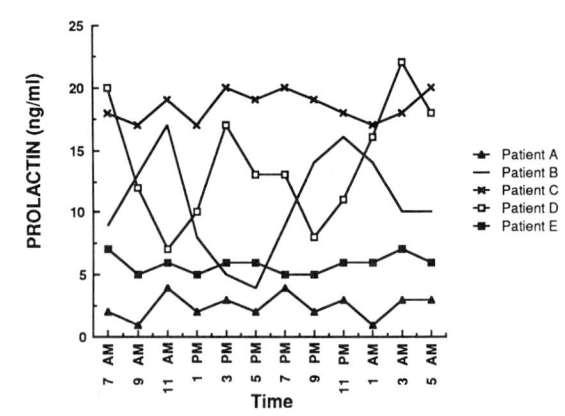

FIGURE 37-1.

7. In the normal patient lactation does not commence until after delivery because

A. prolactin is not secreted until after delivery.
B. placental lactogen is only weakly lactogenic.
C. β-HCG blocks the action of prolactin on the breast.
D. the increase in cortisol associated with the delivery process is important in the initiation of lactation.
E. estrogen inhibits the action of prolactin on the breast.

8. A 33-year-old, who is 5 feet 3 inches tall and weighs 180 pounds, has galactorrhea, oligomenorrhea, a serum prolactin of 18 ng/ml and a normal TSH. At this point you would
    A. do nothing for a year.
    B. order an infusion of Thyrotropin-Releasing-Hormone (TRH) as a provocative stimulus of prolactin.
    C. order a CT (computerized tomography) scan.
    D. order a MRI (magnetic resonance imagery).
    E. order an anteroposterior and lateral coned-down views of the sella turcica.

9. In which of the following patients with galactorrhea, all of whom might have an elevated serum prolactin, are you **most** likely to find that the prolactin actually is elevated?
    A. A 20-year-old with low estrogen and amenorrhea.
    B. A 30-year-old, 8 months postpartum, breast feeding, and with amenorrhea, whose blood is drawn when the woman is in a basal state.
    C. A 25-year-old with normal estrogen and oligomenorrhea.
    D. A 30-year-old with normal estrogen and amenorrhea.
    E. A 25-year-old with normal estrogen and normal menses.

10. A woman who recently has developed trouble breast-feeding her 7-month-old infant has had a basal serum prolactin determination, which is reported to be 10 ng/ml. Having been asked for an opinion, you would state that
    A. this is too low a level for successful lactation.
    B. that she is obviously under stress, and that if she relaxed, the prolactin would increase and she would be able to breast-feed.
    C. the prolactin level is compatible with successful breast-feeding.
    D. without knowing the conditions under which the result was obtained, you cannot offer an opinion.
    E. the patient should be examined for Sheehan's syndrome.

11. A 25-year-old single patient has oligomenorrhea, galactorrhea, and hyperprolactinemia (88 ng/ml). Thyroid function studies are normal. On CT (computerized tomograph) scan a 3 mm microadenoma was noted. The oligomenorrhea and galactorrhea are not of concern to the patient. Recommended therapy for this patient is
    A. bromoergocryptine.
    B. external radiation therapy.
    C. periodic progestin withdrawal.
    D. surgical resection.
    E. implantation of yttrium-90 rods.

12. The major mechanism by which elevated levels of prolactin inhibit ovulation appears to be
    A. a direct action of big-big prolactin.
    B. alterations in normal gonadotrophin-releasing hormone (GnRH) release.
    C. direct inhibition of ovarian secretion of estradiol.
    D. direct inhibition of ovarian secretion of progesterone.
    E. interference with the positive estrogen effect on midcycle LH release.

13. True statements about prolactin include all of the following **EXCEPT**
    A. it is synthesized in chromophobe cells located in the pituitary gland.
    B. it is stored in chromophobe cells located in the pituitary gland.
    C. it is synthesized in decidual tissue.
    D. it is synthesized in endometrial tissue.
    E. it has a half-life of 20 hours.

14. Pituitary tumors that secrete mainly adrenocorticotropic hormone (ACTH) or growth hormone frequently secrete prolactin. Hyperprolactinemia has been reported to occur in about
    A. twenty five percent of patients with Cushing's disease and 10% of patients with acromegaly.
    B. ten percent of patients with Cushing's disease and 25% of patients with acromegaly.
    C. ten percent of patients with Cushing's disease and 10% of patients with acromegaly.
    D. twenty–five percent of patients with Cushing's disease and 25% of patients with acromegaly.
    E. five percent of patients with Cushing's disease and 10% of patients with acromegaly.

DIRECTIONS for questions 15-21: For each numbered item, select the one heading most closely associated with it. Each lettered heading may be used only once.

15–16.
(A) Dopamine
(B) Epinephrine
(C) Serotonin
(D) 2-Br-alpha-ergocryptine mesylate
(E) Estradiol

15. Prolactin-inhibiting factor (PIF)
16. Prolactin-releasing factor (PRF)

17–19. Several pharmacologic agents are associated with galactorrhea and hyperprolactinemia. The pathophysiology depends upon the agent. Match the mechanism with the medication.
(A) Blocks dopamine uptake
(B) Blocks hypothalamic dopamine receptors
(C) Depletes catecholamines
(D) Blocks the conversion of tyrosine to dopa

17. Reserpine
18. Haloperidol
19. Tricyclic antidepressants

20–21.
(A) 10%
(B) 20%
(C) 50%
(D) 80%
(E) >90%

20. Percent of women with hyperprolactinemia who have a prolactinoma.
21. Percent of all pituitary adenomas that secrete prolactin.

DIRECTIONS for questions 22-23: For each numbered item, indicate whether it is associated with
A: only (A).
B: only (B).
C: both (A) and (B).
D: neither (A) nor (B).

22–23.
(A) Prolactin-secreting **Macroadenoma**
(B) Prolactin-secreting **Microadenoma**
(C) Both
(D) Neither

22. Visual field testing
23. Insulin tolerance test

DIRECTIONS for questions 24-35: Each question contains four suggested answers, of which one or more is correct. Choose the answer
A if 1, 2, and 3 are correct
B if 1 and 3 are correct
C if 2 and 4 are correct
D if 4 only is correct
E if all are correct

24. Findings commonly associated with patients who have hyperprolactinemia include
   1. amenorrhea.
   2. anovulation.
   3. oligomenorrhea.
   4. polymenorrhea.

25. Bromoergocryptine (2-Br-alpha-ergocryptine mesylate) is
   1. detectable in the circulation 24 hours after administration.
   2. often (15–25%) a cause of orthostatic hypotension.
   3. has FDA approval for use in patients with infertility, oligomenorrhea, and a prolactin level greater than 10 ng/ml.
   4. a dopamine receptor agonist.

26. A 19-year-old college student developed amenorrhea of 6 months duration. A workup at Student Health revealed a normal physical, including a normal pelvic examination, a FSH in the low normal range, and an early morning serum prolactin of 70 ng/ml. At this point you would order a
   1. quantitative β-HCG.
   2. repeat serum prolactin in mid-afternoon.
   3. LH.
   4. thyroid-stimulating hormone (TSH).

27. A 28-year-old gravida 0 who consulted you because of infertility is found to have a prolactin microadenoma. In discussing bromoergocryptine treatment, you would tell this patient that
   1. she will not get pregnant until her prolactin is less than 20 ng/ml.
   2. she should notify you immediately if she is late for a period so that you can stop the medication since there is some evidence that it is minimally teratogenic.
   3. even with a dose of up to 20 mg/day (about three times the average), 40% of patients with a microadenoma fail to have prolactin levels return to normal.
   4. this medication is not associated with spontaneous abortion or multiple gestations.

28. The patient is a 20-year-old white long-distance track star who consulted you because of amenorrhea. Initially, you felt it was due to her vigorous exercise. Then she developed galactorrhea, and you obtained a serum prolactin. Now, having made the diagnosis of a prolactin-secreting microadenoma, you would inform the patient that if she is not treated she is very likely to develop
    1. adrenal insufficiency.
    2. visual problems.
    3. hypothyroidism.
    4. osteoporosis.
29. Prolactin stimulates the
    1. growth of mammary tissue.
    2. production of milk by mammary tissue.
    3. secretion of milk into the alveoli of breast glands.
    4. release of gonadotrophins.
30. Bromoergocryptine can be used to treat a prolactin-secreting macroadenoma
    1. prior to surgical resection in an effort to alter and shrink the tumor.
    2. instead of either surgery or radiation.
    3. after an irradiation failure.
    4. in a patient who has visual field impairment.
31. A patient has been found to have a prolactin of 55 ng/ml. In discussing the diagnostic workup to rule out a prolactinoma, you inform her about a CT (computerized tomography) scan and an infusion of thyrotropin-releasing-hormone (TRH). You would indicate that
    1. first you will do a CT scan.
    2. a CT scan will expose her to 3 rads.
    3. if the CT is positive, you will order a MRI (magnetic resonance imaging).
    4. a normal response (indicating no tumor) to an infusion of 500 µg of TRH is at least 200% increase in the level of prolactin.
32. Physiologic stimuli that increase prolactin release include
    1. stress.
    2. exercise.
    3. sleep.
    4. nipple stimulation.
33. The rationale for discontinuing bromoergocryptine in a woman who becomes pregnant and has a prolactin-secreting macroadenoma is that
    1. it suppresses fetal prolactin.
    2. less than 1% of such patients have a decrease in visual fields during pregnancy.
    3. if necessary it can always be reinitiated.
    4. it suppresses placental hormone production.
34. An increase in serum prolactin is usually noted with
    1. an infusion of thyrotropin-releasing-hormone (TRH).
    2. a craniopharyngioma.
    3. a macroadenoma.
    4. the empty sella syndrome.
35. A 40-year-old is found to have a prolactinoma. Her serum prolactin is 250 ng/ml, and she gives a history of 3 years of amenorrhea and galactorrhea. The patient has inquired about surgical correction. In discussing the possible outcomes following transsphenoidal microsurgical resection, it would be correct to tell this patient that the likelihood of
    1. hypopituitarism is <2%.
    2. an initial cure is around 35%.
    3. a cure is decreased because of her age.
    4. operative mortality is 2%.

ANSWERS

1. **C**, Page 1002. In cases with borderline elevations of prolactin and an abnormal response to TRH (an increase of less than 200%), a CT scan should be performed. Not all individuals with an abnormal TRH response will have radiologic evidence of a microadenoma, however.
2. **C**, Page 1010. Following delivery, breast feeding may be initiated without adverse effects on the tumor. Following completion of nursing, bromoergocryptine should be ingested for 2 to 3 weeks and then discontinued. At that time a serum prolactin measurement and a repeat CT scan should be performed so that the need for further treatment can be reassessed.
3. **B**, Page 997. Pathologic causes of hyperprolactinemia, in addition to a prolactin-secreting pituitary adenoma, include other pituitary tumors that produce acromegaly and Cushing's disease. Additional causes are hypothalamic disease, various pharmacologic agents, hypothyroidism, chronic renal disease, or any chronic type of breast nerve stimulation, such as may occur with a thoracic operation, herpes zoster, or chest trauma. Ingestion of oral contraceptive steroids can also increase prolactin levels, with a greater incidence of hyperprolactinemia occurring with *higher* estrogen formulations. Nevertheless, galactorrhea does not usually occur during oral contraceptive ingestion because the exogenous estrogen blocks the binding of prolactin to its receptors.
4. **E**, Pages 999, 1012. In most laboratories a normal serum prolactin is under 22 ng/ml. Women with regular menses, galactorrhea, and normal prolactin levels do not have pro-

lactinomas, and therefore radiologic studies do not need to be performed in such women.

5. **D, Pages 994–995.** Big-big prolactin (mol wt >100,000 daltons) may represent an aggregation of many monomeric molecules of prolactin (mol wt = 22,000). The small form is biologically active, and about 80% of the hormone is secreted in the small form. The larger forms of prolactin, big and big-big, are immunoreactive, but most of the immunoassayable prolactin is in the small form. Big-big prolactin has reduced binding to mammary tissue membranes in comparison to the monomeric form and is thus inactive in some bioassays. Specific receptors for prolactin are present in the plasma membrane of mammary cells as well as in many other tissues.

6. **D, Pages 995–996.** Prolactin levels normally fluctuate throughout the day, with maximum levels observed during nighttime while asleep and a smaller increase occurring in the early afternoon.

7. **E, Page 995.** During pregnancy the levels of prolactin increase, reaching about 200 ng/ml in the third trimester, and the rise is directly related to the increase in circulating levels of estrogen. Despite the elevated prolactin levels during pregnancy, lactation does not occur because estrogen inhibits the **action** of prolactin on the breast, most likely blocking prolactin's interaction with its receptor.

8. **E, Page 1002.** A prolactinoma and hypothyroidism have been ruled out in this patient with oligomenorrhea, a normal prolactin, and normal TSH. Because a few patients with galactorrhea, abnormal menstrual function, and normal prolactin levels have been found to have the empty sella syndrome, and very rarely pituitary adenomas, anteroposterior and lateral coned-down views of the sella turcica should be obtained. If this X-ray is abnormal, the diagnosis should be confirmed by CT (computerized tomography) scan.

9. **A, Pages 995–997.** Hyperprolactinemia has been reported to be present in 15% of all anovulatory women and 20% of women with amenorrhea of undetermined cause. The incidence of galactorrhea in women with hyperprolactinemia has been reported to range from 30% to 80%. The incidence of hyperprolactinemia is higher (88%) in those women with galactorrhea who have amenorrhea and low estrogen than in those with galactorrhea and normal menses, oligomenorrhea, or amenorrhea with normal estrogen levels (49%). Basal levels of circulating prolactin decline to the nonpregnant range about 6 months after parturition in nursing women.

10. **C, Page 995.** Prolactin levels reach normal, nonpregnant concentrations in **nonnursing** women in 2 to 3 weeks. Although basal levels of circulating prolactin decline to the nonpregnant range about 6 months after parturition in **nursing** women, prolactin levels increase markedly following each act of sucking and stimulate milk production for the next feeding. A level of 10 ng/ml is in the normal range. Since the patient had established breast feeding, Sheehan's syndrome is not a consideration. Stress should increase, not decrease, the release of prolactin.

11. **C, Page 1004.** Bromoergocryptine therapy is used primarily in women with microadenomas who wish to conceive or who are disturbed by their symptoms. This patient is not married, did not indicate that conception was an objective, and is not bothered by either the galactorrhea or the oligomenorrhea. Since she has some menses, she is producing estrogen. Thus, she does not appear to be at increased risk for osteoporosis and should be treated with periodic progestin withdrawal (medroxyprogesterone acetate 10 mg per day for 10 days of treatment) to prevent endometrial hyperplasia. A barrier type of contraception is advisable. Surgical resection is an option for patients with larger tumors. Radiation is not a primary mode of treatment for this lesion. Results have been inconsistent and there is a delay of several months between treatment and resumption of ovulation.

12. **B, Page 996.** The mechanism which best explains why elevated prolactin levels interfere with gonadotrophin release has not been completely elucidated, but the major factor appears to be alterations in normal gonadotrophin-releasing hormone (GnRH) release. It has also been shown that elevated levels of prolactin directly inhibit basal as well as gonadotrophin-stimulated ovarian secretion of both estradiol and progesterone. However, this mechanism is probably not the primary cause of anovulation, because women with hyperprolactinemia can be stimulated to ovulate with various agents. Some patients with moderate hyperprolactinemia have a greater than normal proportion of the big-big form of prolactin. Because this form of prolactin has reduced bioactivity, these individuals can have normal pituitary and ovarian function.

13. **E, Page 995.** Prolactin is synthesized and stored in the pituitary gland in chromophobe cells called lactotrophs, which are located mainly in the lateral areas of the gland. In addition, prolactin is synthesized in decidual and endometrial tissue. Prolactin circulates in an unbound form and has a 20 minute half-life.

14. **B, Page 999.** Pituitary tumors that secrete mainly adrenocorticotropic hormone (ACTH) or growth hormone frequently secrete prolactin. Hyperprolactinemia has been reported to occur in about 10% of patients with Cushing's disease and 25% of patients with acromegaly.

15–16. 15, **A**; 16, **C**; Pages 995–996. Prolactin synthesis and release are controlled by central nervous system neurotransmitters. The major control mechanism is inhibition. It appears that the major physiologic inhibitor of prolactin release is the neurotransmitter dopamine, which acts directly on the pituitary gland. Dopamine appears to be the prolactin-inhibiting factor (PIF). Both serotonin and thyrotropin-releasing hormone (TRH) stimulate prolactin release. Since the latter stimulates prolactin release only minimally unless infused, it appears that serotonin is a prolactin-releasing factor (PRF). The rise in prolactin levels during sleep appears to be controlled by serotonin. 2-Br-alpha-ergocryptine mesylate, bromoergocryptine, is a semisynthetic ergot alkaloid that is a dopamine receptor agonist and is used to treat hyperprolactinemia. Estrogen stimulates prolactin production and release and is especially important in this regard at the time of puberty and during pregnancy. It is not, however, considered a prolactin-releasing factor.

17–19. 17, **C**; 18, **B**; 19, **A**; Page 997. One of the most frequent causes of galactorrhea and hyperprolactinemia is the ingestion of pharmacologic agents. The tricyclic antidepressants block dopamine uptake, and haloperidol and phenothiazines block hypothalamic dopamine receptors. The antihypertensive agent reserpine depletes catecholamines, and methyldopa blocks the conversion of tyrosine to dopa. Amphetamines stimulate the serotoninergic system.

20–21. 20, **C**; 21, **D**; Page 999. Overall, about 50% of women with hyperprolactinemia have a prolactinoma. The incidence is higher when the prolactin levels exceed 100 ng/ml, and nearly all individuals with prolactin levels greater than 200 ng/ml harbor a prolactinoma. The incidence of an adenoma is greater in those individuals with a more profound disturbance of normal hypothalamic-pituitary-ovarian function, that is, galactorrhea, amenorrhea, and low estrogen levels.

It has been estimated that as many as 80% of all pituitary adenomas secrete prolactin.

Eighty-seven percent of women with a prolactinoma have galactorrhea.

22–23. 22, **A**; 23, **A**; Pages 1001–1002. Visual field determination and tests of adrenocorticotropic hormone (ACTH) and thyroid function are not necessary in patients with microadenomas, as these small tumors do not interfere with overall pituitary function and do not extend beyond the sella. However, these evaluations should be performed in individuals with macroadenomas. An insulin tolerance test is a test of ACTH reserve.

24. **A** (1, 2, 3), Page 996. Hyperprolactinemia can produce disorders of menstrual function, including amenorrhea, oligomenorrhea, and anovulation. Polymenorrhea is not a finding associated with increased serum prolactin.

25. **C** (2, 4), Pages 1005–1006. After ingestion, bromoergocryptine is rapidly absorbed, with peak blood levels reached 1 to 3 hours later. It is not detectable in the serum after 14 hours. For this reason the drug is usually given at least twice daily. The most frequent side effect is orthostatic hypotension, which occurs in about 15% of patients. To minimize the effects of orthostatic hypotension, the initial dose should be taken at bedtime with food. Bromoergocryptine is currently approved by the FDA only for treatment of hyperprolactinemia, which is usually defined as a level greater than 20 to 25 ng/ml. It is a dopamine receptor agonist.

26. **D** (4), Pages 997, 1011. About 3% to 5% of individuals with hyperprolactinemia have hypothyroidism. This is the result of the decreased negative feedback of thyroxine (T_4) on the hypothalamic-pituitary axis. The resulting increase in thyrotropin-releasing hormone (TRH) stimulates prolactin secretion as well as thyroid-stimulating hormone (TSH) secretion from the pituitary. Thus, a TSH assay should be obtained for all individuals with hyperprolactinemia. If the TSH level is elevated, triiodothyronine (T_3) and T_4 should be measured to confirm the diagnosis of primary hypothyroidism, as occasionally the TSH will be elevated as a result of a TSH-secreting pituitary adenoma. In this patient, with a normal pelvic examination, a quantitative β-HCG is not indicated. One might have performed a qualitative β-HCG as an initial screening test. An LH would not be of any help in the differential diagnosis, and the serum prolactin obtained in midafternoon would be about the same or higher, not lower.

27. **D** (4), Pages 1006–1008, 1012. The usual therapeutic dose of bromoergocryptine is 2.5 mg twice or three times a day. About 10% of patients with microadenomas fail to have prolactin levels return to normal despite administration of up to 20 mg per day. Nevertheless, despite the persistently elevated prolactin levels, many of these patients ovulate and conceive. There is no evidence that the drug is teratogenic or adversely affects pregnancy outcome. The incidence of spontaneous abortion and multiple pregnancy is not increased.

28. **D** (4), Pages 1003–1004. Several studies have demonstrated the benign course of untreated microadenomas. These tumors seldom enlarge. Therefore, treatment may not be necessary if the patient is not bothered by the amenorrhea or galactorrhea. In this case, this patient is at increased risk for osteoporosis because of the low estrogen associated with prolactin elevations and her long-

distance running. For this reason she should receive exogenous estrogen.

Macroadenomas can enlarge and cause visual field distortion or disturbance of pituitary function.

29. **A** (1, 2, 3), Page 995. The main functions of prolactin are the stimulation of growth of mammary tissue and the production and secretion of milk into the alveoli. Prolactin interferes with gonadotrophin release. Women with hyperprolactinemia have abnormalities in the frequency and amplitude of luteinizing hormone (LH) pulsations, with a normal or increased gonadotrophin response following gonadotrophin-releasing hormone (GnRH) infusion.

30. **E** (All), Pages 1008–1009. Some authors advocate the use of bromoergocryptine in the management of all patients with macroadenomas. It shrinks 80–90% of all macroadenomas, and although recurrence after cessation of therapy is high, long-term therapy has been successful in some patients. This medication is expensive, however, and a number of women, especially those on higher doses, have unpleasant side effects so that there are patients who prefer surgical treatment. If given preoperatively to shrink the tumor, the drug should be continued until the time of operation because following withdrawal of the drug, the tumor size may increase just as rapidly as it shrank. Bromoergocryptine has been successfully used to treat patients with failure of, or recurrence after, operation or irradiation therapy. Visual field impairment has disappeared with bromoergocryptine treatment.

31. **C** (2, 4), Pages 1000–1002. Also see Shangold GA, Kletzky OA, Marrs RP, et al: Obstet Gynecol 63:771, 1984. If prolactin is measured before and 20 minutes after administration of an intravenous bolus of 500 μg of TRH, normal individuals have at least a 200% increase (three times baseline) of prolactin. All patients with hyperprolactinemia above 20 ng/ml and CT evidence of tumor had less than a threefold increase in prolactin (Shangold et al.). Thus, if a normal response to TRH is found in individuals with mild hyperprolactinemia, there is **no need** to perform a CT scan. However, anteroposterior and lateral coned-down views of the sella turcica should be obtained to rule of the possibility of an empty sella.

Radiation exposure in a CT scan is about 3 rads. With this technique it is possible to assess accurately the presence of a microadenoma 1–2 mm in diameter or larger as well as suprasellar and other extrasellar extensions. The CT scan has virtually replaced hypocycloidal tomography. There would be no reason to do a MRI if the CT were **positive**.

The MRI provides 1 mm resolution and so is felt to be a more sensitive test than a CT. However, this impression is based on limited data.

32. **E** (All), Page 995. Nipple and breast stimulation increase prolactin levels in the non-pregnant female. Other stimuli include stress, exercise, and sleep.

33. **B** (1, 3), Pages 1009-1010. Some advocate surgical treatment of a macroadenoma prior to pregnancy because 20% of patients develop adverse changes in visual fields and polytomographic or neurologic signs during pregnancy. Others feel that following surgery it is more difficult for patients to conceive because of diminished pituitary function and therefore recommend medical management. Bromoergocryptine does suppress fetal prolactin but does not suppress placental hormone production. If stopped at the onset of pregnancy, it should be reinitiated in those pregnant patients who develop visual impairment. During pregnancy women with a macroadenoma should have monthly visual fields and neurologic testing.

34. **E** (All), Pages 994, 999. Thyrotropin-releasing hormone (TRH) can cause the release of prolactin. The normal response to an infusion of 500 μg is greater than three times the baseline prolactin. A craniopharyngioma can produce hyperprolactinemia. A macroadenoma is a type of prolactin-secreting pituitary adenoma (prolactinoma) greater than 1 cm in diameter, usually with extrasellar extension. The empty sellar syndrome is a condition in which there is an intrasellar extension of the subarachnoid space resulting in compression of the pituitary gland and an **enlarged** sella turcica that may be associated with galactorrhea and hyperprolactinemia. Therefore, in patients with radiologic evidence of an enlarged sella, a computerized tomography (CT) scan or pneumoencephalogram should be obtained to establish or rule out the presence of **empty** sella syndrome.

35. **A** (1, 2, 3), Pages 1004–1005. Transsphenoidal operations have a mortality of less than 0.5%. The risk of permanent diabetes insipidus and hypopituitarism is less than 2%. The initial cure rate for microadenomas is about 80% and for macroadenomas 30%, but the long-term recurrence rate is at least 20% for each. Recurrence is greater in persons with an immediate postoperative prolactin of >10 ng/ml. The **initial cure rate** for patients with a serum prolactin **above 200 ng/ml is 35%**. Operative treatment of tumors in patients older than 26 with amenorrhea for more than 6 months carries a poorer prognosis than tumors in younger patients with a shorter duration of amenorrhea.

CHAPTER 38

Hyperandrogenism

DIRECTIONS: Select the one best answer or completion.

1. A 22-year-old, gravida 1 para 1, 125 pound woman is referred with bothersome central hirsutism. She has regular menstrual periods and the referring physician has obtained both serum testosterone and dehydroepiandrosterone sulfate (DHEA-S), which are normal. The most likely source of her problem is
   A. increased *free* testosterone.
   B. increased androstenedione.
   C. increased androsterone.
   D. increased 5-α-reductase activity.
   E. increased etiocholanolone.

2. The best treatment for the patient in question 1 is
   A. spironolactone.
   B. dexamethasone.
   C. conjugated estrogens.
   D. oral contraceptives.
   E. electrolysis.

3. In evaluating a 30-year-old, oligomenorrheic, hirsute woman, a dehydroepiandrosterone sulfate (DHEA-S) of 4 ng/ml is found. (Normal = 0.8 to 3.4 ng/ml.) An ACTH stimulation test is performed to rule out primary adrenal disease, and the DHEA-S is found to triple. This is consistent with the diagnosis of
   A. Cushing's disease.
   B. acromegaly.
   C. an adrenal carcinoma.
   D. polycystic ovarian syndrome.
   E. an androgen-secreting ovarian tumor.

4. Symptoms of androgen excess in patients with congenital adrenal hyperplasia are the result of excessive
   A. adrenal production of free testosterone.
   B. peripheral conversion of C_{19} steroids to testosterone.
   C. adrenal production of free DHEA-S.
   D. adrenal production of free androstenedione.
   E. adrenal cortisol production.

5. A 24-year-old, oligomenorrheic nulligravida is diagnosed as having polycystic ovarian syndrome. Fertility is of no immediate concern. The best treatment is cyclic
   A. medroxyprogesterone acetate.
   B. conjugated estrogens.
   C. norethindrone.
   D. levonorgestrel acetate.
   E. combination oral contraceptives.

6. A 30-year-old, 5 feet 1 inch, 110 pound, gravida 2 para 2 is referred to you for treatment of slowly progressive hirsutism. She has regular monthly menstrual periods. Her serum testosterone is 0.5 ng/ml and serum DHEA-S is 0.2 ng/ml. The most likely diagnosis is
   A. Cushing's syndrome.
   B. idiopathic hirsutism.
   C. polycystic ovarian syndrome.
   D. congenital adrenal hyperplasia.
   E. stromal cell hyperthecosis.

7. The best treatment for the patient in question 6 is
   A. dexamethasone.
   B. combination oral contraceptives.
   C. conjugated estrogen.
   D. medroxyprogesterone acetate.
   E. spironolactone.

8. A 28-year-old, slender, athletic-looking, normotensive woman has an 18 month history of oligomenorrhea and 6 month history of progressive central hirsutism and clitoromegaly. Serum testosterone is 0.8 mg/ml. The DHEA-S is 10 mg/ml. Pelvic examination is normal. This patient should have
   A. computerized tomography (CT) of the adrenal glands.
   B. ACTH stimulation test.
   C. overnight dexamethasone suppression test.
   D. complete dexamethasone suppression test (Liddle's test).
   E. laparoscopic examination of the ovaries.

9. The best laboratory test to confirm the suspected diagnosis of congenital adrenal hyperplasia is
   A. serum testosterone.
   B. serum DHEA-S.
   C. serum pregnanetriol.
   D. serum 17-hydroxyprogesterone.
   E. urinary 17-ketosteroids.

10. A 26-year-old, infertile woman presents with oligomenorrhea. She is 5 feet 7 inches tall and weighs 160 pounds. The ovaries are bilaterally enlarged. She does *not* have hirsutism. Which laboratory test would be expected to be *normal*?
    A. DHEA-S
    B. Adiol-G
    C. Testosterone
    D. Androstenedione
    E. LH

11. A woman delivers a 3200 gram baby at term after an uncomplicated pregnancy. Newborn examination is normal except for the presence of ambiguous genitalia, including an enlarged clitoris, vaginal dimple, and incompletely developed scrotum. The most likely diagnosis is
    A. congenital adrenal hyperplasia.
    B. androgen insensitivity syndrome (testicular feminization).
    C. Cushing's syndrome.
    D. Turner's syndrome.
    E. adrenal carcinoma.

12. A 26-year-old woman is referred for evaluation of bothersome hirsutism. The referring physician has obtained a serum testosterone, which is 1.0 ng/ml. Further information can be best gained by which laboratory test?
    A. Serum androstenedione
    B. Serum androsterone
    C. Serum etiocholanolone
    D. Serum dehydroepiandrosterone sulfate (DHEA-S)
    E. Urinary 17-ketosteroids

DIRECTIONS: For each numbered item, indicate whether it is associated with
A: only (A).
B: only (B).
C: both (A) and (B).
D: neither (A) nor (B).

13–15. (A) Adult onset congenital adrenal hyperplasia
       (B) Polycystic ovarian syndrome
       (C) Both
       (D) Neither

13. Postpubertal onset of oligomenorrhea and hirsutism.
14. Increased free circulating estradiol.
15. Diagnosis confirmed by ACTH stimulation test.

16–18. (A) Testosterone
       (B) Dehydroepiandrosterone sulfate (DHEA-S)
       (C) Both
       (D) Neither

16. Does not have androgenic activity.
17. Major androgen produced by the adrenal gland.
18. Major androgen produced by the ovary.

19–21. (A) Polycystic ovarian disease syndrome (PCOS)
       (B) Stroma cell hyperthecosis
       (C) Both
       (D) Neither

19. Associated with progressively increasing amounts of ovarian testosterone production with age.
20. Gradual onset, anovulation, amenorrhea, hirsutism.
21. Associated with increased rate of ovarian malignancy in fifth decade of life.

22–24. (A) Hirsutism
       (B) Virilization
       (C) Both
       (D) Neither

22. Circulating testosterone of 1.0 ng/ml; coarse hair on upper lip and between breasts.
23. Associated with severe forms of polycystic ovary syndrome.
24. Caused by major enzymatic block.

25–27. (A) Sertoli-Leydig cell tumor
       (B) Hilus cell tumor
       (C) Both
       (D) Neither

25. Androgen-producing germ cell ovarian tumor responsible for rapidly developing virilization.
26. Solid tumor, reproductive age group, palpable adnexal mass.
27. Age 65, markedly elevated serum testosterone, normal serum DHEA-S, normal pelvic examination.

DIRECTIONS: Each question contains four suggested answers, of which one or more is correct. Choose the answer
A if 1, 2, and 3 are correct
B if 1 and 3 are correct
C if 2 and 4 are correct
D if 4 only is correct
E if all are correct

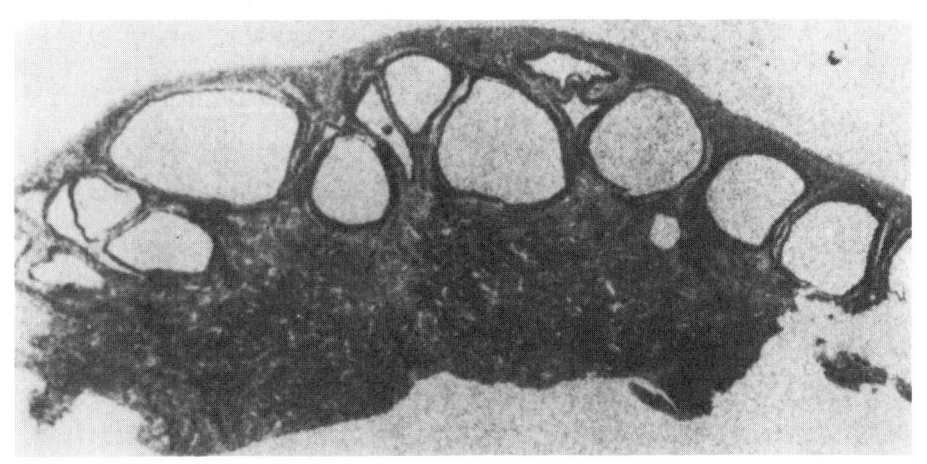

FIGURE 38-1
(From Wilroy RS Jr, Given JR, Wiser WL, Coleman SA, Anderson RN, Summitt RL: Hyperthecosis: An inheritable form of polycystic/ovarian disease. In Bergsma D (ed.): "Genetic Forms of Hypogonadism." Miami: Symposia Specialists for the National Foundation-March of Dimes, BD: OAS XI(4):81, 1975, with permission.)

28. Biochemical characteristics associated with the ovarian histology shown in Figure 38-1 include
   1. increased pulsatility of GnRH.
   2. tonically elevated LH.
   3. increased ovarian androgen.
   4. increased total circulating estrogens.

29. True statements about circulating testosterone include:
   1. The majority is biologically inactive.
   2. It is primarily bound to albumin.
   3. It is metabolized in the periphery to 5-α-dihydrotestosterone.
   4. The measurement reported when a serum testosterone is requested is the concentration of free hormone.

30. True indications regarding the estrogen milieu in women with polycystic ovarian syndrome (PCOS) include
   1. an increase in unbound circulating estradiol.
   2. an increase in total estradiol.
   3. an increase in circulating estrone.
   4. an increase in total estriol.

31. Biochemical characteristics of polycystic ovarian syndrome (PCOS) include
   1. increased GnRH pulse frequency.
   2. an elevation in LH.
   3. increased androgen production.
   4. a decrease in circulating estradiol.

ANSWERS

1. **D,** Page 1020. Idiopathic hirsutism (peripheral disorder of androgen metabolism) is the most common type of androgenic disorder. This usually occurs in regularly menstruating women and is associated with normal levels of serum testosterone and DHEA-S. It has recently been shown that nearly all of these individuals have increased levels of Adiol-G indirectly indicating that the cause of hirsutism could be increased 5α-reductase activity, which converts normal levels of testosterone to increased amounts of biologically active androgens DHT and Adiol-G. If measured, serum androstenedione is usually normal. The other two androgens, androsterone and etiocholanolone, are both 17-ketosteroids and are the metabolic breakdown products of androstenedione.

2. **A,** Pages 1020, 1034. Idiopathic hirsutism is related to abnormalities in the excessive peripheral production of Adiol-G and DHT. It has been shown that there is a localized increase in the activity of 5α-reductase. This is considered a condition of peripheral androgen metabolism in the pilosebaceous apparatus of the skin. Antiandrogens that block peripheral testosterone action or interfere with 5α-reductase activity are moderately effective therapeutic agents. The most widely used agent in this country is spironolactone. Other agents do not exert a direct end organ effect since they are not associated with appreciable changes in 5α-reductase activity. Electrolysis may improve the cosmetic appearance in select areas but does not treat the underlying problem.

3. **D,** Page 1024. Approximately half of the women with polycystic ovary syndrome (PCOS) have elevated levels of dehydroepiandrosterone sulfate (DHEA-S), with one-third of them having levels greater than 4 ng/ml. Although ACTH levels are normal in these women, infusions of ACTH

produce an exaggerated response of DHEA-S, indicating that perhaps the adrenal gland in some patients with PCOS has increased sensitivity to ACTH and that the adrenal gland may be involved in the pathogenesis of this syndrome.

Cushing's disease is the result of excessive adrenal production of glucocorticoids due to increased secretion of ACTH. When the signs and symptoms are due to excessive glucocorticoids secondary to adrenal tumors, the problem is referred to as Cushing's syndrome. These disorders are best evaluated by studies of adrenal suppression such as the overnight dexamethasone suppression test. The findings of androgen excess and exaggerated androgen response in this patient are unrelated to the manifestations associated with acromegaly. Likewise, extremely high levels of DHEA sulfate found with rare adrenal carcinomas are relatively unaffected by the ACTH stimulation test. One would not expect to uncover an androgen-secreting ovarian tumor by this test since ACTH has no effect on the ovary.

4. **B**, Page 1028. Congenital adrenal hyperplasia involves an enzymatic defect of either 21-hydroxylase of 11β-hydroxylase, resulting in decreased cortisone synthesis. ACTH production is thereby increased, and there is a progressive buildup of cortisol precursors, including 17-hydroxyprogesterone and 17-hydroxypregnenolone. These steroids are then converted to DHEA and androstenedione, which in turn are peripherally converted into testosterone, causing hirsutism and/or virilization depending on the severity of the enzymatic block. Testosterone is normally not produced in high amounts directly from the adrenal gland and there is not an excessive amount of endogenously produced (adrenal) DHEA-S. The excessive amount of androstenedione produced is secondary to the enzymatic block and exerts its androgenic effect through peripheral conversion to testosterone.

5. **E**, Page 1032. Treatment of polycystic ovarian syndrome depends on which complaints are most bothersome to the patient. If hirsutism and irregular or infrequent bleeding are most bothersome and if the patient is not desirous of becoming pregnant, combination oral contraceptives using formulations that contain less than 50 μg of estrogen and a progestin other than norgestrel are best. Norgestrel is not used because it is the most potent androgenic progestin in current use. Oral contraceptives are best because these agents inhibit LH secretion, decrease circulating testosterone levels, and increase the levels of sex hormone binding globulin (SHBG), thus binding and inactivating more of the testosterone in circulation. Medroxyprogesterone acetate, conjugated estrogens, and norethindrone acetate do not inhibit LH or decrease circulating testosterone levels to the same extent that cyclic combination oral contraceptives do.

6. **B**, Page 1033. This case exemplifies a patient with idiopathic hirsutism. She has normal adrenal and ovarian androgen levels and is experiencing regular menstrual periods. Fertility has not been a concern. It can be assumed that this patient has increased peripheral androgen activity and if measured, would have a high Adiol-G value. This metabolite is not routinely measured since the presumptive diagnosis is one of exclusion.

This woman did not present with additional findings suggestive of Cushing's disease such as centripetal obesity, dorsal neck fat pads, abdominal striae, or muscle wasting and weakness. Likewise, she does not have the oligomenorrhea that most polycystic ovarian syndrome patients have and does not have the associated modestly elevated serum testosterone. Congenital adrenal hyperplasia is not suspect because of normal DHEA-S levels and an absence of menstrual irregularity and true virilization. Similarly, stromal cell hyperthecosis is ruled out by the lack of menstrual irregularity and a normal testosterone.

7. **E**, Page 1033. The best treatment for idiopathic hirsutism is an agent that inhibits peripheral androgen activity. Of the drugs approved for use in the United States, the most efficacious is Spironolactone. Cimetidine has also been used successfully. In Europe, cyproterone acetate has been used successfully, but this drug is not available in the United States. It has been reported that hair shaft density and the rate of hair growth decreases after two months of spironolactone therapy in doses in excess of 100 mg/day.

8. **A**, Page 1031. Patients with rapidly progressive signs of androgen excess, including virilization, who have modestly elevated testosterone values but markedly elevated DHEA-S values should be suspected of having androgen-producing adrenal tumors. These tumors secrete a large amount of C_{19} steroids, which are normally produced by the adrenal gland, including DHEA-S, DHEA, and androstenedione. The peripheral conversion of these relatively weak androgens to testosterone produces the androgen stigmata. Because of the potential severity of this problem, patients with these laboratory findings and a history of rapid onset signs of androgen excess should undergo computerized tomography (CT) of the adrenal glands to confirm the diagnosis. An ACTH stimulation test would be of little value since one is not concerned with measuring cortisol precursors

secondary to an enzymatic block. Similarly, dexamethasone suppression tests are not indicated since this patient did not present with the stigmata of Cushing's disease.

Since the markedly excessive androgen in this case is of adrenal origin, and since the testosterone level is only mildly elevated, there should be little concern that there is a potential ovarian source, so laparoscopy is not indicated.

9. **D,** Page 1030. The diagnosis of congenital adrenal hyperplasia is established if serum levels of 17-hydroxyprogesterone are greater than 8 ng/ml. This test has replaced the less precise measurement of its metabolite, pregnanetriol. Since one is measuring metabolic products resulting from an enzymatic block, obtaining serum testosterone or DHEA-S will not reveal the source of the problem. Although urinary 17-ketosteroid levels may be elevated, this test is less specific, and awkward collection techniques make interpretation of test results difficult in the newborn.

10. **B,** Pages 1022–1023. Polycystic ovarian syndrome should be thought of as a disorder of hyperandrogenism with chronic anovulation. Serum testosterone levels and serum androstenedione levels are usually mildly to moderately elevated. In addition, about half of the women with this syndrome have elevated DHEA-S. It is estimated that approximately 30% of women with PCOS do not have hirustism even though nearly all of them have elevated circulating androgen levels. The presence or absence of hirsutism depends on whether those androgens are converted peripherally by 5α-reductase to the more potent androgens DHT and Adiol-G. This 5α-reductase activity is reflected by increased levels of Adiol-G. In this patient, with no hirsutism, it would be expected that her Adiol-G level would be normal. In PCOS, LH levels are tonically elevated, usually above 20 mIU/ml.

11. **A,** Pages 1028, 1030. Congenital adrenal hyperplasia (CAH) is the most common cause of sexual ambiguity in the newborn. This is usually caused by a severe 21-hydroxylase block with resultant increased ACTH secretion and increased adrenal production of cortisol precursors proximal to the enzymatic block. These precursors include both 17-hydroxypregnenolone and 17-hydroxyprogesterone. These steroids are then converted to DHEA and androstenedione, which in turn are peripherally converted to testosterone, resulting in masculinization of the female external genitalia. The associated fluid and electrolyte changes occurring in these babies can be severe and lead to death.

Cushing's syndrome results in excessive adrenal production of glucocorticoids due to increased ACTH secretion and is generally not manifest in the newborn. Likewise, androgen insensitivity syndrome and Turner's syndrome are generally disorders appreciated in girls at about the time of menarche or in their mid-adolescence because of their amenorrhea. Adrenal carcinoma is extremely rare in any age group and especially in the newborn. This would be suspected with markedly elevated levels of DHEA-S as opposed to the elevated levels of cortisol precursors one would find in congenital adrenal hyperplasia.

12. **D,** Page 1017. This patient's hirsutism has been partially investigated by the mildly elevated testosterone of 1.0 ng/ml. This is indicative of ovarian androgenic hyperfunction and may be the only source of hyperandrogenism in this patient. However, the other major source for androgen production, the adrenal gland, has not been investigated. The best test to measure the other major androgen source is to obtain a serum dehydroepiandrosterone sulfate (DHEA-S). This will give more complete information as to whether the patient has a combined source of androgen excess. This test is much better than urinary 17-ketosteroids because it gives a direct assessment of potential adrenal androgen excess. Androsterone and etiocholanolone are both 17-ketosteroids and represent metabolic breakdown patterns of androstenedione. This in turn is produced from the metabolism of testosterone, which is not a 17-ketosteroid. Therefore, in investigating patients with complaints of hirsutism, the two basic tests of androgen hyperfunction should represent the two major sources for female androgen production, the adrenal gland and the ovary.

13–15. 13, **C;** 14, **C;** 15, **A;** Pages 1028, 1030, and Figure 38-17 (from Droegemueller). It has been suggested that the mechanism for anovulation in adult onset congenital adrenal hyperplasia is similar to that for polycystic ovarian syndrome. Increased levels of androgen produced by the ovary lower SHBG levels, thus increasing the amount of biologically active circulating estradiol in both conditions. This in turn continues to stimulate tonically high LH levels, which increase ovarian androgen production and delay follicular growth and ovulation. Women with both disorders present with post-pubertal onset of hirsutism and oligomenorrhea.

In patients with levels of 17-hydroxyprogesterone that are elevated but not pathognomonic for adult onset congenital adrenal hyperplasia, the ACTH stimulation test can be performed to confirm this diagnosis

Following overnight suppression with 1 mg of dexamethasone, a morning baseline 17-hydroxyprogesterone is obtained, followed by infusion of 25 IU of synthetic ACTH. One hour later another sample is obtained for 17-hydroxyprogesterone, and if this level increases to more than 20 ng/ml, the diagnosis is established. A similar response is not obtained in women with polycystic ovary syndrome.

16–18. 16, **B**; 17, **B**; 18, **A**; Pages 1016–1017. The ovaries and the adrenal gland are the two sources for androgen production in the female. The major androgen produced by the ovaries is testosterone and that of the adrenal glands is dehydroepiandrosterone sulfate (DHEA-S). In addition to glandular production of androgens, conversion of estrone to androstenedione and DHEA-S to testosterone occurs in peripheral tissues. In itself, DHEA-S does not have androgenic activity but is peripherally converted at a slow rate to a biologically active form of testosterone. Less than 5% of DHEA-S produced by the adrenal glands is converted to testosterone. Other androgens secreted by the ovary are androstenedione and DHEA. These relatively weak androgens have little androgenic activity clinically unless there is significant peripheral conversion to the more potent testosterone. Measurement of the amount of these two steroids (DHEA-S and testosterone) in the circulation provides clinically relevant information regarding the presence and source of increased androgen production in patients who present with disorders involving hirsutism or virilization.

19–21. 19, **B**; 20, **C**; 21, **D**; Pages 1026–1028. Stromal cell hyperthecosis shares certain biochemical and histologic similarities with polycystic ovarian syndrome (PCOS). The capsules of the ovaries in women with stromal cell hyperthecosis are thickened, but unlike the polycystic ovarian syndrome subcapsular cysts are uncommon. The thecal cells in stromal cell hyperthecosis produce large amounts of testosterone, and production of this hormone increases with age. Similar to PCOS, this disease has a gradual onset and is initially associated with anovulation, amenorrhea, and hirsutism. Clinically, stromal cell hyperthecosis is difficult to differentiate from polycystic ovarian syndrome although differences are evident in later life, when serum testosterone levels are often in excess of 2 ng/ml in patients with stromal cell hyperthecosis. Neither disorder is known to be associated with an increased rate of ovarian malignancy.

22–24. 22, **A**; 23, **A**; 24, **B**; Page 1015. Hirsutism and virilization are two clinical signs associated with the production of excess androgens. Knowledge of these two clinical signs and the differentiation of each is important in developing a rationale for the investigation of androgen disorders. True virilization (temporal balding, clitoral hypertrophy, decreased breast size, and increased muscle mass) implies a much more severe disorder and necessitates biochemical investigation through different pathways.

Hirsutism is much more common, and in the absence of other signs of virilization is associated with relatively minor disorders of androgen production. Most commonly, hirsutism is associated with the development of coarse hair in central locations such as the upper lip, the chin and neck, between the breasts, and in the midline abdomen. Circulating testosterone levels are either normal or mildly to moderately elevated (less than 1.5 ng/ml). The symptoms are usually gradual in onset and are not the result of a severe enzymatic block.

Approximately 70% of women with polycystic ovary syndrome have clinically evident hirsutism without any evidence of virilization unless there is a concomitant abnormality involving a major enzymatic block. It depends on whether androgens are converted peripherally by 5α-reductase to the more potent androgen dihydrotestosterone (DHT).

25–27. 25, **C**; 26, **A**; 27, **B**; Page 1028. Many types of ovarian neoplasms are capable of secreting excessive amounts of testosterone from stromal cells. This includes both benign and malignant cystadenomas, Brenner tumors, and Krukenberg tumors. Two germ cell tumors are noted for production of large amounts of testosterone and nearly always cause virilization. Most often, ovarian tumors are associated with normal DHEA-S. The lone exception is the rare adrenal rest tumor, which may produce high levels of both testosterone and DHEA-S.

Sertoli-Leydig cell tumors usually develop during the reproductive age, and by the time they produce detectable amounts of androgen excess, associated with rapidly developing signs of virilization, the tumor is nearly always palpable. Hilus cell tumors most often occur after menopause, are usually small and nonpalpable, and are associated with markedly elevated serum testosterone levels which are responsible for the rapid virilization.

Although these tumors are unusual, appreciation of them is important in order to make the correct diagnosis in patients who present with rapidly developing virilization both in the reproductive age group and in the postmenopausal age group.

28. **E** (All), Pages 1026–1027. This photomicrograph depicts histology typical of polycystic ovarian syndrome. There are characteristic multiple subcapsular cysts, and there are numerous premature atretic follicles. Bio-

chemical associations with these findings include increased pulsatility of GnRH, which produces tonically elevated LH levels and increased ovarian androgen production. In addition, because of increased peripheral conversion of androstenedione to estrone in conjunction with decreased SHBG levels, there is tonic hyperestrogenism.

29. **B** (1, 3), Pages 1017–1018. Most testosterone in the circulation (about 85%) is tightly bound to sex hormone binding globulin (SHBG) and is believed to be biologically inactive. Only about 10 to 15% is loosely bound albumin, with only about 1 to 2% not bound to any protein, representing free testosterone. The measured concentration of free testosterone in a sample is generally reported only upon request. Serum testosterone can be measured in any of these forms. To exert a biologic effect, testosterone is metabolized peripherally in the target tissues to the more potent androgen, 5α-dihydrotestosterone (DHT). It has been shown that although serum levels of total testosterone are similar in normal and hirsute women, there are significant differences in the amount of non-SHBG-bound testosterone, which is elevated in about 60 to 70% of hirsute women.

30. **B** (1, 3), Page 1024. Women with polycystic ovarian syndrome have increased levels of biologically active (non-sex hormone binding globuline, or non-SHBG) estradiol, although total circulating levels of estradiol are not increased. The increased amount of non-SHBG-bound estradiol is caused by a decrease in SHBG, which is produced primarily by increased levels of androgens and secondarily by the obesity present in many of these women. Even though the polycystic ovary does not secrete increased amounts of estrogen or estradiol, the increased levels of androstenedione are peripherally converted to estrone, causing increased circulating estrone levels. Appreciable amounts of estriol are present only in pregnancy as a function of the metabolism of the fetal placenta complex.

31. **A** (1, 2, 3), Pages 1020, 1025. The polycystic ovarian syndrome (PCOS) is a relatively common disorder which begins soon after menarche and consists of a series of endocrinologic abnormalities associated with increased GnRH pulse frequency, tonically elevated levels of LH, and increased androgen production from both the ovaries and the adrenal gland. The polycystic ovary secretes relatively normal amounts of estradiol, but the increased levels of androstenedione are peripherally converted to estrone, causing an increase in circulating estrone.

CHAPTER 39 Infertility

DIRECTIONS: Select the one best answer or completion.

1. During the evaluation of an infertile couple, you receive the husband's initial semen analysis. The report is shown below. The abnormal parameter is
   A. volume: 1.5 ml
   B. viscosity: full liquefaction in 45 min.
   C. sperm density: 60 million/ml.
   D. sperm motility: 3^+–4^+; 75% have good to excellent motility at 1 hour; 50% have good to excellent motility at 3 hours.
   E. sperm morphology: 65% normal.
2. Based on the previous semen analysis results, and assuming that the husband has a normal medical history, your recommendation would be to
   A. repeat the semen analysis immediately.
   B. repeat the semen analysis in 1 month.
   C. begin clomiphene citrate therapy.
   D. begin tetracycline therapy.
   E. have the man examined by a urologist.
3. You are discussing in vitro fertilization with an infertile couple. All of the following statements are true *except*:
   A. Ovarian hyperstimulation is desirable.
   B. Midcycle daily ultrasound is helpful in determining the optimal time for egg retrieval.
   C. Midcycle daily estrogen measurements are helpful in determining the optimal time for egg retrieval.
   D. Midcycle laparoscopy is necessary to retrieve ovum.
   E. The spontaneous abortion rate is high.
4. During a laparoscopy for infertility, you notice three 1 mm superficial implants of endometriosis on each ovary. In addition, there are a few filmy adhesions around both ovaries. Assuming the rest of her workup is normal, you should
   A. perform immediate laparotomy.
   B. perform laparotomy in 6 months.
   C. begin danazol postoperatively.
   D. recommend in vitro fertilization.
   E. fulgurate and then delay medical or other surgical intervention at least 12 months.
5. Of the following, which is associated with the poorest prognosis for conception?
   A. Intrauterine adhesions
   B. Leiomyomata
   C. Bicornuate uterus
   D. In utero DES exposure
   E. Pelvic tuberculosis
6. Donors for artificial insemination (AID) must be screened for all of the following *except*
   A. *Chlamydia trachomatis.*
   B. Herpes simplex II.
   C. *Neisseria gonorrhoeae.*
   D. syphilis.
   E. serum hepatitis B.
7. The likelihood of which of the following is increased when conception occurs following clomiphene treatment?
   A. Spontaneous abortion
   B. Ectopic pregnancy
   C. Multiple gestation
   D. Congenital malformation
   E. Intrauterine fetal death

DIRECTIONS: For each numbered item, select the one heading most closely associated with it. Each lettered heading may be used once, more than once, or not at all.

8–10. (A) Hyperprolactinemia
   (B) Luteal phase deficiency
   (C) Sperm antibodies
   (D) Occult infection
   (E) Abnormality of sperm penetration
8. Bromocriptine
9. Progesterone
10. Corticosteroids
11–13. Match the day of an idealized 28 day cycle with the appropriate test.
   (A) Day 1
   (B) Day 7
   (C) Day 13
   (D) Day 17
   (E) Day 26

11. Postcoital test
12. Hysterosalpingogram
13. Endometrial biopsy
14–17. Match the etiology with its reported frequency in cases of infertility.
    (A) 5%
    (B) 15%
    (C) 35%
    (D) 50%
    (E) 75%
14. Anovulation
15. Abnormal semen production
16. Impairment of tubal motility
17. Abnormal sperm transport through cervix

DIRECTIONS: For each numbered item, indicate whether it is associated with
A: only (A)
B: only (B)
C: both (A) and (B)
D: neither (A) nor (B)

18–19. (A) Distal tubal disease
       (B) Proximal tubal blockage
       (C) Both
       (D) Neither
18. Use of microsurgery has improved subsequent pregnancy rates.
19. Repeat surgical procedure recommended if occlusion reoccurs.
20–23. Treatment for properly selected cases in which anovulation is the sole cause of infertility.
       (A) Human menopausal gonadotrophin
       (B) Clomiphene citrate
       (C) Both
       (D) Neither
20. Ovulatory rate >95%.
21. Pregnancy rate per cycle is 20%.
22. Ovarian enlargement in 1% of treatment cycles.
23. Overall conception rate ≤ 50%.

DIRECTIONS: Each question contains four suggested answers, of which one or more is correct. Choose the answer
A if 1, 2, and 3 are correct
B if 1 and 3 are correct
C if 2 and 4 are correct
D if 4 only is correct
E if all are correct

24. True statements concerning the postcoital test include:
    1. The test should be performed 6–12 hours after coitus.
    2. The test should be scheduled on day 14 of the cycle.
    3. Cervical mucus should be thick and cloudy.
    4. At least five motile sperm per high-powered field should be seen.
25. Of the following, which are *not* direct evidence of ovulation?
    1. Serum progesterone
    2. History of regular menstrual cycles
    3. Endometrial biopsy
    4. Basal body temperature chart
26. A 30-year-old female lawyer and her 31-year-old accountant husband seek advice regarding the possibility of needing an infertility workup. Neither has been married previously. Both are healthy, with no significant past medical history. You would advise them that
    1. up to 15% of married couples in the U.S. are infertile.
    2. in 50% of infertile couples, the only abnormal factor found is in the semen.
    3. the incidence of infertility increases with increasing age of the woman.
    4. the etiology of infertility can be determined in over 95% of cases.
27. You have just performed a hysterosalpingogram on a 22-year-old patient as part of her infertility evaluation. You and the radiologist interpret the test as normal. You can tell the patient that
    1. the next step in her evaluation should be hysteroscopy.
    2. there is no evidence of salpingitis isthmica nodosa.
    3. there are no pelvic adhesions.
    4. both fallopian tubes are patent.
28. Indications for washed intrauterine insemination include
    1. cervical stenosis.
    2. oligospermia.
    3. inadequate mucus.
    4. small semen volume.
29. A 25-year-old patient has undergone infertility investigation, including serum progesterone, semen analysis, postcoital test, and hysterosalpingogram. All tests were normal. A diagnostic laparoscopy is now scheduled. Test(s) performed at the time of laparoscopy that would likely provide additional information as to the etiology of infertility include(s)
    1. D&C.
    2. hysteroscopy.
    3. cervical culture.
    4. transcervical insufflation with indigo carmine.

30. Although numerous abnormalities are treated in the management of the infertile couple, some treatments have never been shown to be effective in prospective double-blind studies. Treatment of which of the following abnormal findings have been shown to significantly increase fertility?
   1. Zona-free hamster egg penetration test (no penetration).
   2. Late luteal phase endometrial biopsy (luteal phase defect).
   3. Serum prolactin (30 ng/ml).
   4. Postcoital test (25 WBCs/HDF).
31. In response to a patient's inquiry regarding the use of gonadotrophin-releasing hormone for ovulation induction, you should tell her that
   1. it cannot be administered orally.
   2. ovulation rates exceed those of HMG.
   3. the overall pregnancy rate is less than that for HMG.
   4. hyperstimulation is more common than with HMG.
32. A recently married, healthy 23-year-old patient comes to your office inquiring how she and her husband might maximize their chance of conception as soon as possible. Assuming that she and her husband are both normal, you should tell her that
   1. sperm are capable of fertilization for only a few hours after coitus.
   2. among fertile couples who have coitus just before ovulation, there is only a 25% chance of achieving a clinical pregnancy in each ovulatory cycle.
   3. the basal body temperature chart is prospectively useful to predict the time of ovulation.
   4. the optimal time to have intercourse is a few hours before ovulation.

ANSWERS

1. **A,** Page 1043. Although there are no absolute standards for a normal semen sample, there are some recommended guidelines, shown in Table 5. Using these recommendations, this man's volume is abnormally low.
2. **B,** Page 1043. Given a semen sample that shows normal parameters except for a low volume, one might suspect an incomplete collection or a specimen that merely reflects one extreme in the wide variability normally seen in a man's semen sample. Repeating the test in 1 month with an appropriate abstinence period of 2–3 days preceding collection would be the appropriate next step.

   Immediately repeating the test might be stressful or provide an abnormally low value.

TABLE 5 Recommended Standards for Semen Analysis

Parameter	Recommended Normal Value
Volume	2–6 ml
Viscosity	Full liquefaction within 60 minutes
Sperm density	20–250 million/ml*
Sperm motility	
Progressive	Good to very good†
Quantitation	First hour ≥60%, 2–3 h ≥50%
Vital staining	≤35% dead cells
Sperm morphology	≥60% within normal configuration

Modified from Eliasson R: Parameters of male fertility. In Hafez ESE, Evans TN, eds: Human reproduction. New York, Harper & Row, Publishers, 1973.
*20 million/ml is low normal, in contrast to 40 million/ml. International Society of Andrology.
†3 to 4+ quality.

It should be recalled that it takes 74 days for germ cells to become mature sperm. Therefore, appropriate timing of a repeat semen analysis is important. Clomiphene citrate and tetracycline therapy would be inappropriate until a specific diagnosis is made. A physical examination by a qualified urologist or reproductive gynecologist is a part of the workup of a male with a semen abnormality, but at this point there is no evidence that it is needed.

3. **D,** Pages 1072–1074. Although in vitro fertilization (IVF) was originally intended for women with severe tubal disease, it is now being used for women with severe endometriosis and couples with male factor or unexplained infertility. Nearly all centers utilize some type of ovarian hyperstimulation because the rate of pregnancy is related to the number of embryos placed in the uterine cavity. Because of the use of hyperstimulation, daily ultrasound and estrogen measurements must be done. Originally, oocyte retrieval was accomplished with laparoscopy. The development of an advanced vaginal ultrasound probe now allows oocyte retrieval to be accomplished either transvaginally or transabdominally. Unfortunately, there is a high spontaneous abortion rate (30%) for pregnancies after IVF.
4. **E,** Pages 1064–1065. Based on the American Fertility Society classification of endometriosis, the patient has minimal endometriosis (Stage I). No therapy, either medical or surgical, has been shown to be efficacious in patients with less than moderate endometriosis (Stage III). Since no other cause of infertility has been identified, it is advisable to delay medical or surgical intervention for at

least 12 months. In all likelihood, at the time of laparoscopy, the laparoscopist would fulgurate both the implants and the adhesions.

5. **E**, Pages 1058–1059. Women with pelvic tuberculosis should be considered sterile because pregnancies after chemotherapy are rare. On the other hand, if intrauterine adhesions are the sole abnormality and not overly extensive, prognosis for conception after lysis of adhesions is good. Congenital uterine defects such as bicornuate uterus are a rare cause of infertility. Maternal ingestion of DES has not been clearly shown to be a cause of infertility. There are circumstances, fairly uncommon, in which leiomyomata can be associated with infertility. In selected cases, myomectomy has been reported to achieve a 50% pregnancy rate.

6. **B**, Page 1058. Donors for AID should be carefully screened to ascertain that they are in good health, do not have a potentially inheritable disorder, and will not transmit an infectious agent in the semen. Screening must be performed to rule out hepatitis B, syphilis, *Neisseria gonorrhoeae*, and *Chlamydia trachomatis*. Since cultures for the human immunodeficiency virus (HIV) may not turn positive for 2–3 months after the disease is acquired, it is suggested that only frozen semen of over 2 months' storage be used. The donor is then tested for HIV.

7. **C**, Page 1051. When conception occurs after ovulation has been induced with clomiphene, the incidence of multiple gestation increases to 5%. The rates of spontaneous abortion, ectopic gestation, intrauterine fetal death, and congenital malformation are not significantly increased over the general population.

8–10. 8, **A**; 9, **B**; 10, **C**; Pages 1068–1072. There is no evidence that treatment of the secondary infertility factors significantly improves pregnancy rates when compared with withholding therapy. Nevertheless, if hyperprolactinemia is discovered, it would be reasonable to begin bromocriptine anticipating good results. Progesterone is advocated for the treatment of luteal phase defects. Antisperm antibodies can be treated with condoms to prevent the woman's exposure to sperm or corticosteroid immunosuppressive therapy with variable results.

11–13. 11, **C**; 12, **B**; 13, **E**; Pages 1044, 1046, 1069. Certain infertility tests should be performed at specific times of the cycle in order to avoid potential complications and/or to maximize the information obtained. The postcoital test is performed on the day prior to ovulation (day 13) in order to assess maximal estrogen effect on cervical mucus. The hysterosalpingogram should be performed during the week after menses in order to avoid irradiating a possible pregnancy. An endometrial biopsy late in the luteal phase will reflect the maximal effect from the sex steroids produced by the corpus luteum.

14–17. 14, **B**; 15, **C**; 16, **C**; 17, **B**; Pages 1039. Currently available techniques are able to identify the etiology of infertility in 85–90% of couples. In the United States, 10–15% of cases are due to anovulation, 30–40% to an abnormality of the semen, 30–40% to pelvic disease interfering with normal tubal motility, and 10–15% to abnormalities of sperm transport through the cervical canal.

18–19. 18, **B**; 19, **D**; Pages 1059–1062. The prognosis for fertility after tubal reconstruction depends on the extent of damage to the tube as well as the location of obstruction. If both proximal and distal obstructions exist, operative repair should not be undertaken. Similarly, if obstruction reoccurs, a second surgery is not advised because subsequent pregnancy rates are less than 10%. Rates for conception after initial salpingostomy are about 30%, whereas after salpingolysis and fimbrioplasty for only partial obstruction they are 65%. Unlike results for distal disease, the use of microsurgery has improved pregnancy rates for proximal tubal obstruction. Term pregnancy rates of 50% have been reported after tubo-cornual reanastomosis for proximal blockage when the interstitial portion of the tube is not damaged and less than 1.5 cm of occluded tube is removed.

20–23. 20, **A**; 21, **C**; 22, **B**; 23, **D**; Pages 1048–1054. Both clomiphene citrate and human menopausal gonadotrophin (HMG) are used to induce ovulation. Typically, HMG is withheld unless the patient fails to respond to clomiphene or she is amenorrheic with low estrogen levels. The ovulatory rate with HMG approaches 100%. With clomiphene, 90% of women with oligomenorrhea and 66% with secondary amenorrhea have presumptive evidence of ovulation. Both drugs achieve a pregnancy rate per cycle of approximately 22%. Ovarian enlargement is detectable in 1% of clomiphene cycles and up to 10% of HMG treatment cycles. Overall, conception rates are 60% for HMG and up to 85% with clomiphene. Pregnancy and conception rates are interesting, but the patient should be aware of the percentage of live births following treatment.

24. **D** (4), Pages 1045–1046. The postcoital test (PCT) is the only in vivo test that provides information about both partners in an infertility workup. *Ideally* the test is performed on the day prior to ovulation, when there is maximal estrogen stimulation. The exact day of ovulation is anticipated, not known. Realistically a PCT is scheduled properly if the mucus has a good estrogen effect. This results in clear, watery cervical

mucus with a spinnbarkeit of at least 6 cm. If the mucus is cloudy and thick, either the timing of the test was poor or the woman has a cervical problem.

For a PCT to be normal, at least five motile sperm should be seen in each high-powered field. The number of motile sperm seen is directly related to the time interval between the test and coitus. Thus, a standard different from the one stated should be used if the test is more than 2–3 hours after coitus.

25. **E** (All), Pages 1042, 1068–1069. The first diagnostic step in the evaluation of infertility is to obtain presumptive evidence that the woman is ovulating. A history of regular menses constitutes presumptive evidence of ovulation, and a midluteal serum progesterone above 10 ng/ml is also indirect evidence of adequate ovulation. Both endometrial biopsy and basal body temperature charts reflect response to progesterone but are not direct evidence of ovulation. Therefore, all four choices provide indirect rather than direct evidence of ovulation. The only direct evidence of ovulation is pregnancy.

26. **B** (1, 3), Page 1039. The inability to conceive is one of the most common problems for which women seek gynecologic care. It is estimated that 10–15% of married couples in the United States are infertile (usually defined as inability to conceive within 1 year). The incidence of infertility increases with increasing age of the woman. For example, in the 20–24-year-old age group, 80% of nonsterile married women will conceive within 12 months of unprotected intercourse, whereas the percentage drops to 63% for the 30–34-year-old age group. An abnormality in semen production is identifiable in 30–40% of infertile couples. In up to 10% of cases, the etiology of infertility cannot be determined by currently available techniques.

27. **C** (2, 4), Page 1047. A normal hysterosalpingogram (HSG) demonstrates bilateral tubal patency and thus excludes the presence of salpingitis isthmica nodosa (diverticula of the endosalpinx into the muscularis of the isthmic portion of the tube). The finding of a normal endometrial cavity obviates the need for hysteroscopy unless the cavity was overfilled with dye and the pathology obscured. Although tubal patency is documented, the presence of peritubal pelvic adhesions cannot be completely ruled out by HSG alone.

28. **E** (All), Page 1055. Washed intrauterine insemination is a technique in which sperm are inseminated into the uterus after they have been separated from the semen by centrifugation. It is used in several different circumstances: if the amount of mucus is small or the mucus is not thin and watery with good spinnbarkeit; if the patient has undergone conization; if the male is oligospermic; if the semen volume is small (less than 2 ml) or large (greater than 8 ml); or if the serum is of high viscosity.

29. **D** (4), Page 1047. When performing diagnostic laparoscopy for infertility, indigo carmine should be introduced through the cervix to confirm tubal patency. If the hysterosalpingogram was normal, neither D&C nor hysteroscopy is indicated. A cervical culture should have been performed earlier in the workup had there been any suspicion of cervical infection. A normal postcoital test, in which no white cells were seen and there were ample numbers of motile sperm, negates the need for a cervical culture.

30. **D** (4), Page 1048. The five primary investigative steps for the infertile couple are evidence of regular ovulatory cycles, semen analysis, postcoital test, hysterosalpingogram, and laparoscopy. Correction of an abnormal finding results in an increased incidence of pregnancy as compared to withholding therapy. Studies comparing the secondary tests (zona-free egg penetration, late luteal phase endometrial biopsy, serum prolactin and thyroid stimulating hormone, immunologic tests for sperm antibodies, and bacteriologic cultures of the sperm and cervical mucus) with placebo or no treatment have not been carried out.

31. **B** (1, 3), Page 1054. Because gonadotrophin-releasing hormone (GnRH) is a peptide, it cannot be given orally and must be administered either intravenously or subcutaneously. The ovulation rate (75–85%) and pregnancy rate (25%–30%) appear to be slightly lower than for HMG, although no comparative studies are available. GnRH is less frequently associated with hyperstimulation than is HMG.

32. **C** (2, 4), Pages 1040–1042. Often a young, healthy couple requires only education and/or specific instruction rather than a costly medical evaluation in order to achieve pregnancy. The patient described should be instructed to have intercourse a few hours prior to ovulation because sperm are capable of fertilization for 1–2 days after coitus, whereas the egg probably degenerates a few hours after it reaches the ampulla of the oviduct if fertilization does not occur. Ovulation cannot be predicted in a current cycle by use of a basal body temperature chart since it demonstrates a biphasic temperature shift only after levels of progesterone have increased. Reassurance that a fertile couple has only a 25% chance of getting pregnant each ovulatory cycle may help relieve patient anxiety. In telling the patient to have coitus at the time of ovulation, one should not neglect the marital aspects of the act by focusing only on conception.

CHAPTER 40 Menopause

DIRECTIONS for questions 1–7: Select the one best answer or completion.

1. A 45-year-old diabetic, hypertensive patient complains of severe hot flushes following a recent hysterectomy and bilateral salpingo-oophorectomy for large uterine leiomyomata. Without medication, the patient's blood pressure is 145/95. This woman has a past history of thrombophlebitis at age 30 and a myocardial infarction at age 44. Prior to surgery, blood lipids were measured. This woman's LDL cholesterol was high, and her HDL cholesterol low. You would
   A. prescribe estrogen.
   B. not prescribe estrogen because of her hypertension.
   C. not prescribe estrogen because of her blood lipid profile.
   D. not prescribe estrogen because of her past history of thrombophlebitis.
   E. not prescribe estrogen because of her past history of a myocardial infarction.

2. The increase in facial hair noted in postmenopausal women is the consequence of
   A. increased levels of testosterone.
   B. increased levels of androstenedione.
   C. increased sensitivity of the hair follicles.
   D. a decrease in the estrogen-androgen ratio.
   E. none of the above.

3. When considering the addition of progestin therapy in an attempt to lessen the chance of adenocarcinoma of the endometrium developing in a woman who is on postmenopausal estrogen replacement, the most important factor to take into account is
   A. the formulation of the progestin.
   B. the dose of the progestin.
   C. the route of administration of the progestin.
   D. The length of progestin administration each month.

4. A 67-year-old gravida 5 para 5 has urgency, urge incontinence, and stress incontinence. The stress incontinence is confirmed by urodynamic testing. Urinalysis is normal, and urine culture is negative. She has a pale atrophic vagina. The patient takes no medication, or vitamin supplementation, and otherwise feels well. At this point you would
   A. do a retropubic suspension.
   B. do a vaginal hysterectomy and anterior colporrhaphy.
   C. start a beta-adrenergic.
   D. start an anticholinergic.
   E. start vaginal estrogen.

5. The mean age for the menopause is
   A. 45.
   B. 47.
   C. 49.
   D. 51.
   E. 53.

6. In a patient whose major complaint is hot flushes that greatly interfere with her daily life, you would expect to find all of the following **EXCEPT**
   A. less than ideal body weight.
   B. decreased estrone.
   C. decreased estradiol.
   D. increased sex hormone binding globulin (SHBG).
   E. increased FSH.

7. In those women at risk for the development of osteoporosis who are not properly treated, the percent loss of bone mass each year after the menopause is
   A. 0.25–0.75
   B. 1.00–1.50
   C. 2.00–2.50
   D. 3.00–3.50
   E. 4.50–5.00

DIRECTIONS for questions 8–13: For each numbered item, select the one heading most closely associated with it. Each lettered heading may be used once, more than once, or not at all.

8–10. (A) 5
      (B) 10
      (C) 15
      (D) 20
      (E) 25

8. Percent of Caucasian or Asian women who develop spinal compression fractures by age 60.
9. Percent of 80-year-old women who die from a hip fracture or its complications within 6 months.
10. Percent of 80-year-old white women who will develop hip fractures.

11–13. (A) 0.3 mg
(B) 0.625 mg
(C) 2.5 mg
(D) 1.0 g
(E) 2.0 g

11. In patients who are taking adequate calcium supplementation, the minimum amount of conjugated equine estrogen that when given on a cyclic basis is necessary to prevent osteoporosis.
12. The amount of medroxyprogesterone acetate given daily for 10 days, along with 0.625 mg of conjugated equine estrogen, necessary to reduce nuclear estrogen receptor levels to a normal luteal phase level.
13. The minimum recommended amount of daily elemental calcium that should be ingested by a menopausal woman.

DIRECTIONS for questions 14–19: For each numbered item, indicate whether it is associated with

A: only (A)
B: only (B)
C: both (A) and (B)
D: neither (A) nor (B)

14–16. Studies support the effect listed below.
(A) Diminishes severity of hot flushes
(B) Prophylaxis against osteoporosis
(C) Both
(D) Neither

14. Conjugated equine estrogens
15. Intramuscular medroxyprogesterone acetate
16. Clonidine

17–19. (A) Estrogen
(B) Progesterone
(C) Both
(D) Neither

17. Increases the synthesis of estrogen receptors.
18. Increases the synthesis of progesterone receptors.
19. Decreases the synthesis of progesterone receptors.

DIRECTIONS for questions 20–35: Each question contains four suggested answers, of which one or more is correct. Choose the answer

A if 1, 2, and 3 are correct
B if 1 and 3 are correct
C if 2 and 4 are correct
D if 4 only is correct
E if all are correct

20. Estrogen replacement therapy **CAUSES**
    1. adenocarcinoma of the endometrium.
    2. hypertension.
    3. thrombosis.
    4. a thickened vaginal epithelium.

21. There are multiple prospective and retrospective studies that look at the likelihood of developing cancer if the woman has been on estrogen replacement. The conclusions reached are that postmenopausal estrogen is associated with
    1. a relative risk of more than 5.0 of developing adenocarcinoma of the endometrium.
    2. an increased risk of adenocarcinoma of the endometrium which is dependent on the length of therapy.
    3. an increased risk of adenocarcinoma of the endometrium which is dependent on the dose of estrogen prescribed.
    4. a relative risk of more than 5.0 of developing breast cancer.

22. A 42-year-old woman complains of hot flushes. Her periods are fairly regular every 26 to 30 days. Flow lasts 3 to 7 days. In the past, periods were exactly 28 to 29 days, and flow lasted 3 to 4 days. A serum LH and estradiol were within normal limits, but the FSH was elevated. A serum progesterone was 10 ng/ml. Your advice would be that this patient should
    1. stop worrying about contraception.
    2. use progestin supplementation.
    3. consider herself menopausal.
    4. take estrogen.

23. Of the several women listed below, which are likely to experience hot flushes?
    1. A 50-year-old 45X who had been taking 1.25 mg of premarin 25 days each month until 6 months ago.
    2. A 60-year-old white, 5 feet 2 inch tall, 100 pound woman.
    3. A 38-year-old white, 5 feet 4 inch tall, 180 pound woman who has just undergone a total abdominal hysterectomy with a bilateral salpingo-oophorectomy.
    4. An 18-year-old woman who has pure gonadal dysgenesis.

24. The mechanism by which estrogen is thought to retard the development of osteoporosis involves
    1. direct inhibition of bone resorption.
    2. direct inhibition of parathyroid hormone.
    3. stimulation of 1-alpha-hydroxylase.
    4. stimulation of calcitonin.
25. The histologic appearance of the ovaries of a woman 49 years of age who had her last normal menstrual period 1 year ago would reveal
    1. lack of ovarian follicles.
    2. degeneration of the theca.
    3. degeneration of the granulosa.
    4. degeneration of the stroma.
26. A typical 52-year-old woman who has hot flushes describes them to you. She is likely to tell you that they
    1. are worse at night.
    2. come on suddenly.
    3. usually occur no more than once in 24 hours.
    4. last 10 to 15 minutes.
27. The early diagnosis of osteoporosis in trabecular bone is accurately accomplished by
    1. computerized tomography (CT) scans.
    2. single photon absorptiometry.
    3. dual photon absorptiometry.
    4. X-ray.
28. Compared to nonusers, postmenopausal conjugated equine estrogen users have increased
    1. triglyceride.
    2. cholesterol.
    3. LDL cholesterol.
    4. HDL cholesterol.
29. The addition of 10 to 12 days of synthetic progestin to a cyclic postmenopausal estrogen regimen
    1. renders it less effective in the prevention of hot flushes.
    2. causes a slight increase in bone density because it acts synergistically with estrogen.
    3. enhances the beneficial effect that estrogen has on serum lipids.
    4. in a woman who just reached the menopause will cause that woman to have predictable menstrual-like withdrawal bleeding each month.
30. Factors that appear to affect the age of a woman's menopause include
    1. weight.
    2. use of oral contraceptives.
    3. number of term pregnancies.
    4. smoking.
31. The obese postmenopausal woman is **less likely** to
    1. have significant hot flushes.
    2. have elevated levels of circulating estrone.
    3. develop osteoporosis.
    4. develop endometrial hyperplasia.
32. Factors known to increase the risk of osteoporosis include
    1. diet high in alcohol.
    2. early spontaneous menopause.
    3. cigarette smoking.
    4. reduced weight for height.
33. A patient who is given an estrogen-progestin combination for 5 days (Monday through Friday) each week and no supplementation on the weekend will have
    1. breakthrough bleeding frequently.
    2. more hot flushes than a woman on a 25 day regimen.
    3. less of a risk of developing breast cancer.
    4. an atrophic endometrium.
34. In the postmenopausal woman androstenedione is
    1. secreted primarily by the ovary.
    2. secreted by the adrenal.
    3. estrogenic.
    4. converted to estrone in peripheral body fat.
35. Arguments against the postmenopausal use of estrogen include that women on this treatment
    1. have an increased risk of developing ovarian carcinoma.
    2. who develop adenocarcinoma of the endometrium are more likely to die.
    3. have a relative risk of 5 of developing cholelithiasis when compared to women who do not take estrogen.
    4. can develop vaginal bleeding or spotting which is related entirely to hormone replacement.

ANSWERS

1. **A**, Pages 1097–1101. This patient's hot flushes are an indication for estrogen replacement. There is no contraindication given in the history to its application. Although the use of oral contraceptive agents has been associated with the development of hypertension and thrombophlebitis, postmenopausal estrogen therapy has not. This is due in part to the potency and formulation of the estrogens involved. Because of the theoretic possibility, one should consider carefully the risk-benefit ratio in the face of severe hypertension or recent thrombophlebitis. Studies demonstrate that postmenopausal estrogen

users have improved lipid profiles. Both retrospective and prospective cohort studies have shown that postmenopausal estrogen users have a decreased likelihood of death due to myocardial infarction. In fact, the age-adjusted all-cause mortality rate is lower in estrogen users.
2. **D**, Page 1085. The postmenopausal levels of testosterone and androstenedione are not elevated. The physiologic process of a decrease in the estrogen-androgen ratio is the cause of the increased facial hair growth that frequently occurs after menopause.
3. **D**, Page 1103. Studies have shown that the duration of progestin therapy is more important than the dosage. Small amounts of progestin administered for more than 10 days each month have been shown to reduce the incidence of endometrial carcinoma. No one has reported differences that indicate that either the route or formulation of the progestin is important in the prevention of endometrial hyperplasia. The formulation might be important in maintaining normal blood lipids, however.
4. **E**, Page 1085. The trigone of the bladder and the urethra are embryologically derived from estrogen-dependent tissue, and estrogen deficiency can lead to their atrophy, producing symptoms of urinary urge incontinence, dysuria, and urinary frequency. With a decrease of elastic tissue around the vagina, due to estrogen deficiency, a urethrocele may develop. Although surgery may ultimately be needed, local estrogen should be tried first since it may relieve the symptoms. It should be given before surgery to thicken the vaginal mucosa. This patient might also benefit from Kegel exercises.
5. **D**, Page 1082. The mean age of menopause is 51.4 years. The 95% confidence limits are between ages 45 and 55 years. Menopause is defined as the cessation of menstruation for at least 6 months due to depletion of ovarian follicles.
6. **D**, Pages 1085, 1087, 1104. Postmenopausal women with hot flushes have lower circulating estrone and estradiol levels, less total body weight, and a lower percentage of ideal body weight as compared to those without hot flushes. They also have less sex hormone binding globulin (SHBG).
7. **B**, Page 1090. In short, frail, thin-skinned, sedentary women about 1% to 1.5% of bone mass is lost each year after the menopause.
8–10. 8, **E**; 9, **B**; 10, **D**; Page 1091. By age 60, 25% of Caucasian and Asian women develop spinal compression fractures. Loss of bone mass in **cortical** bone occurs at a much slower rate, so osteoporotic fractures of the femur usually do not begin to occur until about age 70 or 75. By age 80, 20% of all Caucasian women will develop hip fractures, and of these about 10% will die from the fracture itself or from complications within 6 months.
11–13. 11, **A**; 12, **C**; 13, **D**; Pages 1093, 1095, 1103, and 1105. The minimum dosage of estrogen needed to prevent osteoporosis is 0.625 mg of conjugated equine estrogen. In addition to estrogen replacement, calcium supplementation and weight-bearing exercises are of ancillary benefit in preventing postmenopausal osteoporosis. It is recommended that in addition to estrogen, 1 to 1.5 g of elemental calcium be ingested daily. With adequate calcium supplementation the dosage of estrogen supplement may be reduced to 0.3 mg conjugated equine estrogen. A 55-year-old produces more estrogen than an 80-year-old. Does that mean that the older woman should be given more exogenous estrogen? The addition of Vitamin D has not been shown to be useful in the prevention of osteoporosis.

In patients receiving 25 days each month of 0.625 mg of conjugated equine estrogen, 2.5 mg of medroxyprogesterone acetate given daily for the last 10 days of the cycle reduced nuclear estrogen receptors to levels normal for the luteal phase.
14–16. 14, **C**; 15, **C**; 16, **A**; Pages 1087–1089. The most effective treatment for the hot flush is estrogen, and conjugated equine estrogens are the most frequently prescribed estrogen for the menopausal population. Its use appears to retard the development of osteoporosis. Depomedroxyprogesterone acetate has been compared with conjugated equine estrogens in the treatment of hot flushes and was as effective as estrogens in relieving the symptoms of the hot flush. Depomedroxyprogesterone acetate decreases markers of bone resorption to an extent similar to that of 0.625 mg of conjugated equine estrogen. Other agents shown to reduce hot flushes include clonidine, naloxone, and methyldopa (Aldomet).
17–19. 17, **A**; 18, **A**; 19, **B**; Pages 1102–1105. Estrogen increases the synthesis of both estrogen and progesterone receptors in the endometrium; progesterone and synthetic progestins decrease the synthesis of both these receptors and thus have an antiproliferative and antimitotic action.
20. **D** (4), Pages 1096–1097. An association between the use of estrogen and adenocarcinoma of the endometrium, hypertension, and thrombosis has been established. This is not the same as cause and effect. Furthermore, the development of these complications is highly dependent on the dosage, mode of administration, length of treatment, and type of estrogen. For example, 2.5 mg of conjugated equine estrogen causes less of an increase in the liver's production of bind-

ing globulin than does 30 μg of ethinyl estradiol, the estrogen used in many contraceptive pills. One such globulin is angiotensinogen, which when converted to angiotensin is associated with an increase in blood pressure. The potency of an estrogen depends upon the effect used to measure potency, that is, vaginal thickness, lipid concentration, etcetera. In all probability patient predisposition is also a factor in the development of these complications.

21. **A** (1, 2, 3), Pages 1101–1103. Since 1975 many studies have addressed the question: What is the relative risk for estrogen users of developing adenocarcinoma? These have been both prospective and retrospective investigations. There are several reviews that critique these studies. Given all of this, it would appear that the relative risk for patients who taken an estrogen without a progestin is 3 to 7. The risk increases with increasing duration of use of estrogen as well as with increased dosage. Only a few of many epidemiologic studies investigating the relation of estrogen use and breast cancer have shown an increased risk of breast cancer in some postmenopausal estrogen users. None have indicated a relative risk as high as 5. The possibility exists, however, that estrogen can stimulate a nonpalpable breast cancer.

22. **D** (4), Pages 1083–1084. About 5 years before the actual menopause, FSH is elevated because of lack of negative feedback due to the fact that although a serum estradiol may be in the normal range, the total estrogens from cycle to cycle are decreased. The low estrogen is responsible for this patient's hot flushes. Since her progesterone is normal, this patient is still ovulating, and although unlikely, she can still become pregnant. This woman would benefit from low dose estrogen supplementation, 0.3 mg of conjugated equine estrogen or 0.3 mg of estrone sulfate.

23. **B** (1, 3), Pages 1086–1088. A woman who has had low estrogen levels throughout her life, such as an 18-year-old with pure gonadal dysgenesis, will not have hot flushes. If a woman without any ovaries, the 50-year-old 45X, were to receive estrogen, she would probably experience hot flushes when the estrogen is stopped. The change in estrogen levels leads to alterations in the hypothalamus that are probably mediated through the central nervous system. Hot flushes do not persist in most women for more than 2 to 3 years, and it is uncommon for a woman to have hot flushes that last more than 5 years after the menopause. Ninety-five percent of women will be menopausal by the age of 55 years. When the change in estrogen levels is not gradual but sudden, such as occurs after castration, the individual is more likely to develop symptomatic hot flushes.

24. **D** (4), Pages 1091–1093. Parathyroid hormone increases serum calcium levels by three mechanisms: bone resorption, tubal resorption of calcium in the kidney, and production of an enzyme (1-alpha-hydroxylase) that changes vitamin D from its inactive form to its active form and thereby increases calcium absorption from the gut. It has been postulated that estrogen, androgens, and progestins block the action of parathyroid hormone on bone resorption, reducing the amount of calcium resorbed from the bone. Since there are no estrogen receptors in bone, estrogen cannot inhibit the action of parathyroid hormone directly. However, estrogen increases calcitonin levels, and calcintonin prevents bone resorption. Bone formation in women with osteoporosis is normal.

25. **A** (1, 2, 3), Pages 1083–1085. The basic feature of menopause is depletion of ovarian follicles with degeneration of the granulosa and theca cells. As theca cells degenerate, they fail to react to endogenous gonadotrophins. As a result, less estrogen is produced, and there is a decrease in the negative feedback on the hypothalamic-pituitary axis. In contrast to the follicular cells, the stroma cells of the ovary continue to function and are the major source of androgens.

26. **A** (1, 2, 3), Pages 1087–1088. About one-half of women with flushes have at least one a day, and about 20% have more than one a day. These flushes frequently occur at night, awaken the individual and then produce insomnia. A hot flush is a sudden explosive systemic physiologic phenomenon that takes place over a period of 30 seconds to 5 minutes.

27. **B** (1, 3), Page 1091. At least 25% of the bone needs to be lost before osteoporosis is diagnosed by routine X-ray examination. Dual photon absorptiometry and computerized tomography (CT) scans effectively measure bone density in trabecular bone. The technique of single photon absorptiometry can only be used to measure the density of structures composed primarily of cortical bone—bones in the axial skeleton such as the radius, femur, or os calcis. Since postmenopausal osteoporosis affects trabecular bone more rapidly than it does cortical bone, utilization of single photon absorptiometry on bones in the limbs can fail to detect the presence of loss of trabecular bone in the thoracic spine because the density of the bone being measured may remain within the normal range.

28. **D** (4), Pages 1100–1101. Compared to nonusers, postmenopausal estrogen users have decreased cholesterol, triglyceride, LDL cholesterol, and increased HDL cholesterol levels.

29. **C** (2, 4), Page 1103. The addition of a progestin to estrogen therapy does not appear to cause an increase of any other systemic disease and acts synergistically with estrogen to cause a slight increase in bone density. The use of synthetic progestins may reverse the beneficial effect of estrogen upon serum lipids. The epidemiologic data showing a reduction in heart attacks in estrogen users were derived from women taking estrogen without a progestin. Whether the addition of a progestin to the regimen will reverse the beneficial action of estrogen upon cardiovascular disease remains to be determined. Progestin is active alone in the treatment of hot flushes. Estrogen and progestin together do not cancel each other and constitute effective treatment for hot flushes. In a woman who has just reached the menopause, the addition of both progesterone and estrogen will cause that woman to have predictable menstrual-like withdrawal bleeding each month.
30. **D** (4), Page 1082. The age at which the menopause occurs is genetically predetermined. It is not related to the number of prior ovulations; that is, it is not affected by pregnancy, lactation, use of oral contraceptives, or failure to ovulate spontaneously. It is also not related to race, socioeconomic conditions, education, height, weight, age at menarche, or age at the last pregnancy. The age of menopause may be affected by smoking, as it has been reported that cigarette smokers experience an earlier spontaneous menopause than do nonsmokers.
31. **B** (1, 3), Page 1085. A slim postmenopausal woman converts about 1.5% of androstenedione to estrone, while an obese woman converts as much as 7%. For this reason obese women are less likely to develop symptoms of estrogen deficiency, are less likely to develop osteoporosis, and are also more likely to develop endometrial hyperplasia and adenocarcinoma of the endometrium.
32. **E** (All), Page 1091. Factors known to increase the risk of osteoporosis include
    - Race: white or Asian
    - Reduced weight for height
    - Early spontaneous menopause
    - Early surgical menopause
    - Family history of osteoporosis
    - Diet: low calcium intake, low vitamin D intake, high caffeine intake, high alcohol intake, and high protein intake
    - Cigarette smoking
    - Sedentary life-style
33. **D** (4), Pages 1103–1104. A treatment regimen of 0.625 mg of conjugated equine estrogen or estrone sulfate together with 2.5 to 5 mg of medroxyprogesterone acetate administered every day Monday through Friday reduces the chance of developing breakthrough bleeding and also avoids a week off treatment during which symptoms may appear. Preliminary data indicate that most women do not bleed with this regimen, and their endometrium remains atrophic. There are no well-controlled epidemiologic studies that provide evidence that use of progestins reduce the risk of breast cancer.
34. **C** (2, 4), Page 1085. Ninety-five percent of postmenopausal androstenedione is produced by the adrenal while 5% comes from the ovary. Androstenedione is an androgen and is converted in the peripheral body fat to estrone. This rate of conversion increases as individuals age.
35. **D** (4), Pages 282, 835, 1097, 1101–1103. Estrogen treatment has not been implicated in the development of ovarian carcinoma. The risk of developing endometrial cancer is 3 to 7 times greater in postmenopausal women who are ingesting estrogen without progestins as compared with nonestrogen users. The endometrial cancer that develops in estrogen users is usually well differentiated and so is usually cured by performing a simple hysterectomy. Menopausal patients do bleed whether on or off estrogen. Since those taking estrogen could be bleeding because of withdrawal, the responsible physician may feel that it was his or her fault that the patient has bled. In measuring relative risks, this line of thinking should receive little weight.

    Oral contraceptives appear to accelerate the process of cholelithiasis but do not increase its overall incidence. Although some studies have shown a statistically increased risk of gallbladder disease in postmenopausal estrogen users, others have reported no such risk. Estrogens may accelerate the formation of cholelithiasis in susceptible individuals.